WALTER REED
ARMY MEDICAL CENTER

Centennial

A Pictorial History
1909-2009

Borden Institute Staff

Director and Editor in Chief: Martha Lenhart, MD, PhD, COL, MC, US Army
Managing Editor: Joan Redding
Senior Volume Editor: Vivian Mason
Volume Editor: Marcia Metzgar
Senior Layout Editor/ Information Technology: Douglas Wise
Visual Information Specialist: Bruce Maston
Administrative Officer: Ronald Wallace, Master Sergeant (Ret), US Air Force
Executive Assistant: Narvin Gray

Contributing Editors

John R. Pierce, MD
COL, MC, US Army (Ret)
Historian
Walter Reed Society

Kathleen Stocker, MLS
Assistant Archivist
Otis Historical Archives
National Museum of Health and Medicine
Armed Forces Institute of Pathology

Michael G. Rhode
Archivist
Otis Historical Archives
National Museum of Health and Medicine
Armed Forces Institute of Pathology

Catherine F. Sorge, MSLS
Archivist
Walter Reed Army Medical Center

Marylou Gjernes
Picture Research Consultant
OTSG Office of Medical History

Douglas Wise
Layout, Design, and File Manager
Borden Institute

Martha K. Lenhart, MD, PhD
COL, MC, US Army
Director
Borden Institute

The opinions or assertions contained herein are the private views of the authors and are not to be construed as official or as reflecting the views of the Department of the Army or the Department of Defense.

Use of Trade or Brand Names:

Use of trade or brand names in this publication is for illustrative purposes only and does not imply endorsement by the Department of Defense.

Neutral Language:

Unless this publication states otherwise, masculine nouns and pronouns do not refer exclusively to men.

Published by:
Borden Institute
Office of the Surgeon General
US Army Medical Department Center and School
Walter Reed Army Medical Center
Washington, DC 20307-5001
www.bordeninstitute.army.mil

Library of Congress Cataloging-in-Publication Data

Walter Reed Army Medical Center centennial : a pictorial history, 1909-2009 / edited by John R. Pierce ... [et al.].
  p. ; cm.
  ISBN 978-0-9818228-3-9
   1. Walter Reed Army Medical Center--History--20th century--Pictorial works. I. Pierce, John R., 1947-
  II. Walter Reed Army Medical Center. III. Borden Institute (U.S.)
  [DNLM: 1. Walter Reed Army Medical Center. 2. Hospitals, Military--history--District of Columbia.
  3. History, 20th Century--District of Columbia. 4. History, 21st Century--District of Columbia.
  WX 28 AD6 W234 2009]

UH474.5.W3W34 2009
355.3'4509753--dc22

978-0-9818228-3-9

WALTER REED
ARMY MEDICAL CENTER

Centennial

A Pictorial History
1909-2009

Edited by

John R. Pierce, MD
COL, US Army (Ret)

Michael G. Rhode

Marylou Gjernes

Kathleen Stocker, MLS

Catherine F. Sorge, MSLS

Douglas Wise

Martha Lenhart, MD, PhD
COL, US Army

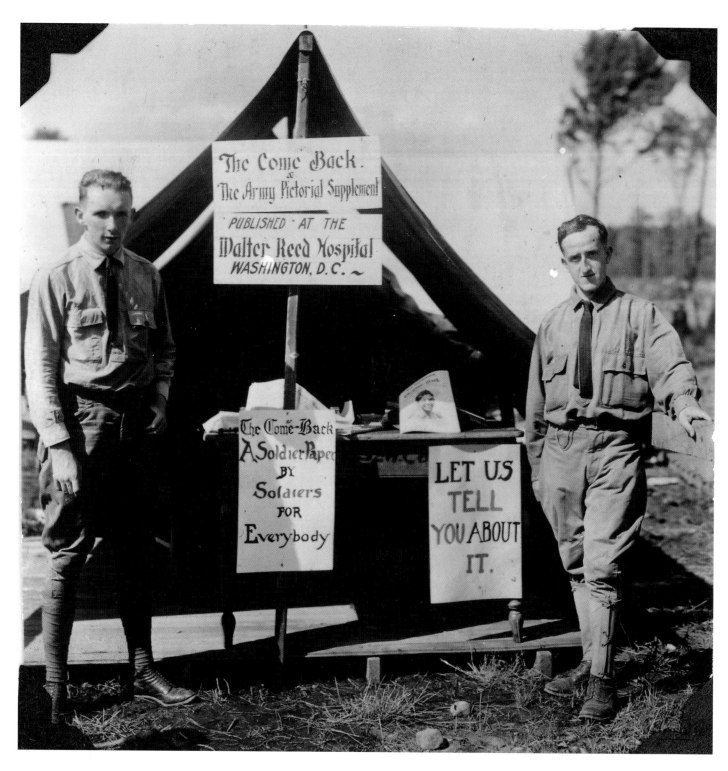

Source: Walter Reed Army Medical Center, Directorate of Public Works Archives.

Contents

Acknowledgments vii

Foreword ix

Preface xi

Introduction xiii

First Decade: 1909–1919 1

Second Decade: 1920–1929 25

Third Decade: 1930–1939 59

Fourth Decade: 1940–1949 75

Fifth Decade: 1950–1959 101

Sixth Decade: 1960–1969 137

Seventh Decade: 1970–1979 165

Eighth Decade: 1980–1989 195

Ninth Decade: 1990–1999 213

Tenth Decade: 2000–2009 241

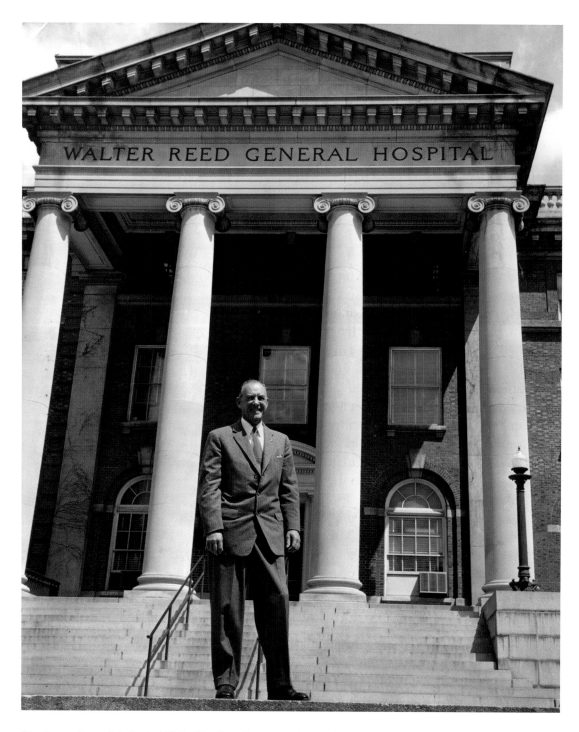

Standing on the walk in front of Walter Reed's main entrance Homer Greenfield smilingly recalls that he was the hospital's 1st, though unofficial, patient. He had been hunting strawberries and cut his finger rather badly on some barbed wire. Running to the hospital for help, he collapsed near the front steps. A hospital corpsman took him into the freshly prepared operating room and repaired his finger. At that time the hospital had not been officially opened. He was a patient a second time, this time officially, when he returned from France with shell fragments in his leg and suffering from poison gas effects. Later on, he spent a short time as head of the Quartermaster Commissary. (Original caption)
Source: Walter Reed Army Medical Center, Directorate of Public Works Archives.

Acknowledgments

This assemblage of images depicting Walter Reed Army Medical Center (WRAMC) was compiled from resources at the National Archives and Records Administration, the National Museum of Health and Medicine, the editorial office of WRAMC's newspaper Stripe, the WRAMC Public Affairs Office, the WRAMC History Office, the WRAMC Department of Public Works, WRAMC Medical Library (*Borden's Dream*), Library of Congress, OTSG - Office of Medical History, and several private collections. The images presented here — pictures, newspaper clippings and memorabilia — were selected to highlight ten decades at the medical center. While this book does not provide a detailed or comprehensive history of WRAMC, its personnel, or its patients, we believe it captures the essence and spirit of the WRAMC campus through the years.

As with any publication, this work would not be possible without the work of numerous contributors. We are sincerely grateful to all those who supported this publication. Dr. John Greenwood, former Chief Historian to the US Army Surgeon General, proposed a photographic history of Walter Reed Hospital in time for its 100th anniversary and has provided valuable input in reviewing the manuscript. Many photographs and Kodachrome slides were made available by Don Chory, Master Planner, in the WRAMC Directorate of Public Works. The slides were scanned and preserved by Donna Rose and Lori Hamrick of Information Manufacturing Company. Sherman Fleek, Command Historian for the North Atlantic Regional Medical Command and WRAMC, provided access to many files with photographs that were ultimately incorporated in the book. Bernard Little, Editor; Craig Coleman, Assistant Editor; and Stripe staff writers Kristin Ellis and Sharon Taylor-Conway were very generous with their time and resources. We are also grateful for image research assistance from WRAMC Public Affairs Officer Chuck Dasey, Deputy Public Affairs Officer Terry Goodman, and Community Relations Officer Thom Cuddy. We are eternally indebted to WRAMC staff and the thousands of patients and their families. Without them, there would be no history of the Walter Reed Army Medical Center.

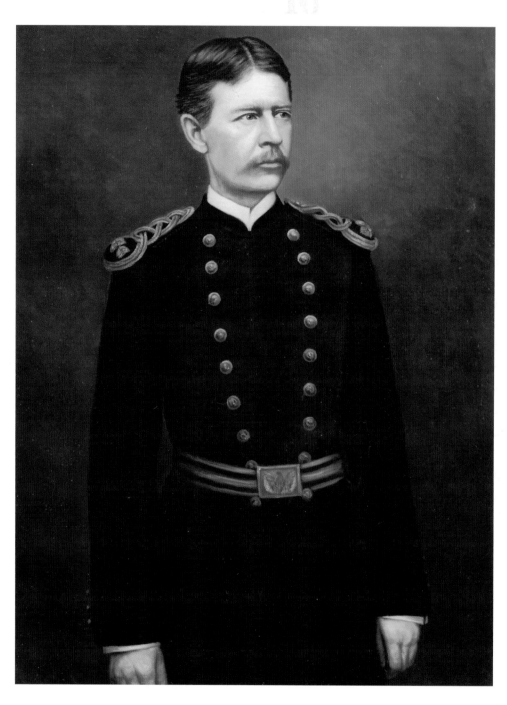

Major Walter Reed

Foreword

On May 1, 1909, Walter Reed General Hospital opened its doors, with ten patients treated on that first day. The original hospital, Building 1, expanded over the decades to provide care for thousands of service members during World War I, World War II, and the Korean and Vietnam wars. On September 26, 1977, the current Walter Reed Army Medical Center inpatient facility opened. Today, more than 600,000 outpatients and 13,000 inpatients per year receive care at Walter Reed.

In 2009, Walter Reed Army Medical Center's centennial year, we commemorate the hospital center's legacy of medical care and innovation. As we celebrate the expert healthcare provided by the physicians, nurses, and allied staff who have served before us, we also take pride in our continued excellence in clinical medicine, advances in knowledge and techniques, and implementation of leading-edge rehabilitation services.

Our ability to provide advanced care for service members injured at home or during deployment has endured nearly 100 years, and has earned this hospital its reputation as the world's premier military medical facility. Ultimately, the character of Walter Reed Army Medical Center is a testament to the men and women who strive (to paraphrase Abraham Lincoln) to care for those who have borne the battle and for their dependents. During this centennial, as you relive this hospital's past through the images presented here, it is my hope that this book will serve as a tribute to the accomplishments of Walter Reed's dedicated team of healthcare providers throughout its 100-year legacy. We are Walter Reed!

Carla Hawley-Bowland
Major General, US Army
Commander, North Atlantic Regional Medical Command
and Walter Reed Army Medical Center

Washington, DC
March 2009

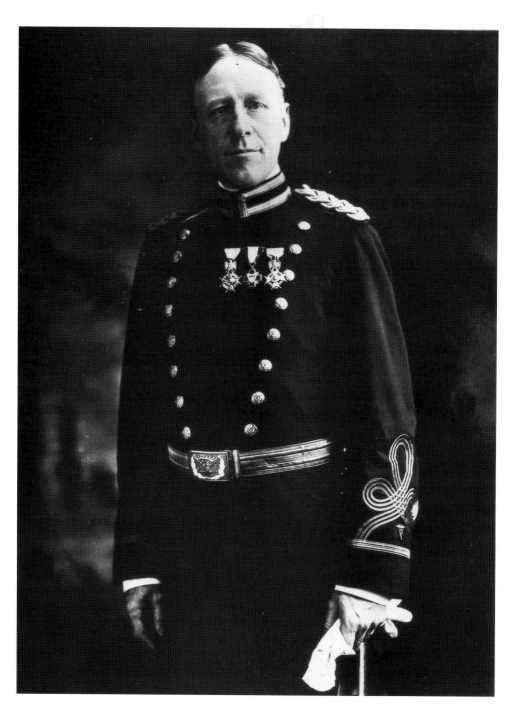

Lt. Colonel William Cline Borden

Preface

As I reflect upon the history of this great health care organization I can not help but wonder what Major (later Lt. Colonel) William Borden, who first envisioned a hospital complex named for Walter Reed, and Colonel (later Brigadier General) William Arthur, the first commander, would think today when looking across the 113 acres of buildings, across the top of Building 1, the original Walter Reed General Hospital, to that great grey edifice that is Building 2, the Heaton Pavilion, and the home of the current hospital. I wonder what they, and other former commanders, many now members of that ghostly assemblage, would think of the changes that have occurred throughout the years and across the wars, the advances in the practice of medicine, the thousands of research protocols conducted, the addition of family member care, and of the creation of residency training programs and fellowships, and not all just for physicians, but for nurses, administrators, technicians, and chaplains as well. I think that he, and the others, would say simply, "Well done; after all, we are Walter Reed!"

When completed in December 1908, the hospital was state of the art for the time, and, in essence, defined "world class" for military facilities. This is the true legacy of Walter Reed, the organization, for we are still, to this day, helping to define what it means to be world class. We are, and have always been, leaders in military medicine, and in medicine in general. We continue to serve as a medical education powerhouse, graduating some of the best physicians and health care professionals in America. We continue to serve as a research powerhouse, with some 800+ protocols on-going at any time. We continue to serve as an innovator in military medicine through the creation of the Warrior Transition Unit, the Warrior Clinic, the Military Advanced Training Center, our numerous Centers of Excellence, our one-of-a-kind Executive Medicine Service, and our renewed focus on Healthcare Hospitality and Customer Service. In short, our motto sums it all up, for at Walter Reed, "We are warrior care, and so much more."

The legacy of this great institution, and the people who have served in it, and have been treated by it, will live on as we move forward into the future with the creation of the Walter Reed National Military Medical Center at Bethesda. The legacy of Major Walter Reed himself will live on; for just as he, through his landmark discovery of the transmission of yellow fever, lives on in the lives that have been saved from this disease, so too shall the legacy of Walter Reed Army Medical Center live on in the warriors and their family members whose lives it has touched.

Norvell Vandervall Coots, MD
COL, MC, US Army
Commander (2008–2011)
Walter Reed Health Care System
Walter Reed Army Medical Center

Washington, DC
March 2009

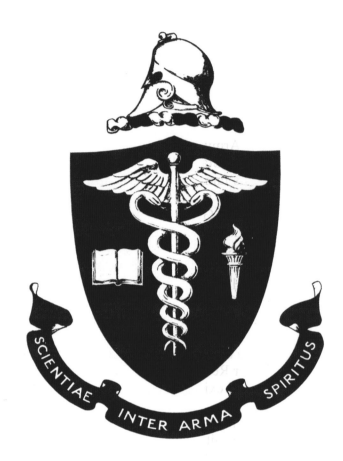

Regrouping of the Walter Reed General Hospital and the Army Medical School as the Army Medical Center resulted in the adoption of a shield, used for a number of years without a motto. The caduceus on the shield represented the Medical Department; the yearbook and flaming torch represents knowledge. The crest is the helmet of Minerva — patroness of medicine. The Medical Department colors, maroon and white, form the relief.

The motto was selected from suggestions of officers, nurses, aides, dieticians, and enlisted men of the troop command of the Army Medical Center. The one proposed by the late Lieutenant Colonel Henry J. Nichols, once a member of the Army Medical School faculty, was selected: "to the spirit of science and the instinct of service."

The wise and beloved Jefferson Randolph Kean, Medical Department sage for over a half-century, suggested that "to the spirit of science and instinct of service" be revised to read "the spirit of science among arms." – a dedication for a great military hospital responsible for the care and prevention of casualties of war.

Adapted from Mary Standlee's *Borden's Dream*

Introduction

The first time I heard of Walter Reed Army Medical Center was in early elementary school. Dwight D. Eisenhower was President of the United States and it was probably related to one of his visits to the hospital as a guest or patient, perhaps his famous admission in June 1956. He was nearing the end of his first term and there was speculation as to whether the former general and World War II hero would run again. Walter Reed commander Major General Leonard Heaton led the team of surgeons who successfully operated on the President; Eisenhower recovered, ran, and was elected to a second term.

I came to Walter Reed in 1985 as Assistant Chief, Department of Pediatrics, and Consultant in Pediatrics to the Surgeon General. I remained here for 15 years, half of my 30 years on active duty, and served in a number of positions, including Chief, Department of Pediatrics, Director of Medical Education, and Deputy Commander for Clinical Services. Walter Reed provided me (as I am sure it did many of you reading this) a remarkable opportunity for professional growth and contribution, both personally and collectively.

The visibility of our medical center in the consciousness of the American public has been tied to the American soldier. In a great sense Walter Reed has earned its reputation and fame from the wounded warriors it so proudly serves. Walter Reed exists to relieve their suffering and to restore their lives as completely as possible.

Major Walter Reed won fame by leading the US Army Yellow Fever Board in Cuba in 1900–1901, proving that the deadly scourge was transmitted by the common domestic mosquito, *Aedes aegypti*. In Cuba, under occupation by the US Army following the Spanish American War, the results of this research were quickly applied by Major William C. Gorgas with remarkable success, essentially ending yellow fever's long reign of terror.

Major Reed returned to Washington to assume other military duties; over the course of the next year he received recognition and acclaim for his scientific work. However, in the fall of 1902, he felt ill and made the self-diagnosis of appendicitis. He visited his friend Major William C. Borden, commander of the Army General Hospital in Washington, DC, who after a period of observation operated on Reed on November 17. Borden was shocked to find his condition much worse than expected. Reed developed peritonitis; without antibiotics, it was hopeless.

Borden, devastated by Reed's death, dedicated himself to honoring his friend. Borden worked for several years to raise funds for a new hospital to replace the inadequate one at Washington Barracks (now Fort Lesley J. McNair). Borden also worked to have the new hospital named for his friend. In his desire to honor Reed, Borden succeeded in ways he could not have imagined.

Opened in May 1909, Walter Reed General Hospital, the US Army's first named permanent general hospital, was built with a capacity for about 80 patients. Within the hospital's first decade, World War I brought rapid and tremendous growth as wounded "doughboys" poured in from the trenches of Europe; the patient census swelled into the thousands. Many temporary buildings were constructed to accommodate the new patients. It was almost a decade after the war that additional significant permanent construction took place, as the large wings were added to the east and west ends of "old main." Walter Reed hosted one venue of the Army School of Nursing, established in 1918 to meet war needs. The first graduating class in

1921 of over 400 is reputed to be the largest graduating class of nursing students in American history.

During World War II wounded "GIs" flooded in from the European, Pacific, and China-Burma-India theaters; additional space was needed and the Forest Glen Annex was purchased and converted into a patient care and convalescent area. Following the war, the introduction of physician residency training programs at Walter Reed mirrored the civilian physician education system and filled a need for specialty training for Army physicians.

In September 1951, to mark the 100th anniversary of the birth of Walter Reed, the installation name was changed to Walter Reed Army Medical Center. During the 1950s, when General Heaton was commanding officer, the institution came to national and international prominence as world figures came to WRAMC for care and to visit the sick and wounded. Following his command at Walter Reed, General Heaton became surgeon general of the US Army and served more than 10 years as the leader of Army medicine. During his tenure as surgeon general, he made plans to ensure the future of WRAMC well beyond his lifetime and into the next century.

In 1967, with the assistance of Senators Everett Dirksen, Richard Russell, and John Stennis, General Heaton procured funds from Congress to start planning for a new hospital facility. On August 26, 1972, after more than 5 years of planning, groundbreaking ceremonies were held. Five years later, on September 26, 1977, the new facility was dedicated. The completed building had 5,500 rooms, 28 acres of floor space, 1,280 beds, and 16 operating rooms. In 1994 the building was rededicated and named the Heaton Pavilion.

During the time of planning and constructing the new facility, wounded "grunts" from the Vietnam War were sent to Walter Reed. One of the orthopaedic wards, infamously known as "the snake pit," became the temporary home of many wounded warriors, some of whom later became leaders in the Army (4-star Generals Norman Schwarzkopf and Barry McCaffrey) and government (Senator Max Cleland and Judge Jack Farley). The global war on terror brought more wounded soldiers. Deployed intensive care units and critical care air transport have made it commonplace for severely wounded warriors to arrive at WRAMC within days of being injured. It is interesting to consider who among this generation will become leaders of the Army and the country.

Warren G. Harding, the first sitting president to visit wounded warriors at Walter Reed, began a tradition of paying respect and providing comfort to the wounded soldiers and their families continued today by former President George W. Bush and President Barack Obama. In addition to presidents and other American and world political leaders, celebrities of all kinds have visited Walter Reed during time of war to visit and to cheer up the troops. Today, movie stars, musicians, singers, and famous athletes visit the newest generation of wounded warriors to show support for their sacrifices.

Throughout its almost century of providing care, Walter Reed's patients have included presidents, vice-presidents, cabinet secretaries, senators, congressmen, federal judges, generals and high-ranking officers of all grades, Medal of Honor winners, former prisoners of war, sergeant majors, and foreign heads of state; but none have been more important than the lowest ranking wounded warrior. To those who have shed their blood in defense of America and its ideals, a special respect is due: respect and honor for their deeds, sacrifice, and courageous examples in overcoming often grievous wounds, and a duty to provide the best and most comprehensive care available, to give them the best chance possible to return to full function.

Walter Reed Army Medical Center is a monument to a long tradition of patient care, medical research, and educational development and a tribute to the vision, intelligence, and dedication of the men and women who have worked here through the years. The next century in its history is waiting to be written, as the changes mandated by the Base Closure and Realignment Commission in 2005 loom in the immediate future. Whatever the future brings, the American people can be assured that the dedicated personnel of Walter Reed will remain true to the values of loyalty, duty, respect, selfless service, honor, integrity, and personal courage in providing US soldiers and their families the best of compassionate care.

John R. Pierce, MD
COL, MC, US Army (Ret)
Historian
Walter Reed Society

Washington, DC
2009

WALTER REED ARMY MEDICAL CENTER

Centennial

A Pictorial History
1909-2009

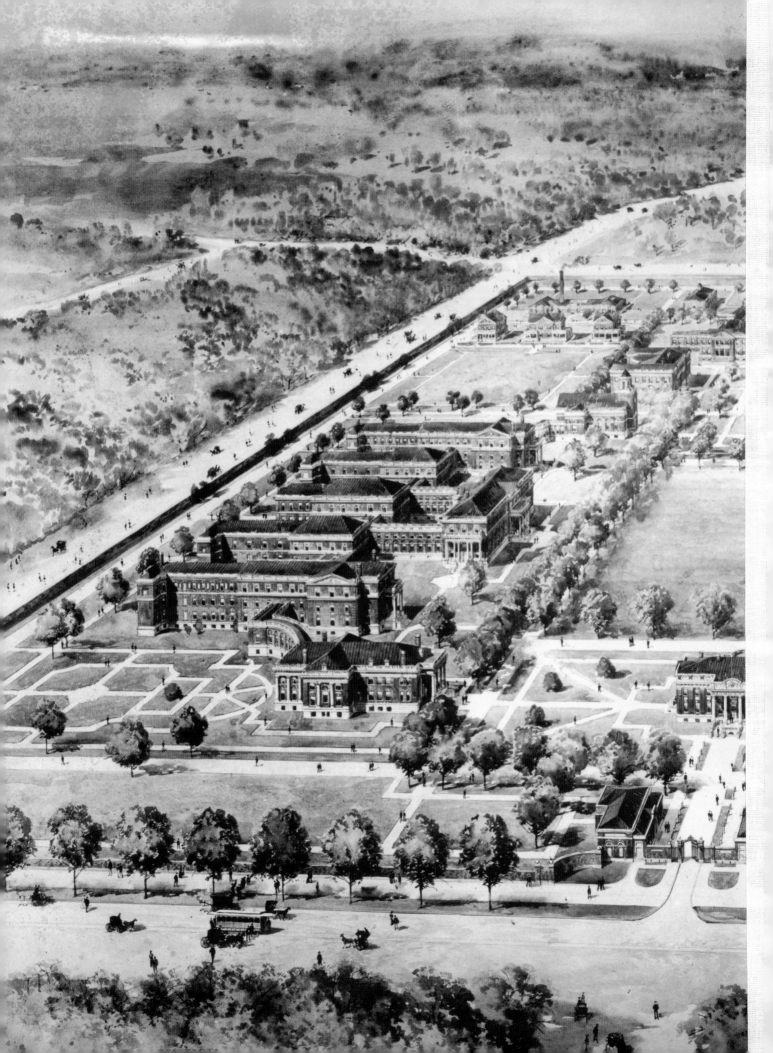

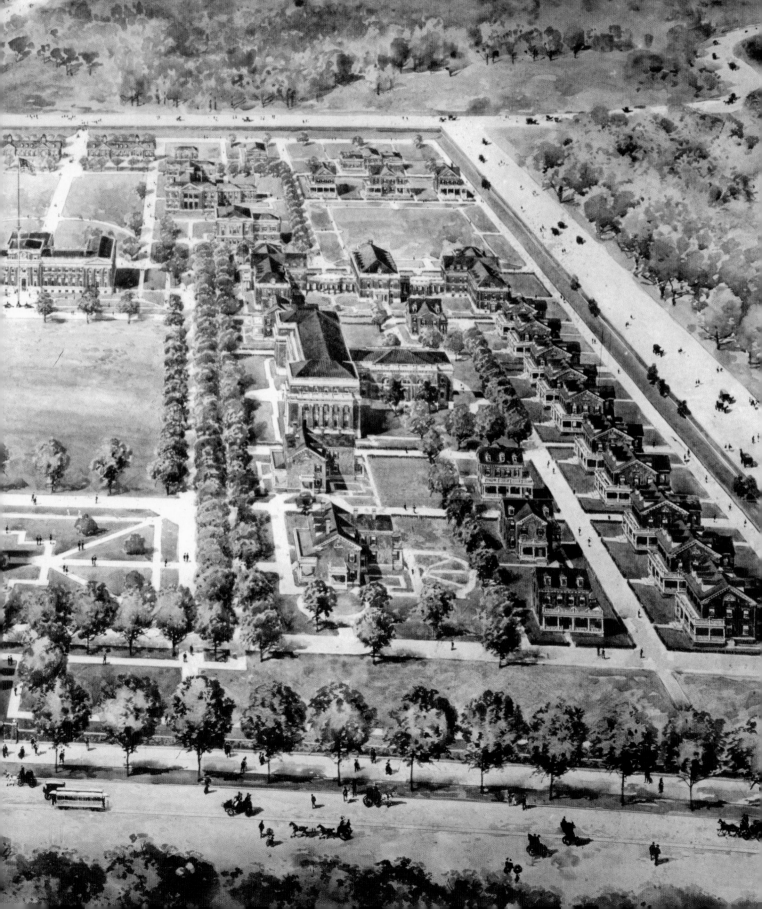

1909–1919

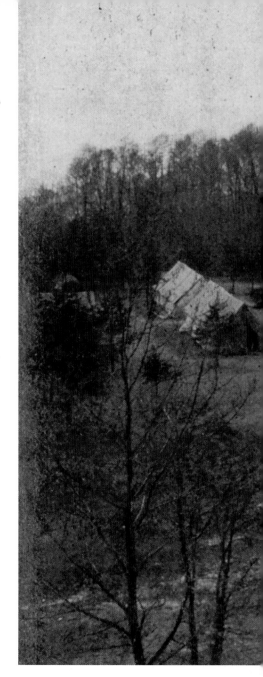

▶ The first medical department unit to occupy Walter Reed Hospital Reservation was Company C of the Hospital Corps. The area that they bivouacked had been used by Confederate General Jubal Early on July 11-12, 1864 in his attack on Washington. This same site was used for the Army Medical School building in 1923.
Source: *Military Surgeon,* Vol. 64, No. 4, April 1929

The early history of Walter Reed General Hospital begins here with a few details to set the stage for the photographs in this volume. Limited by an initial appropriation of $100,000 for the land, which purchased a little over 43 acres known as the Cameron Tract, and $200,000 for the buildings, the nascent campus of 1909 contained only the main hospital building for administration, 65–80 beds for inpatient care (reports vary), and two double sets of sergeant's quarters. During the first two years, support buildings were added to include a quartermaster storehouse and commissary, a stable, a wagon shed and garage, a barracks for the Hospital Corps (Building 7), and two sets of Captain's quarters (currently the General Officer quarters). In 1911, the Army Nurse Corps Home (Building 12) for 20 nurses was completed. The original clinical facility of Building 1 was soon outgrown, and new additions were added. A separate building for an "isolation hospital" of 12 beds opened in 1913, a west addition to Building 1 was completed in 1914, and an east addition was completed in 1915.

World War I would, of course, change everything. The Post Return for April 1917, the month the United States entered the war, reported an active duty staff of 15 officers and 158 enlisted men, with 121 inpatients and an approximately 180-bed capacity. A total of 173 personnel for 121 patients may seem like excessive staffing, but, at the time, there were only a few civilian employees and active duty personnel who did almost all the work, including clinical care, maintenance of the facility and equipment, minor construction projects, feeding of all personnel, and maintaining the animals.

To care for the war wounded, construction of temporary buildings started on June 15, 1917, and, by the end of the year, the hospital had a capacity of 950 beds. An additional land purchase of a little more than 25 acres was made from several surrounding landowners and along with the original purchase of 43 acres brought the total reservation to 69 acres. By the end of 1918, the total bed capacity was 2,500 beds, and admissions for 1918 were the highest

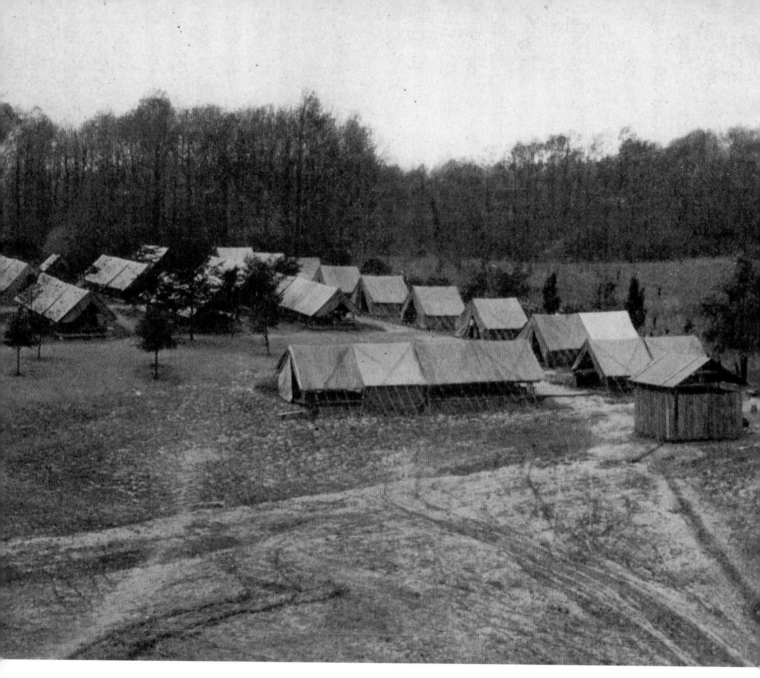

for the World War I period at 13,752. If the war was not enough, the great influenza pandemic swept the country and world in the fall of 1918, leading to over 2,000 admissions for influenza and more than 150 deaths at Walter Reed during a difficult 6-month period.

In addition to the wounded, war brought volunteers to the hospital to assist in their care and recovery. Edith Oliver Rea, a wealthy Pittsburgh philanthropist temporarily residing in Washington with her husband who came to assist with the war effort, became a benefactor to Walter Reed. Mrs. Rea was asked by the American Red Cross to be the Field Director at Walter Reed. She did so for 1 year, and then turned the title over to Miss Margaret

Lower; but, she stayed on as the leader of the volunteers who, because of their soft pearl-gray uniforms, became known as the Red Cross Gray Ladies, a moniker that spread nationally and continues to this day.

The war generated the need for additional trained nurses, which led to the establishment at Walter Reed and other locations of the Army School of Nursing (ASN) in August 1918. Planned for three years of training, the ASN was the Army's first adventure into training its own female nurses. Its charter class at Walter Reed swelled to over 400 students and is reputed to be the largest in American history; subsequent classes were significantly smaller. Although trained at government expense, there

was no statutory service obligation and less than one-third of the graduates actually elected to enter active duty. The war ended in November 1918, but the ASN remained at Walter Reed until it was phased out in the early 1930s. The ASN was unusual for nursing schools of its day because the purpose of ASN was to train nurses, not to provide a pool of inexpensive skilled labor for its hospital.

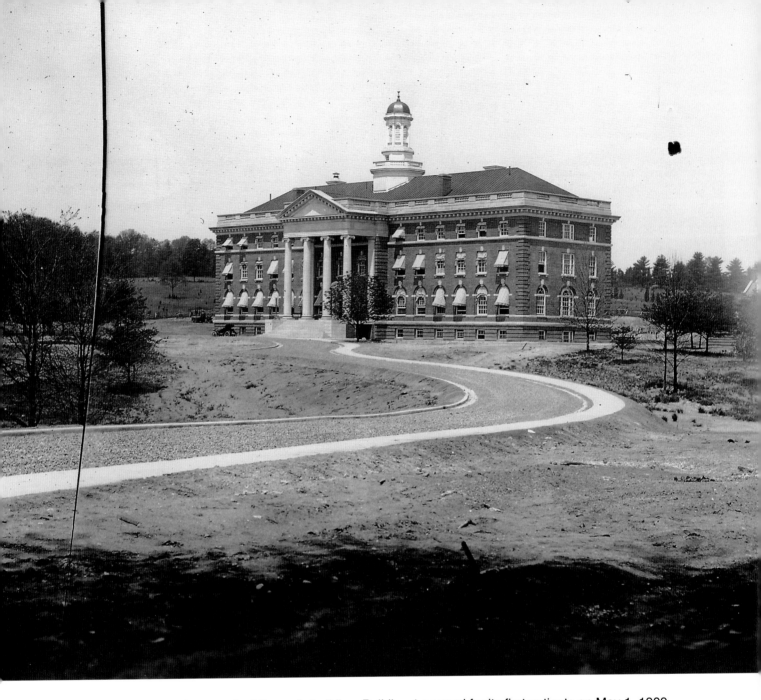

This is the oldest known photograph of the main building. Building 1 opened for its first patients on May 1, 1909.
Source: National Museum of Health and Medicine, AFIP, AMM 484

▶ Originally designed for 65–80 patients, the hospital was expanded to 2,500 beds for servicemembers from World War I.
Source: National Museum of Health and Medicine, AFIP, 65-12603

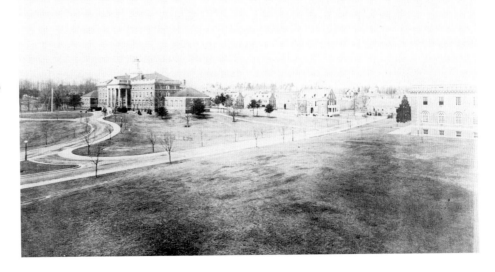

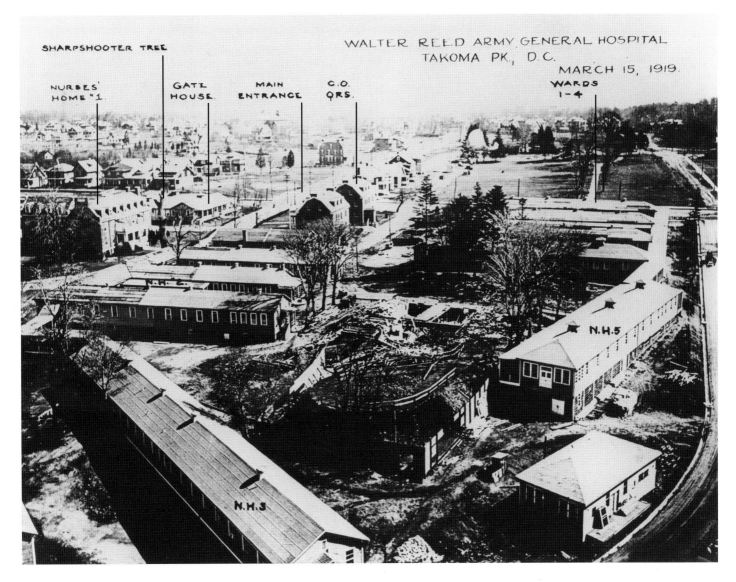

SHARPSHOOTER TREE

WALTER REED ARMY GENERAL HOSPITAL
TAKOMA PK., D.C.
MARCH 15, 1919.

NURSES'   GATE   MAIN   C.O.   WARDS
HOME *1   HOUSE.   ENTRANCE   QRS.   1-4

N.H.C.

N.H.5

N.H.3

▲ Aerial view of the campus is dated March 15, 1919. The annotated photograph identifies three nurses homes, the gate-house, main entrance, Commander's Quarters, and Wards 1 through 4. This view is looking toward present-day Georgia Avenue. The Sharpshooter's Tree can be seen between nurses' home 1 and the gatehouse. This chaotic picture was typical of the temporary expansion of the campus in World War I. Note the address is Takoma Park, D.C.
Source: National Museum of Health and Medicine, AFIP, WRAMC History Collection

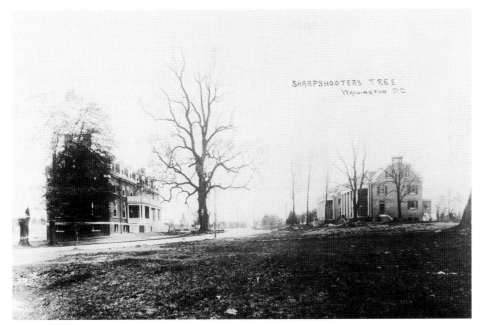

SHARPSHOOTERS TREE
Washington D.C.

◀ In July of 1864 the Sharpshooter Tree was used by Confederate soldiers during the Battle of Fort Stevens. General Jubal Early commanded the Confederate Army's II Corps in its advance on Washington. They used this tulip tree to position sharpshooters to take shots at Union soldiers stationed at Fort Stevens located half a mile to the south.
Source: Library of Congress

7

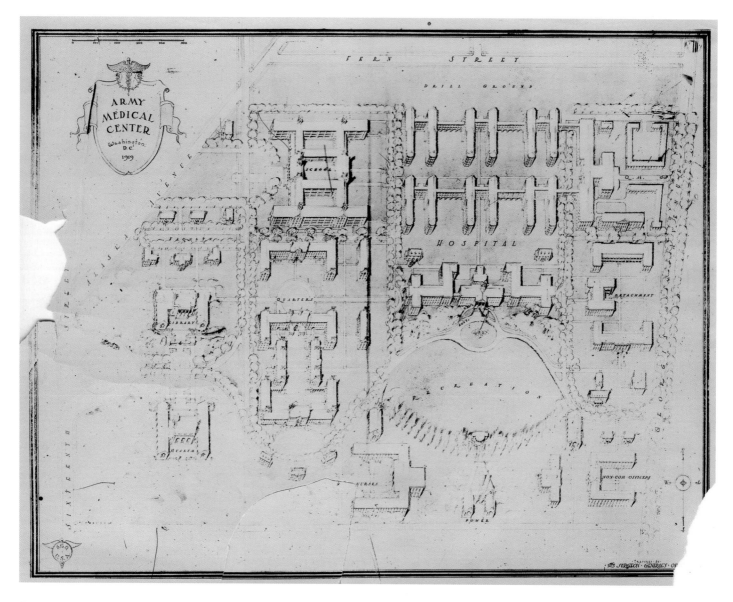

Artist's conception of the proposed Army Medical School and Army Medical Center dated 1919.
Source: National Museum of Health and Medicine, AFIP, Reeve 2398

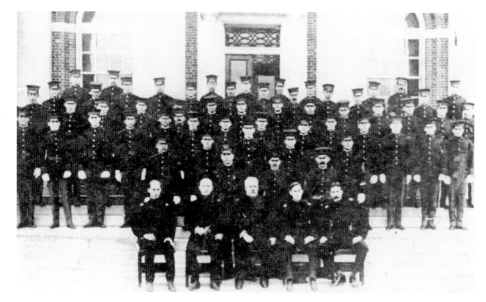

◄ Photograph of detachment of medical personnel that opened Walter Reed Hospital on May 1, 1909. Seated in the front are (left to right) Capt. Walter Huggins, acting Quartermaster; Maj. Thomas L. Rhodes, adjutant and surgeon; Col. William Arthur, commanding officer; Capt. William Pipes, Capt. Percival L. Jones.
Source: Signal Corps

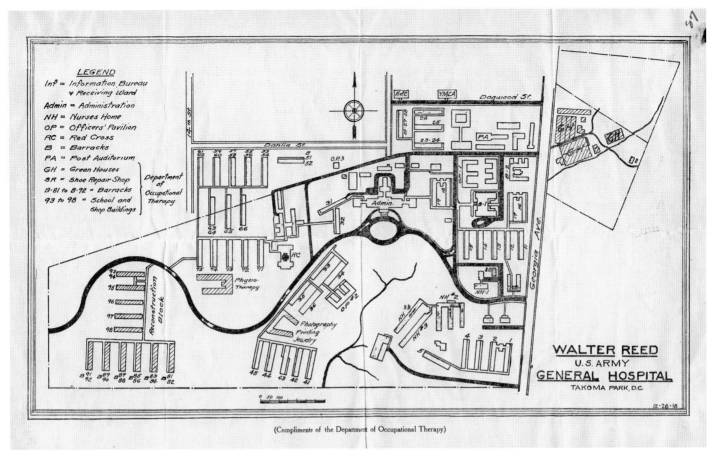

(Compliments of the Department of Occupational Therapy)

This 1918 map (top) of the grounds of the hospital shows the increase in temporary buildings required to serve the returning veterans. Note the greenhouses on the east side of Georgia Avenue. The reverse of the map (bottom) encourages the patients to be active. As the poster says, "something to do" may be things in leather, decorative bookbinding, drawing, block printing, stenciling, metal work, beadwork, or twine work.

Source: National Museum of Health and Medicine, AFIP, WRAMC History Collection

IF YOU ARE A PATIENT

You want your health and strength and your hospital discharge as soon as possible. Doing something with your hands and your head will greatly aid in these. What you do here may help you to know and to do your old job better or may lead to a job you like better and thus give you a happier life. The "Reconstruction Aides" will bring you something to do while you have to stay in your ward. This "Something to do" may be things in leather, decorative woodwork, basketry, book-binding, drawing, block-printing, stenciling, metal work, bead work, twine work; or it may be some of the subjects listed below.

Social Service Aides in Building 93, Room 6 are ready to discuss any problem you may have.

If you can leave the ward, you can visit the building named at the top of each list and try the kind of work you would like to do. The map will show you the way to the buildings. Come and see. Look over the lists.

Buildings 93 and 94:	Building 95:	Building 96:	Building 97:	Building 98:	Greenhouse and Farm:
English French, Spanish	Toy Making Working Drawings	Automobile Repairing	Artificial Limb Work Special Leather Wark	Carpentry	
Arithmetic, Geometry Algebra, Trigonomerty	Tracing Blueprinting Reading Blueprints	Tractor Instruction Machine Shop Practice	Cement and Concrete Work	Cabinet Making Wood Turning	Truck Farming
Penmanship Lefthand Writing	Architectural Drawing Perspective	Engine Lathe	Lathing	Pattern Making	Vegetable Raising (Greenhouse)
Civil Service History	Freehand Sketching Topographical Drawing	Drill Press	Plastering	Wood Carving	
Commercial Arithmetic Commercial English Commercial Law	Slide Rule Use Gas Engine Study Steam Engine Study	Sensitive Drill Drill Grinder	**Building 40:** South Wing Basement	Rug Weaving	Flower Growing
Shorthand, Stenotypy Typewriting	Power Plants Electricians Course	Shaper	Printing Hand Composition	Loom Weaving	Text Book Studies in Agriculture
Filing and Recording Duplicating Machine Calculating Machine	Dynamo Tending Electrical Engineering	Handwork in Filing	Linotype Operating Press Work Proof Reading	Gobelin Tapestry	Poultry Keeping
Bookkeeping Salesmanship Journalism	Wireless Telegraphy Radio Work Blacksmithing	Motion Picture Operation	**Building 40:** North Wing Basement	Sign Painting	Breeding Farm Management
Telegraphy Citizenship	Oxy-Acetelyne Welding Forging		Jewelry Making	Clay Modeling	Horticulture Bee-Keeping, Etc.

The American Library Association has a library room in Building 94. In it are many books on many subjects for your information and study. There is also a chance to read and write. Call in.

Agent of the Federal Board for Vocational Training—Building 93, Room 11.

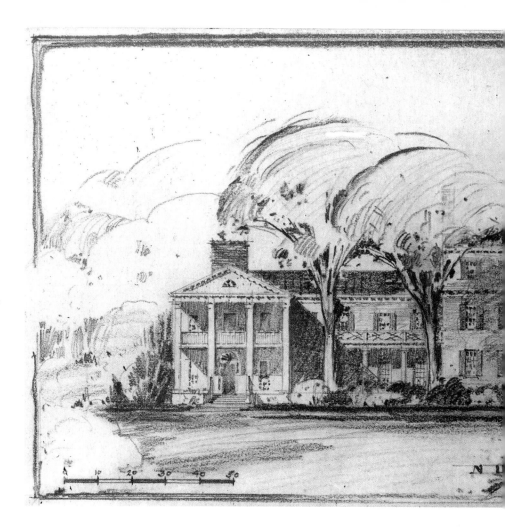

▶ Artist's conception of the Nurses Quarters and Training School dated February 14, 1919. The Army School of Nursing at Walter Reed opened in 1918. Delano Hall was later built to house the nurses.
Source: National Museum of Health and Medicine, AFIP, Reeve 3146

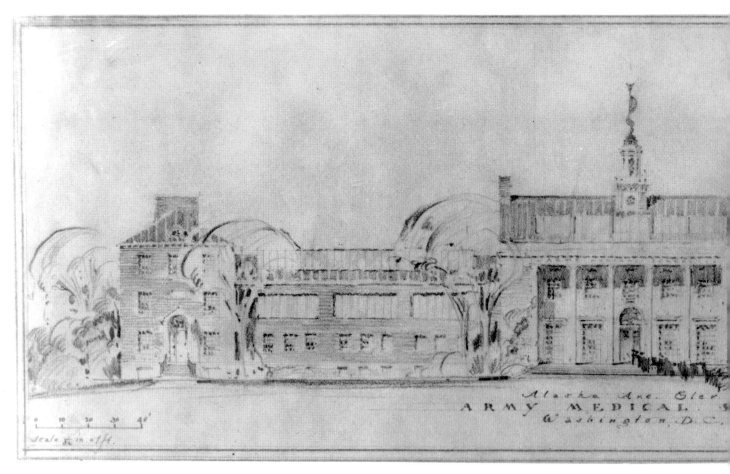

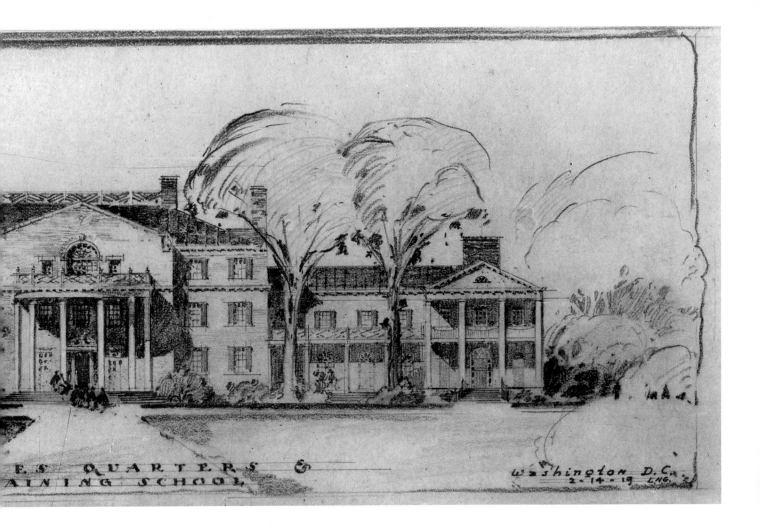

ES QUARTERS &
AINING SCHOOL.

Washington D.C.
2-14-19 LNG.

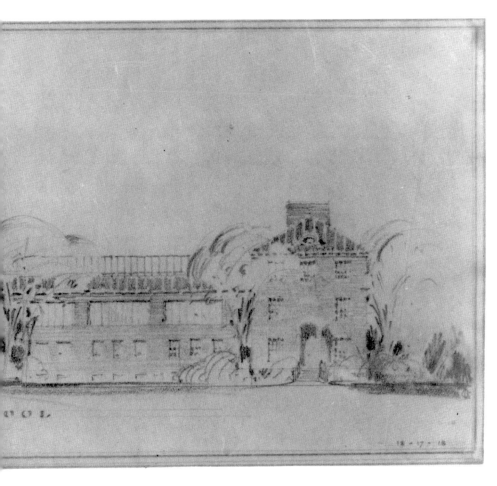

◄ This 1918 artist's conception is a plan for the Army Medical School. The Army Medical School moved to the hospital campus in 1923 from its location in downtown Washington. A building to house the school was built to the west on a direct line with Building 1. The architecture was compatible with the permanent buildings, the exterior being of brick with limestone trimmings. The main entrance to the south wing lead into a large central lobby. When completed a decade later, the building would consist of two long wings connected by a central portion that housed a large auditorium.
Source: National Museum of Health and Medicine, AFIP, WRAMC History Collection, Reeve 2211

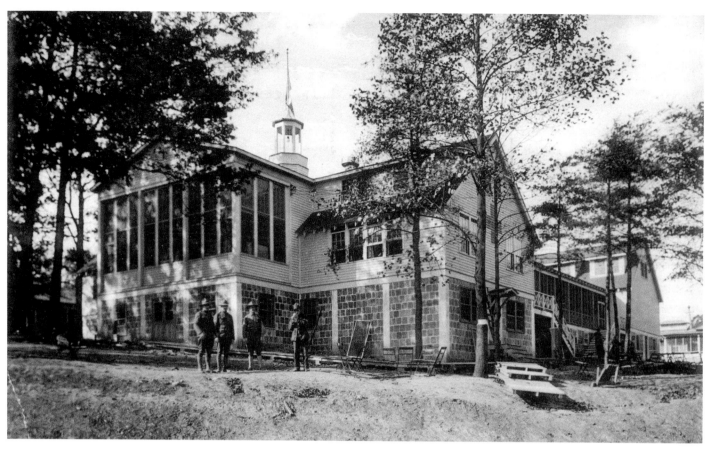

▲ Red Cross House and Post Exchange.
Source: National Museum of Health and Medicine, AFIP, NCP 15008

▼ Red Cross volunteers.
Source: Walter Reed Army Medical Center, Directorate of Public Works Archives

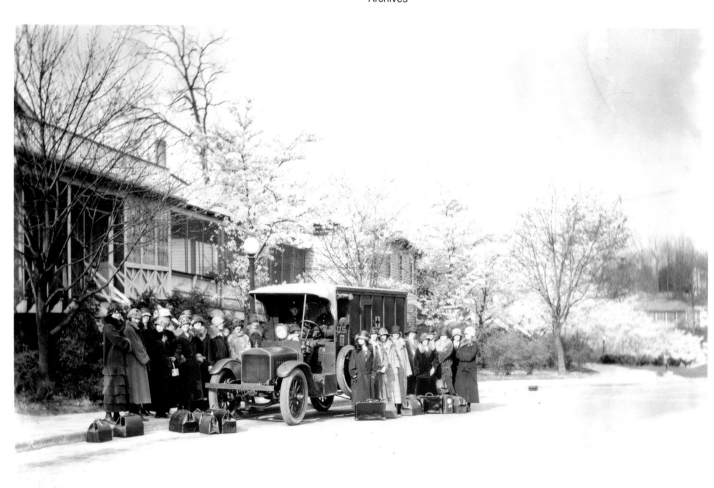

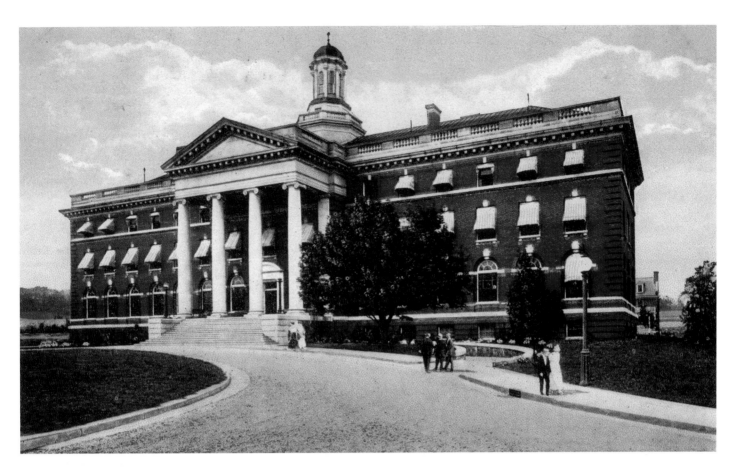

▲ The Walter Reed Army General Hospital is located on Georgia Avenue, near Takoma Park, and is on the ground where the battle with General Early's army was fought during the Civil War. It honors the name of Maj. Walter Reed, Medical Corps, U.S.A., whose life ended on November 23, 1902. (Postcard)
Source: Pierce Collection

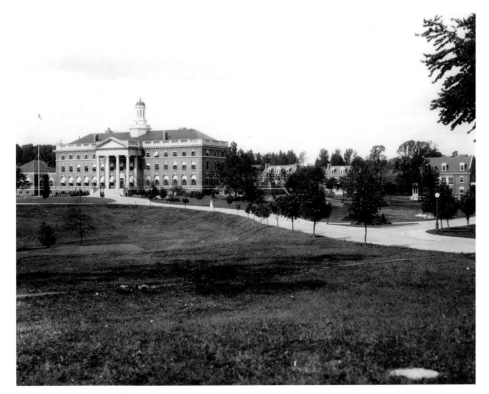

◄ A view of the hospital and some of the support buildings probably taken in 1915 as the west addition (left) to Building 1 is completed and the east addition is under construction.
Source: National Museum of Health and Medicine, AFIP, Reeve 3080a

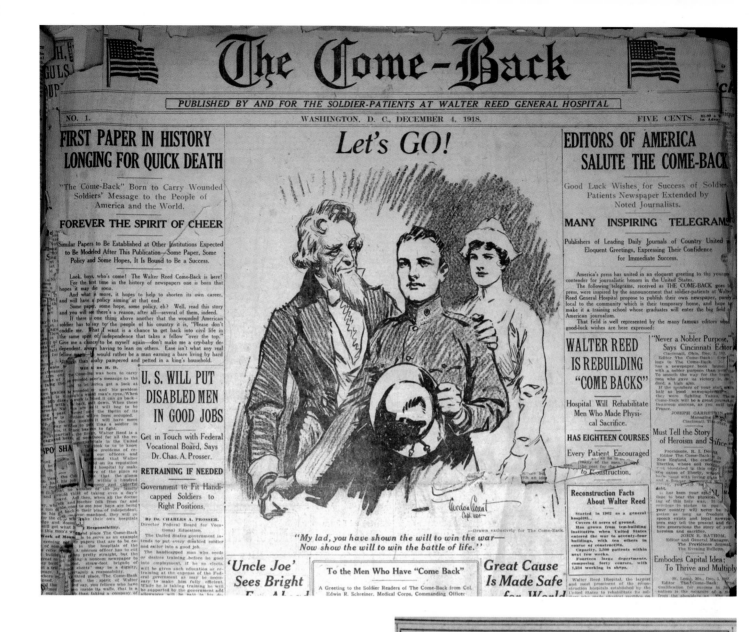

► Radio communication played a major role in connecting the wounded veterans with the world outside the hospital grounds. In February 1919, the Telegraphy School, with assistance from the Signal Corps, installed two complete sets of wireless instruments. This apparatus consisted of a long-wave receiving set for handling the high-powered overseas stations, and a commercial wave set for recording signals sent out by ship and shore stations. The set could also tune as low as 100 meters, thus enabling the operator to handle the amateurs on the waves of 200 meters. By June 1920, it was considered one of the most up-to-date radio stations of its size on the East Coast. *The Come-Back,* June 26, 1920.
Source: National Museum of Health and Medicine, AFIP, WRAMC History Collection

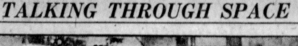

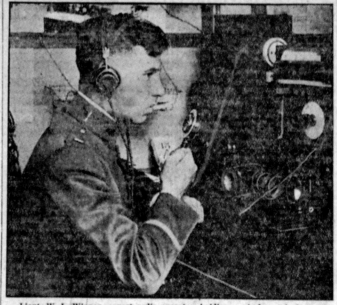

Lieut. W. L. Winner, expert radio operator, holding a wireless telephone conversation in the radio room of the Walter Reed Hospital Reconstruction Department, using apparatus constructed by himself and Mr. Leroy Chichester.

◀ *The Come-Back,* published from December 4, 1918 to September 17, 1926 strengthened the morale of the soldiers and soldier-patients of the hospital. It was one of approximately 50 newspapers published at military hospitals around the country. *The Come-Back* was sold on the streets of Washington and sales to the community were encouraged. To cover the cost of production, advertising space was sold to local businessmen, and the paper itself cost five cents. Because of the audience, general news was covered in addition to news of happenings at the hospital. Initially four pages, within a year it was 12 pages, and its circulation doubled and then tripled. The paper became an effective crusader for soldiers successfully fighting for reduced rates on rail travel.
Source: National Museum of Health and Medicine, AFIP, WRAMC History Collection

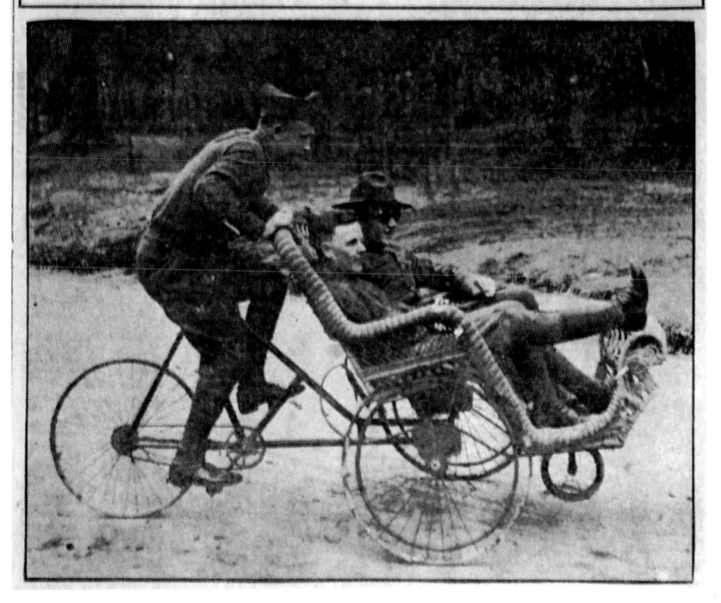

N-C's Have Nothing on This
Sixty Per at Walter Reed

▲ This rickshaw wheelchair combination was perfect for negotiating paths around the hospital grounds. *The Come-Back,* Vol. 1, May 21, 1919.
Source: National Museum of Health and Medicine, AFIP, WRAMC History Collection

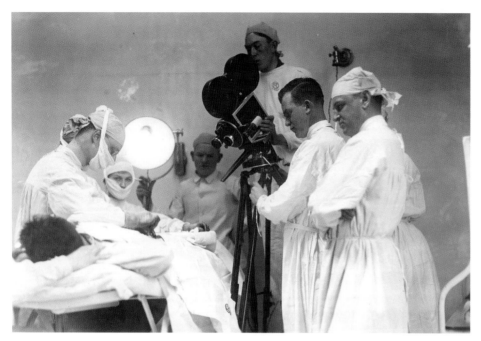

◀ Here, a camera is recording an operation. The motion picture camera became a critical part of the teaching mission of the hospital.
Source: National Museum of Health and Medicine, AFIP, Reeve 562

▼ Pneumonia ward in 1919. There were more than 150 patient deaths due to the influenza pandemic in the fall and winter of 1918–1919.
Source: National Museum of Health and Medicine, AFIP, Reeve 604-2

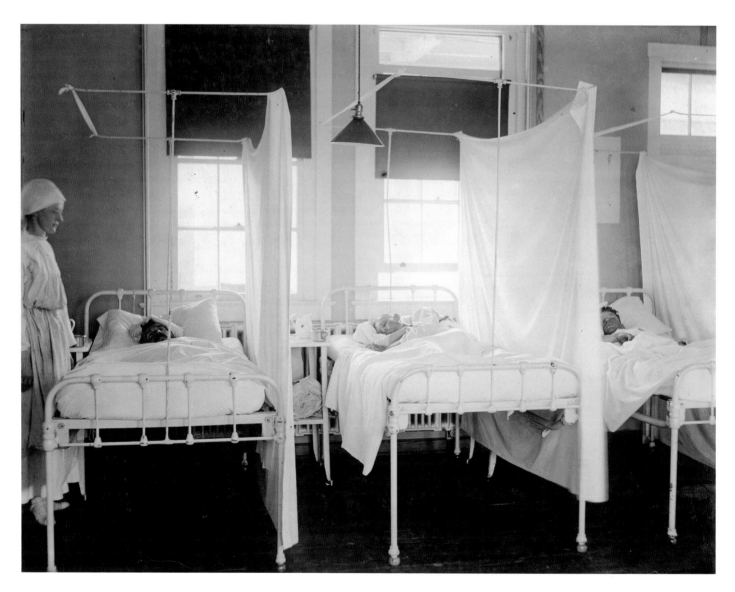

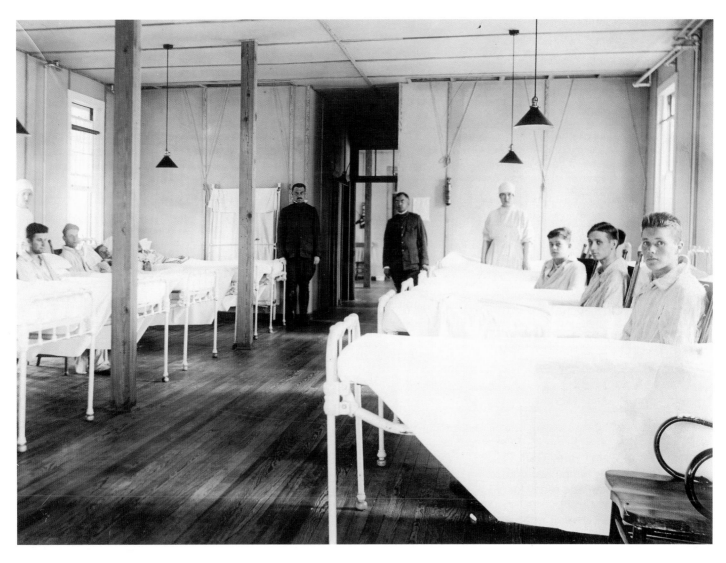

▲ Observation Ward.
Source: National Museum of Health and Medicine, AFIP, Reeve 602

▶ Mess Hall Ward, Ward Y for patients.
Source: National Museum of Health and Medicine, AFIP, Reeve 743

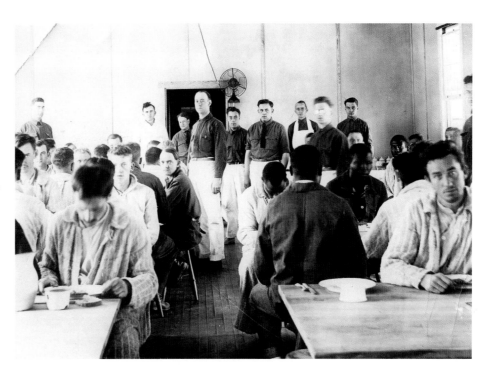

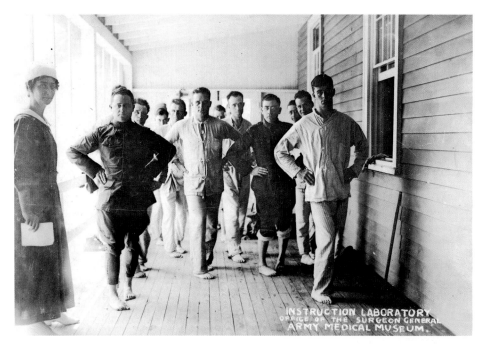

◀ Foot gymnastics for soldiers from Army camps, Walter Reed Hospital.
Source: National Museum of Health and Medicine, AFIP, Reeve 279

▶ Amputees at Walter Reed General Hospital whose stumps were massaged daily and made ready for prosthetics.
Source: National Museum of Health and Medicine, AFIP, Reeve 273

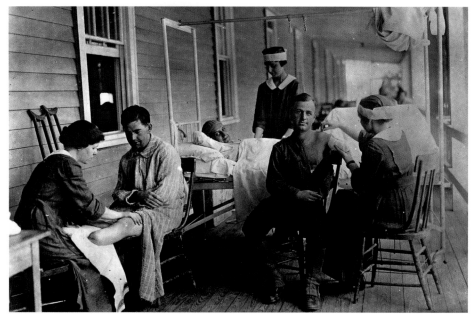

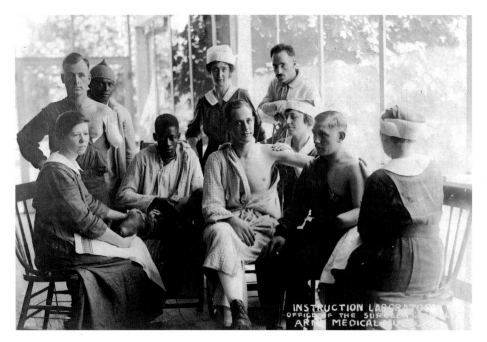

◀ Massaging residual limbs of soldiers preparatory to prosthetic fitting.
Source: National Museum of Health and Medicine, AFIP, Reeve 278

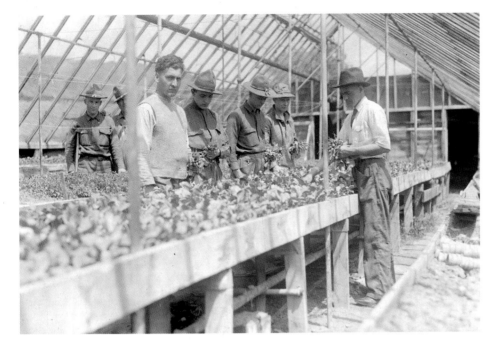

◀ When a second greenhouse was needed, there was no funding available. Used and about to be discarded, glass X-ray plates were cleaned, set into frames, and reused as window panes in construction of the new greenhouse. The two original greenhouses and a third donated by the U.S. Park Service in 1943 were demolished in 1998.
Source: National Museum of Health and Medicine, AFIP, Reeve 275

▶ Soldier-patients working in the garden at Walter Reed Hospital, Reconstruction Division.
Source: National Museum of Health and Medicine, AFIP, Reeve 469

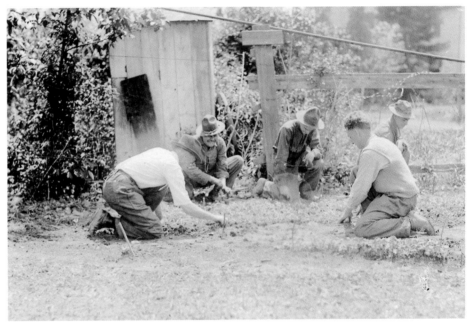

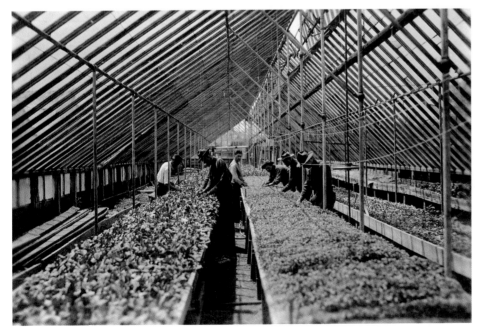

◀ Horticultural therapy involves the use of gardening, landscaping, flower arranging, nature crafts, and related activities. The purpose is to boost the patient's self-esteem, develop a sense of accomplishment, and overcome stress. In addition to the therapy, the greenhouses produced plants and holiday flowers used for programs and activities at the hospital.
Source: National Museum of Health and Medicine, AFIP, Reeve 276

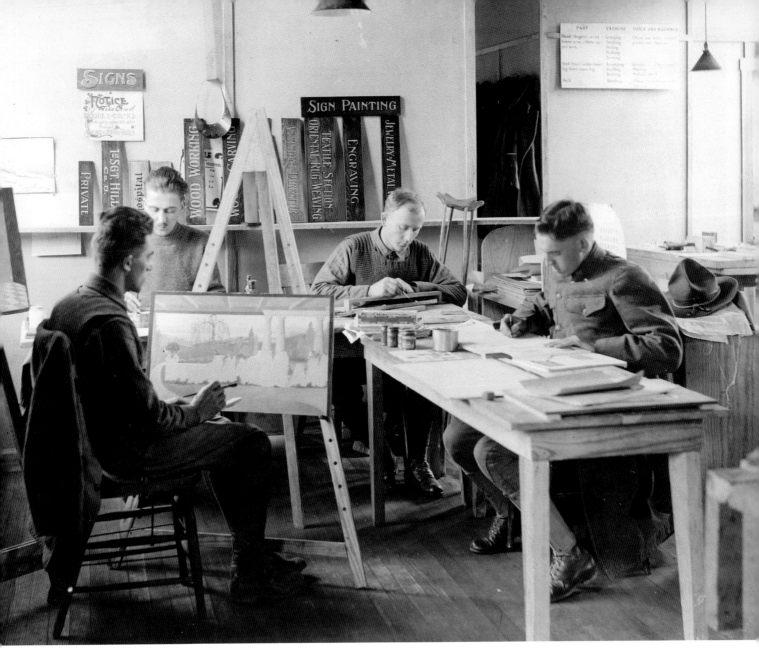

▲ Sign painting class provided re-education of the wounded. Walter Reed Hospital, Reconstruction Division.
Source: National Museum of Health and Medicine, AFIP, Reeve 2011

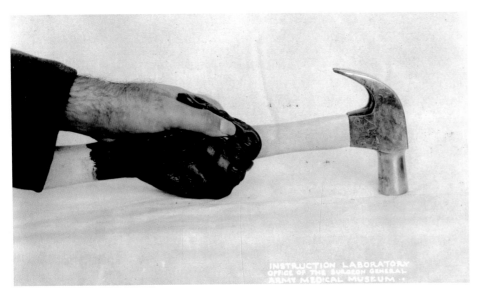

◄ Hammer with hand mold for wounded hand. Used by Pvt. John Aver (37th Division, U.S. Infantry), World War I.
Source: National Museum of Health and Medicine, AFIP, Reeve 1789

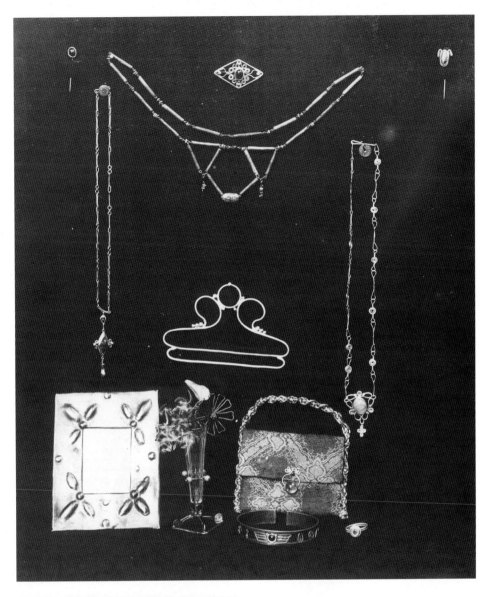

◄ Making jewelry provided re-education opportunities for wounded soldiers.
Source National Museum of Health and Medicine, AFIP, Reeve 2022

▼ Pvt. Ralph Grimm, who became an expert Silversmith in the Walter Reed occupational therapy shop. (Original caption)
Source: Pierce Collection

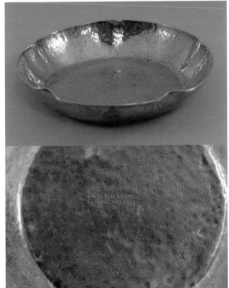

▲ A silver ashtray made by a patient undergoing therapy at Walter Reed. Stamped on the bottom is "Walter Reed General Hospital"
Source: Pierce Collection, Douglas Wise - photographer

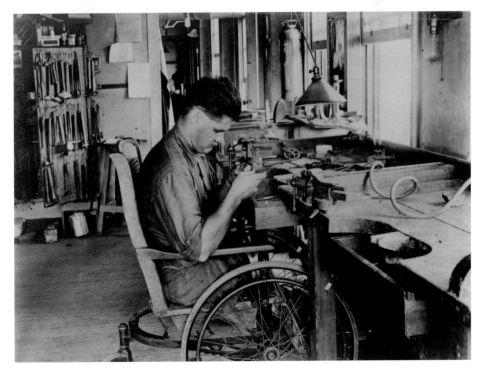

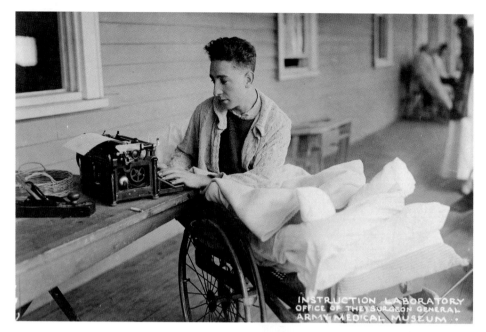

◀ Wounded soldier learning to type.
Source: National Museum of Health and Medicine, AFIP, Reeve 285

▶ Patient working at his old trade as a draughtsman.
Source: National Museum of Health and Medicine, AFIP, Reeve 277

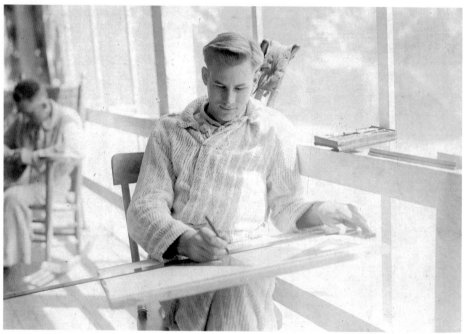

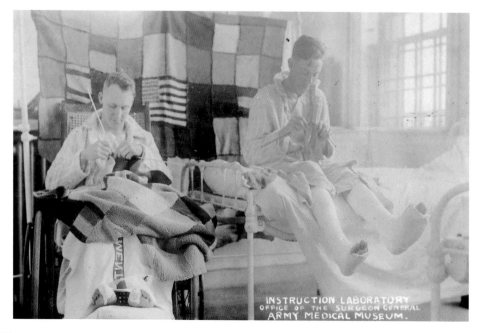

◀ Injured soldiers learning to knit. Walter Reed General Hospital, Reconstruction Division.
Source: National Museum of Health and Medicine, AFIP, Reeve 305

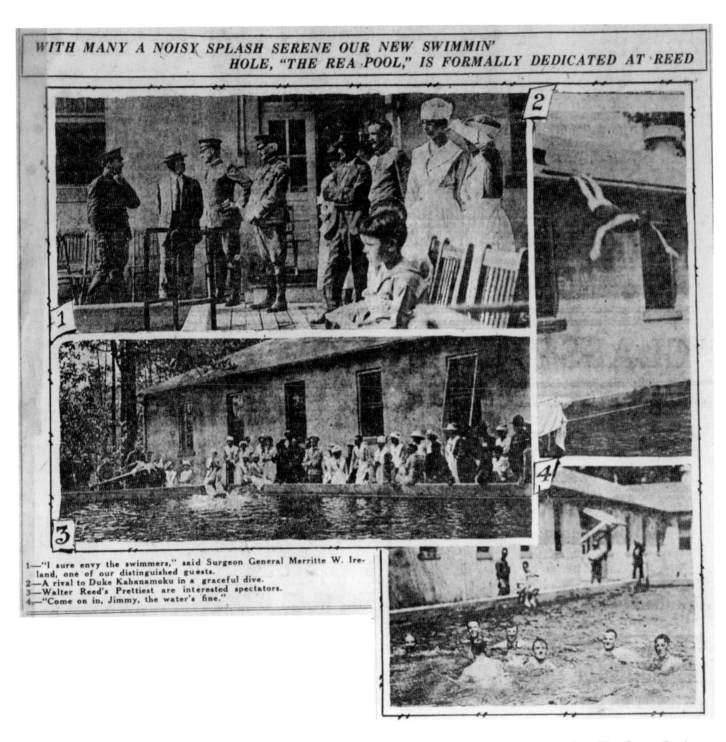

WITH MANY A NOISY SPLASH SERENE OUR NEW SWIMMIN'
HOLE, "THE REA POOL," IS FORMALLY DEDICATED AT REED

1—"I sure envy the swimmers," said Surgeon General Merritte W. Ireland, one of our distinguished guests.
2—A rival to Duke Kahanamoku in a graceful dive.
3—Walter Reed's Prettiest are interested spectators.
4—"Come on in, Jimmy, the water's fine."

The new swimming pool, donated by Mrs. Rea, was used for physical therapy and soldier recreation. *The Come-Back,* July 9, 1919.
Source: National Museum of Health and Medicine, AFIP, WRAMC History Collection

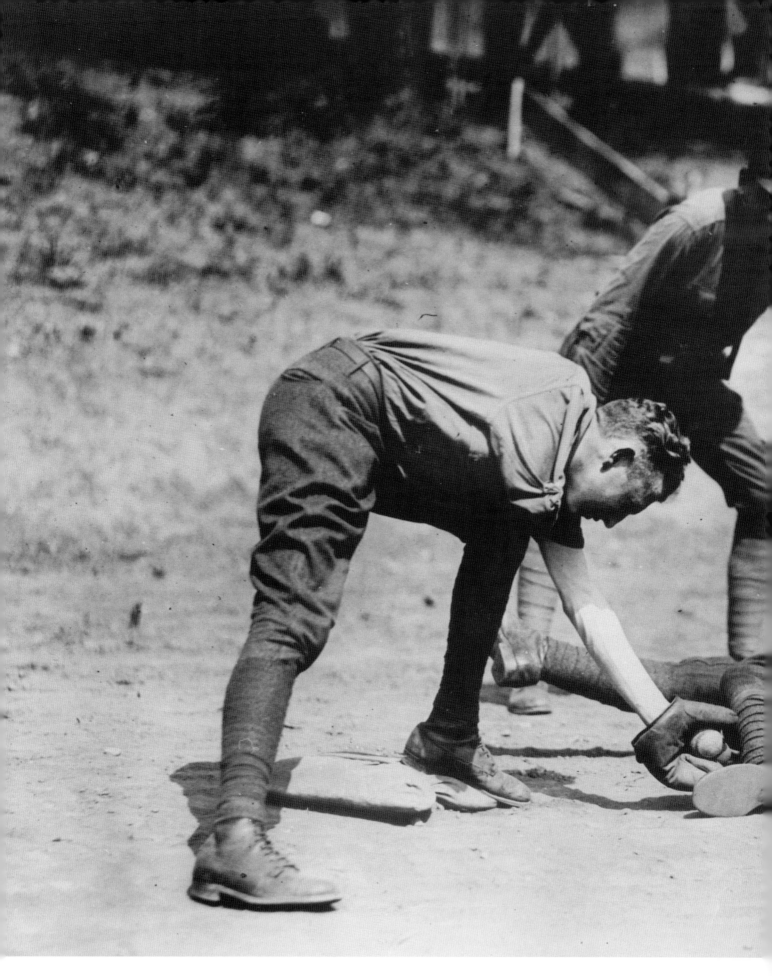

Patient rehabilitation. Playing baseball.
Source: National Museum of Health and Medicine, AFIP, WRAMC History Collection

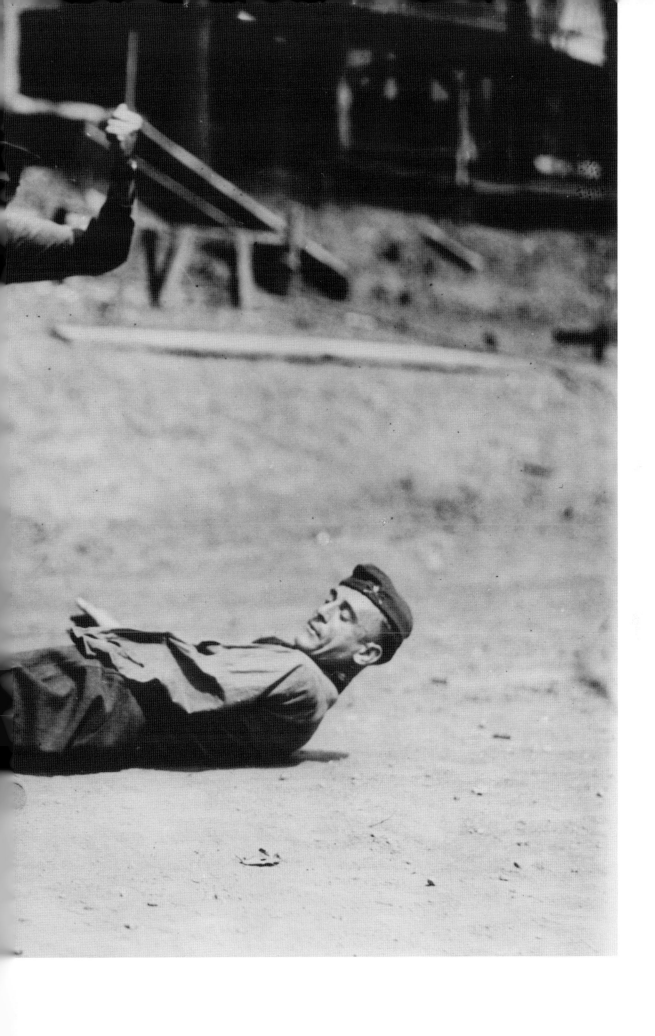

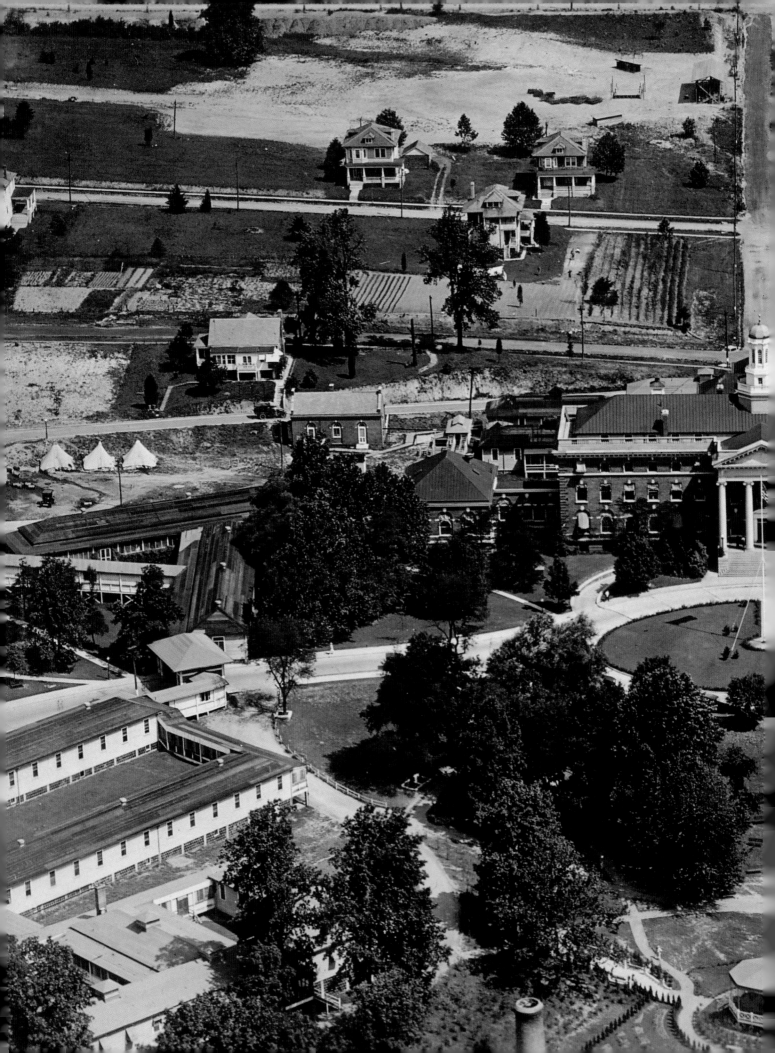

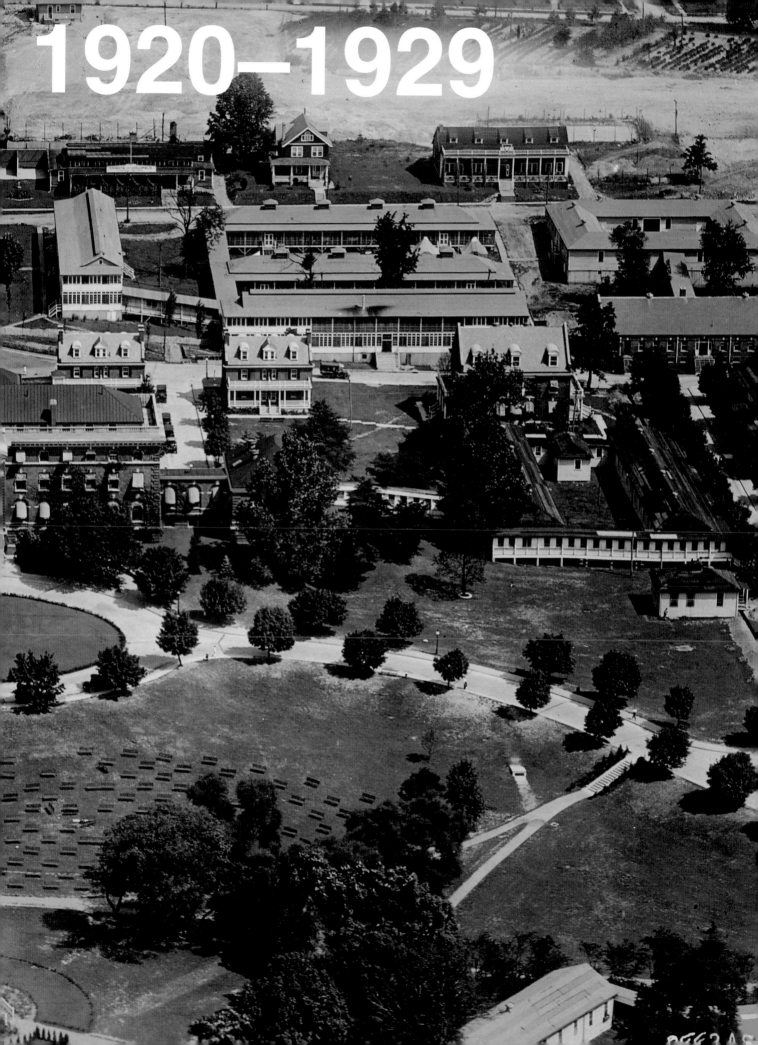

1920–1929

Title page - This aerial view, taken in the summer of 1921, looks north toward Building 1, the main administration and clinical building, which was completed in 1908 and occupied in 1909. The new Wards A (west) and B (east, hidden behind the trees) were completed in 1914 and 1915, respectively. Directly north of the east portion of Building 1 are two identical double sets of Sergeant's quarters, Buildings 2 and 3. To the east of Building 3 (right in the photo) is the larger "Isolation Hospital" of 12 beds completed in 1913. Temporary wards for World War I are seen in the foreground (left and right). The YMCA building is seen in the upper right of the photograph. Also north of Building 1, in the upper portion of the photos, are former private homes that were on the property that was purchased for the facility. These were used as officer's quarters.
Source: National Archives and Records Administration, 9882AC

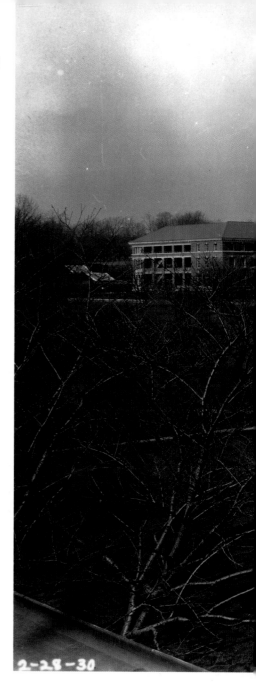

▶ Building 1 as it appeared late in the second decade after two major additions.
Source: National Museum of Health and Medicine, AFIP, WRAMC History Collection

The war was over, but the care and rehabilitation of war wounded continued at Walter Reed during the early years of its second decade. Closure of temporary Army hospitals that were opened during the war lead Congress to provide additional funds to Walter Reed to purchase additional property and to replace many of the temporary buildings added during the war with permanent structures. Between 1920 and 1922, the Army purchased 44 acres of land north of the Post that was part of the Sixteenth Street Heights subdivision. This brought the campus to its present size of approximately 116 acres. Later in the decade, major east and west additions were added to "old main," bringing Building 1 to essentially what is seen today.

Warren G. Harding, elected President of the United States in 1920, was the first President to personally visit Walter Reed. Mrs. Rea and Miss Lower from the Red Cross at Walter Reed were at the White House making arrangements to bring wounded soldiers there for a garden party when the President approached them and asked if he could come out for a visit. He said how about this Sunday, and they said "of course." Concerned that they had committed to the President of the United States without the knowledge of the hospital commander, they rushed back to the hospital hoping that everything would be alright. It was of course and the President's visit on a beautiful Sunday afternoon in May was a rousing success.

The rolling of Easter eggs on the Monday following Easter was a Washington children's tradition long before it began at Walter Reed in 1923. In 1927, Walter Reed held Washington's first Easter Sunrise Service soon becoming an annual event interrupted only during World War II.

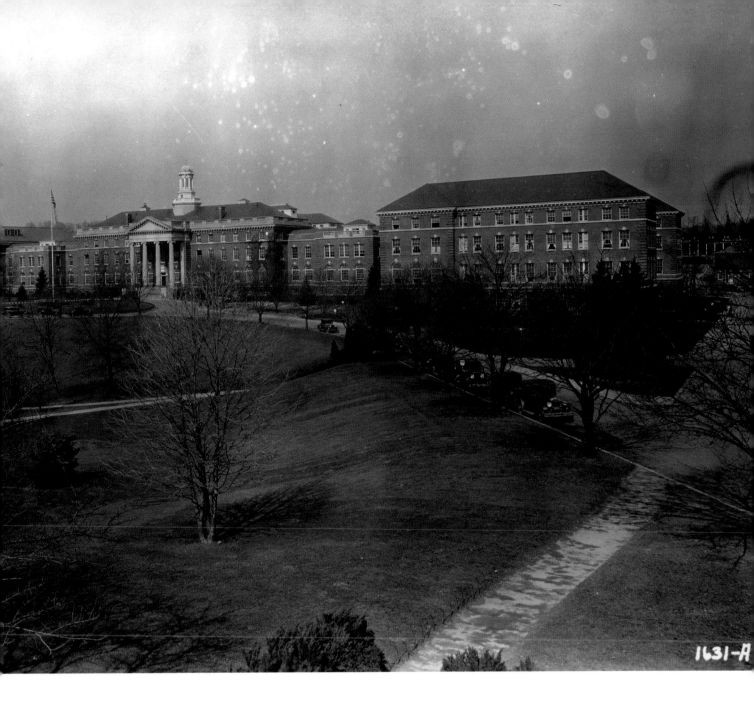

1631-A

The Army Medical School's new permanent building was built on the little knoll to the west of Building 1 that had been the location of the tent-sheltered Hospital Company C in April 1909, the first medical unit to occupy the grounds. The Army Medical School, founded by Surgeon General George Miller Sternberg in 1893, was not a four-year medical school as we know it today, but was a course of variable length depending on the needs of the Army that was an introduction to military medicine for physicians who had no prior service. The new building (Bldg. 40) opened in 1923 and also housed the Army Dental School and Army Veterinary School.

Over the years, Building 40 would undergo significant additions in the 1930s and 1960s. With the arrival of the Army Medical School, the installation was now named the Army Medical Center, which encompassed the schools (Army Medical School, Army Dental School, and Army Veterinary School), Walter Reed General Hospital, and all other activities on Post.

James D. Glennan, Walter Reed General Hospital (1919-1923) and Army Medical Center (1923-1926) commander was an avid garden enthusiast and had much to do with developing the formal garden south of Building 1. He

is credited with acquiring a number of Japanese cherry trees that were surplus from over 3,000 sent from Japan for planting around the tidal basin and Potomac River and having them planted on the upper rim of the rose garden basin.

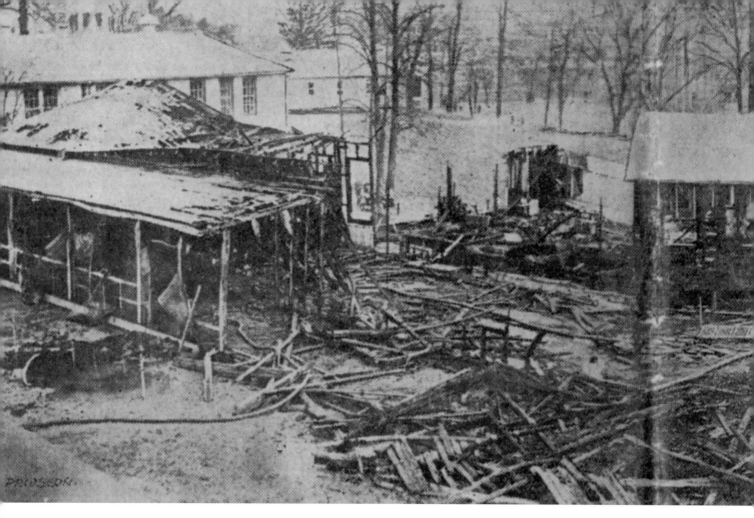

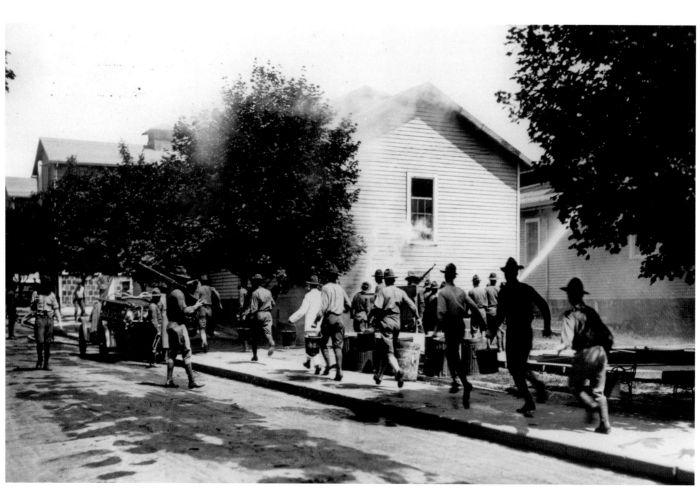

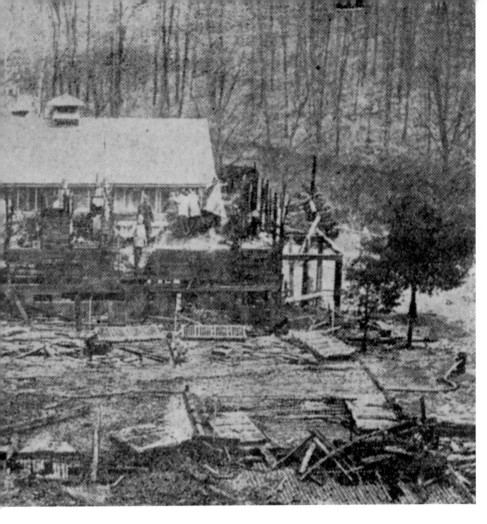

On December 12, 1920, a fire in Ward 43, the ward for neuropsychiatric patients under observation, caused $25,000 damage and the death of one patient. Wards 43 and 44 were completely destroyed. Thirty-eight patients were helped to safety, earning the staff a collective special commendation for conspicuous and meritorious conduct. The destroyed buildings were long low structures, part of a number erected to care for the wounded veterans from World War I. *The Come-Back,* Vol. 2, No. 27, December 18, 1920.

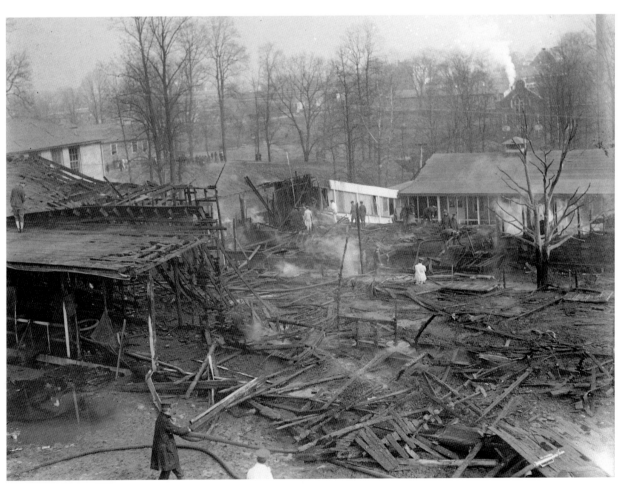

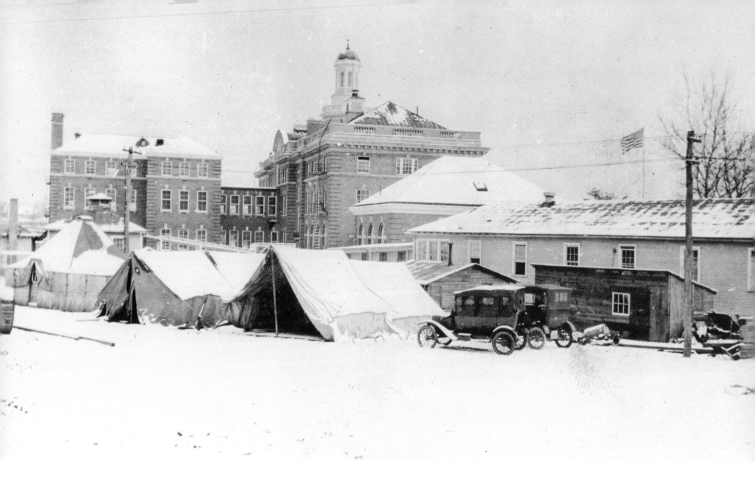

▲ The great influx of patients during and after World War I contributed to crowded conditions on the campus. Temporary buildings and tents filled the grounds around the main building.
Source: National Museum of Health and Medicine, AFIP, Reeve 30624

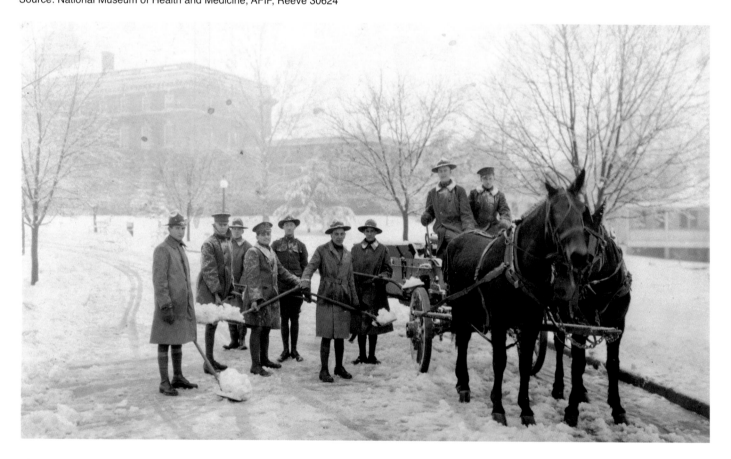

▲ Snow removal team taking quick action.
Source: Walter Reed Army Medical Center, Directorate of Public Works Archives

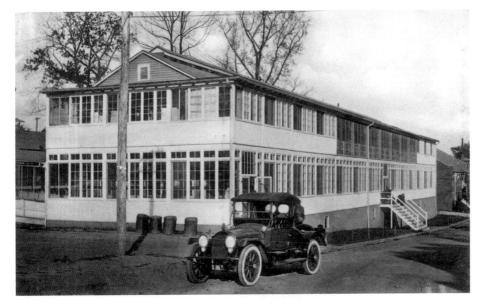

◀ Convalescent Wards 23 and 24 with sunporches.
Source: National Museum of Health and Medicine, AFIP, NCP 15001

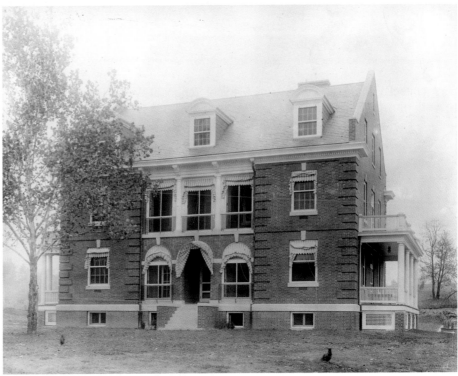

▶ The 12-bed isolation ward was built in 1913. This building was razed in the 1970s to make way for the new hospital building.
Source: National Museum of Health and Medicine, AFIP, Reeve 4176

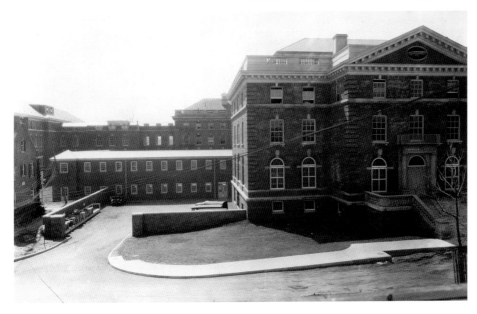

◀ 1927, Entrance to Kitchen Area. Right: first floor, Mess II; second floor, Library; third floor, Eye, Ear, Nose and Throat Wards.
Source: *Borden's Dream* by Mary W. Standlee, p. 218

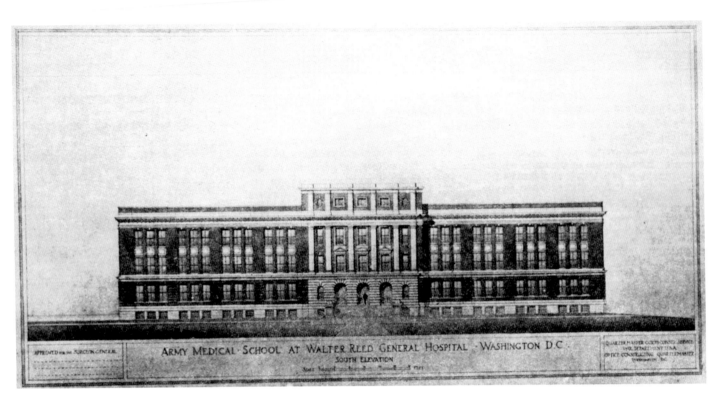

▲ Architect's rendering of the Army Medical School at Walter Reed Hospital. South Elevation. The Army Medical School moved from 7th Street in downtown Washington, D.C., to a location on a knoll west of Building 1, site of the original Company C Hospital Corps encampment.
Source: *The Come-Back*, March 17, 1922

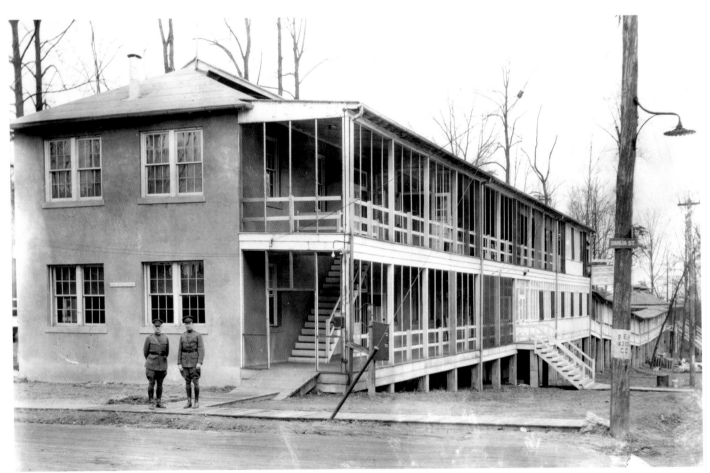

▲ The Army Dental School was located in these temporary WWI buildings from 1922 to 1930 when these buildings were condemned and torn down. March 23, 1923.
Source: Walter Reed Army Medical Center, Directorate of Public Works Archives

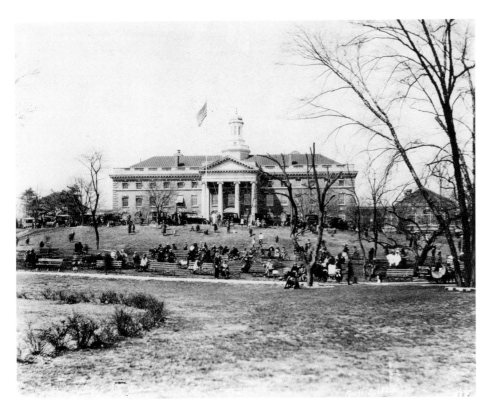

◀ The First Easter Egg Roll at Walter Reed was held the Monday after Easter on April 2, 1923 in the formal gardens.
Source: National Museum of Health and Medicine, AFIP, WRAMC History Collection

▼ The first Easter Sunrise Service in Washington, D.C., was held at Walter Reed in 1927. More than 8,000 people attended the second Easter Sunrise Service in 1928. The services were broadcast live by local Radio Station WRC. The initial Service, co-sponsored by the Washington Federation of Churches and the U.S. Army, featured an impressive "Living Cross" formed by Walter Reed personnel with music by the U.S. Army Band. This annual event, held every year except 1942–1944, has attracted thousands of participants.
Source: *Borden's Dream* by Mary W. Standlee. p. 215

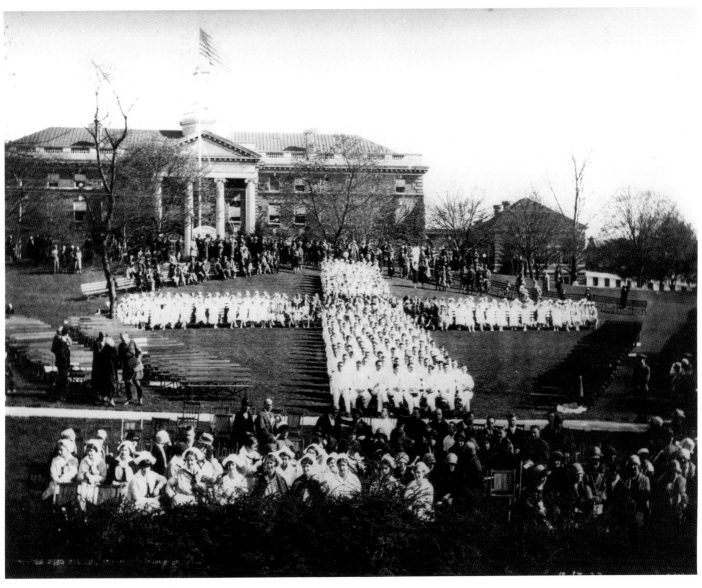

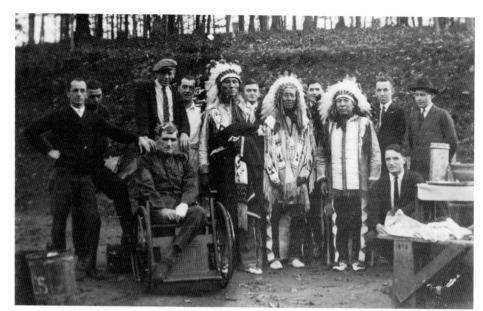

▶ Native Americans with patients.
Source: National Museum of Health and Medicine, AFIP, WRAMC History Collection

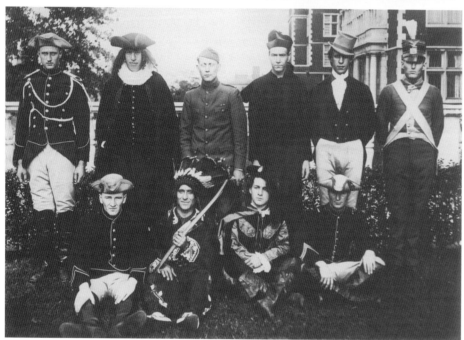

◀ Thanksgiving pageant.
Source: National Museum of Health and Medicine, AFIP, Montgomery Collection

▶ 4th of July pageant.
Source: National Museum of Health and Medicine, AFIP, Montgomery Collection

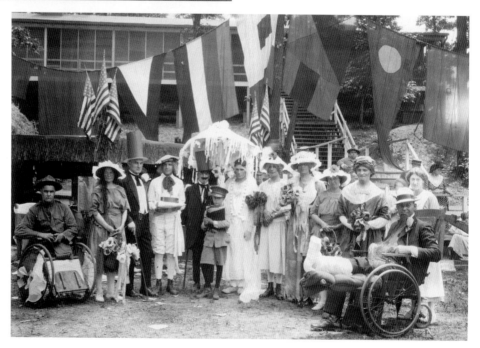

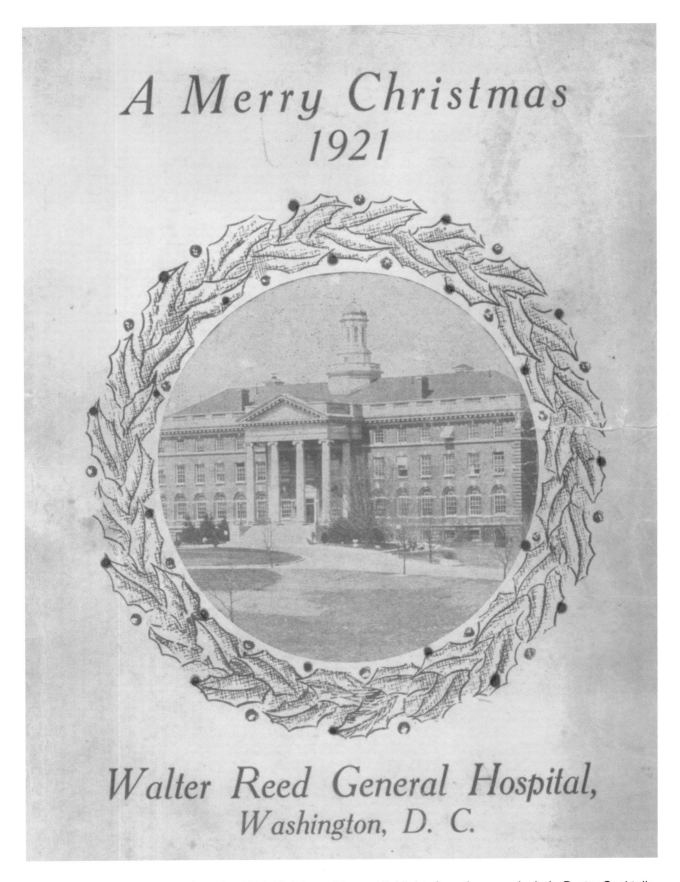

A Merry Christmas
1921

Walter Reed General Hospital,
Washington, D. C.

Front of the Christmas Menu from the 1921 Christmas Dinner. Highlights from the menu include Oyster Cocktails, Roast Virginia Turkey, Skookum Apples, and English Plum Pudding.
Source: Pierce Collection

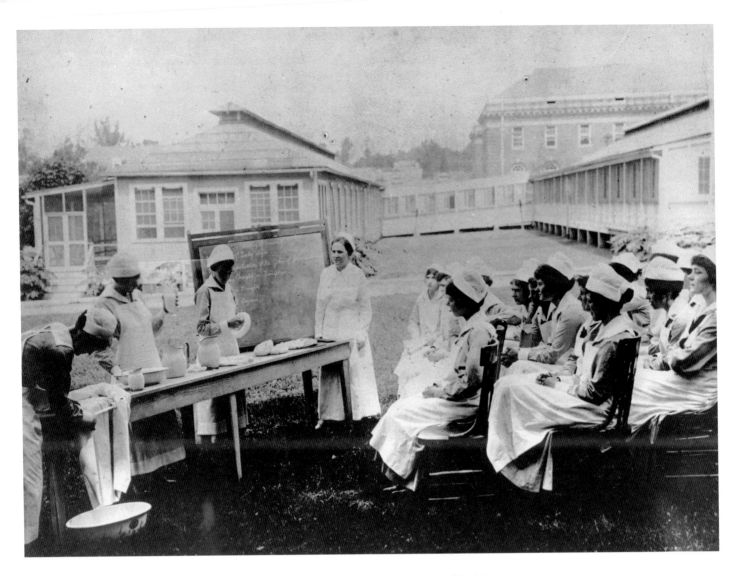

▲ Outdoor class for the nurses. Notice the temporary ward construction behind them.
Source: National Museum of Health and Medicine, AFIP, WRAMC History Collection

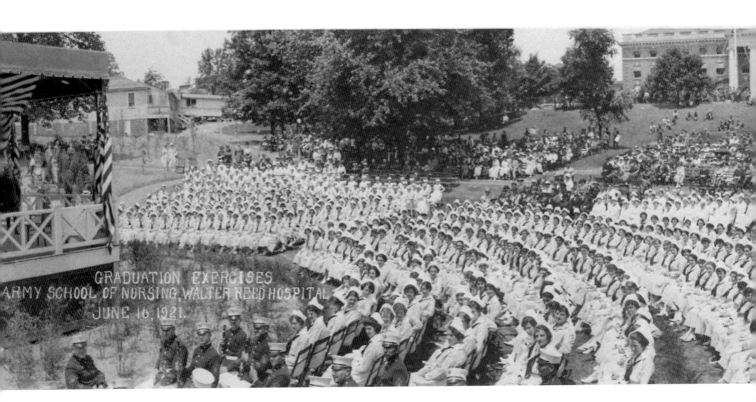

GRADUATION EXERCISES
ARMY SCHOOL OF NURSING, WALTER REED HOSPITAL
JUNE 16, 1921.

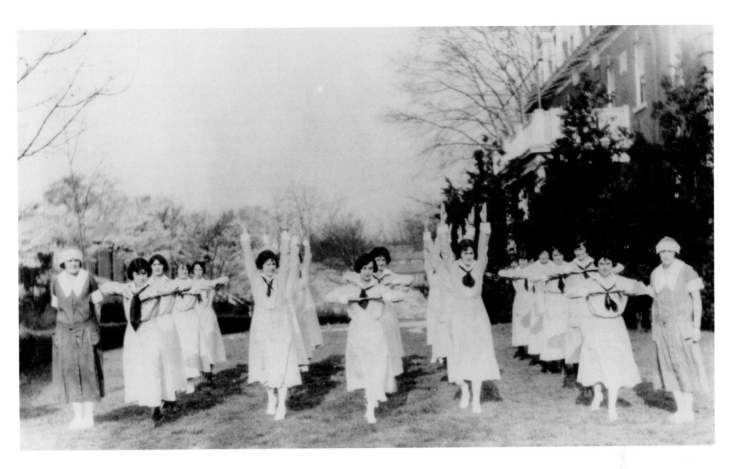

▲ Nurses doing their morning exercises.
Source: Office of The Surgeon General, Office of Medical History

▼ Maj. General Merritte W. Ireland, U.S. Army Surgeon General, presided at the graduation ceremonies for more than 400 students from the Army School of Nursing at Walter Reed. It was said to be the largest graduating class from any similar institution in the United States. June 16, 1921.
Source: National Museum of Health and Medicine, AFIP, 65-12604

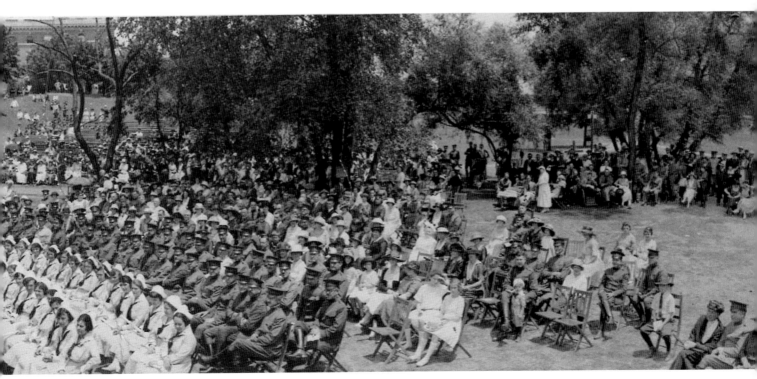

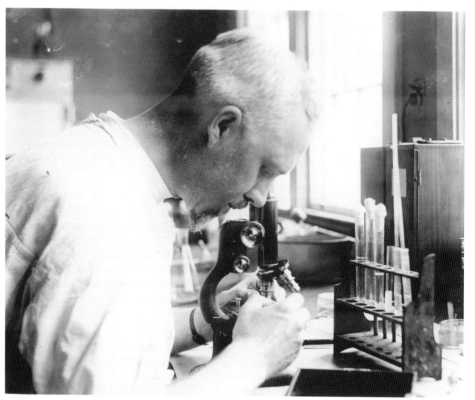

► The study of bacteriology has been important from the beginning of Walter Reed Hospital's history. Here, one of the specialists is studying a slide.
Source: National Museum of Health and Medicine, AFIP, Reeve 608

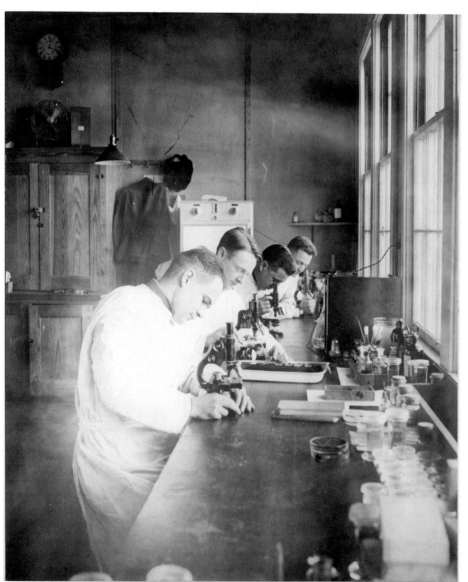

◄ A long view of the bacteriology lab where physicians trained in the Army Medical School.
Source: National Museum of Health and Medicine, AFIP, Reeve 2313

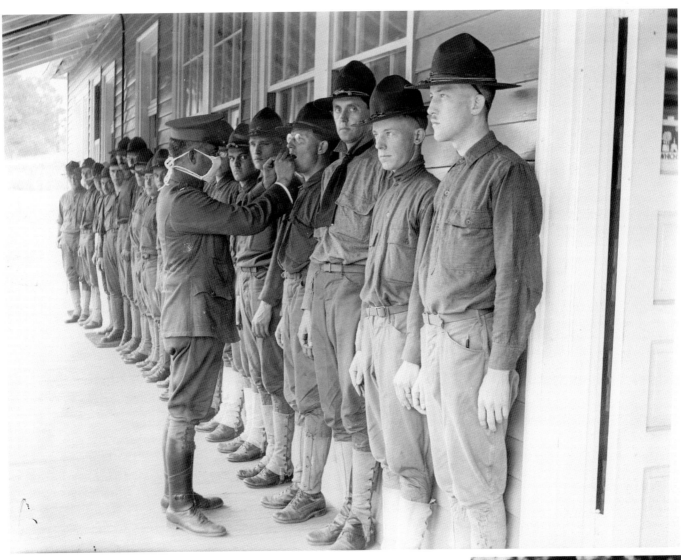

▲ Army officer examining men's teeth.
Source: National Museum of Health and Medicine, AFIP, Reeve 607

▶ (Left) Mrs. Henry (Edith Oliver) Rea, the original Red Cross Gray Lady. She was appointed by the American Red Cross to coordinate the Red Cross activities at Walter Reed during World War I. (Right) Shown is Mrs. Rea wearing the uniform of the day that gave the volunteer women their unofficial name based on the pearl gray color of their dress.
Sources: (Left) Pierce Collection; (Right) National Museum of Health and Medicine, AFIP, WRAMC History Collection

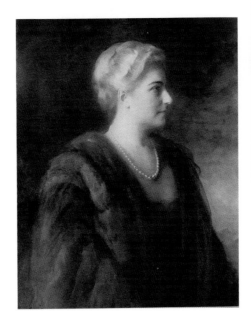

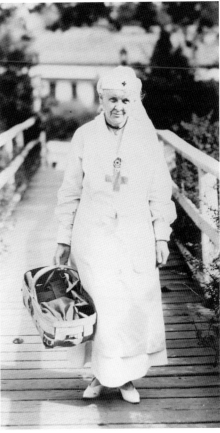

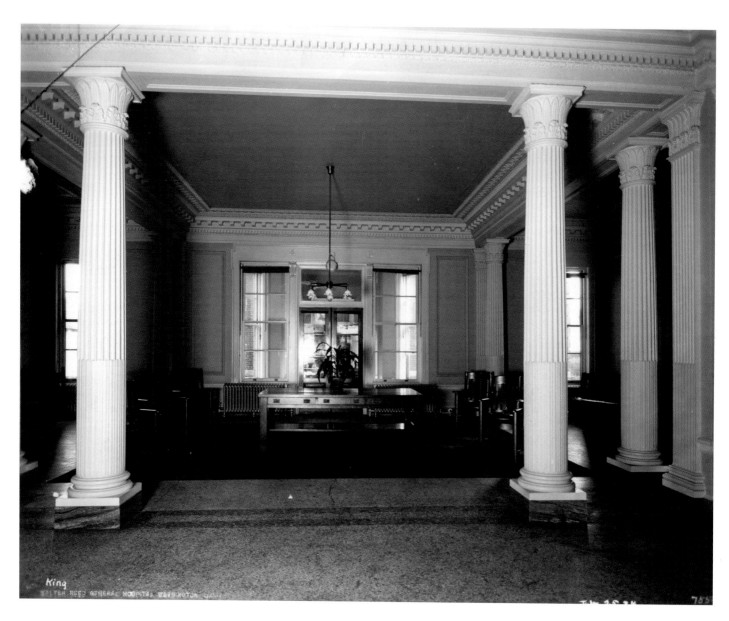

Inside the main entrance to the main hospital (Building 1), July 25, 1924.
Source: Walter Reed Army Medical Center, Directorate of Public Works Archives

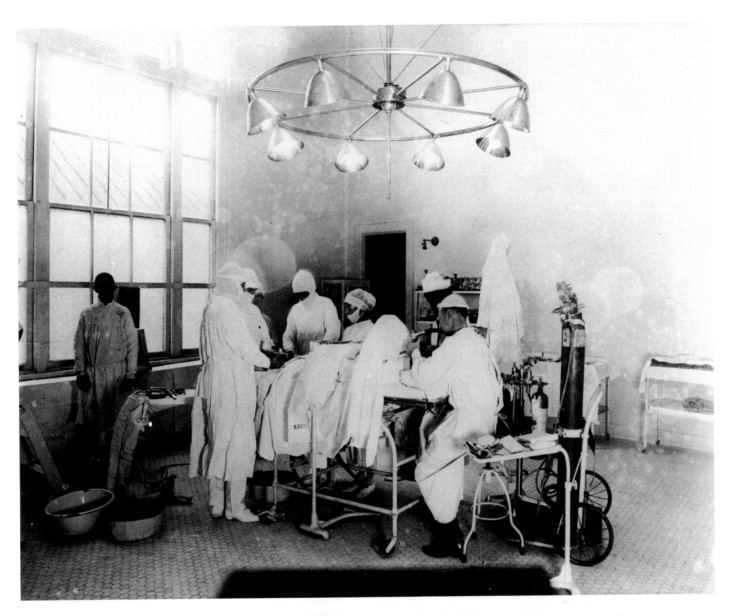

▲ Col. William L. Keller, Chief of Surgery, at work.
Source: *Borden's Dream* by Mary W. Standlee, p. 163

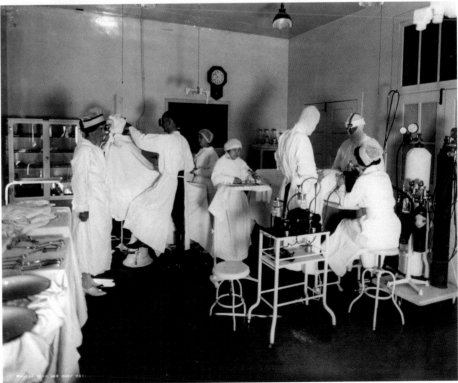

▶ Inside of the Operating Room of the Eye, Ear, Nose, and Throat Clinic, 1922.
Source: Walter Reed Army Medical Center, Directorate of Public Works Archives

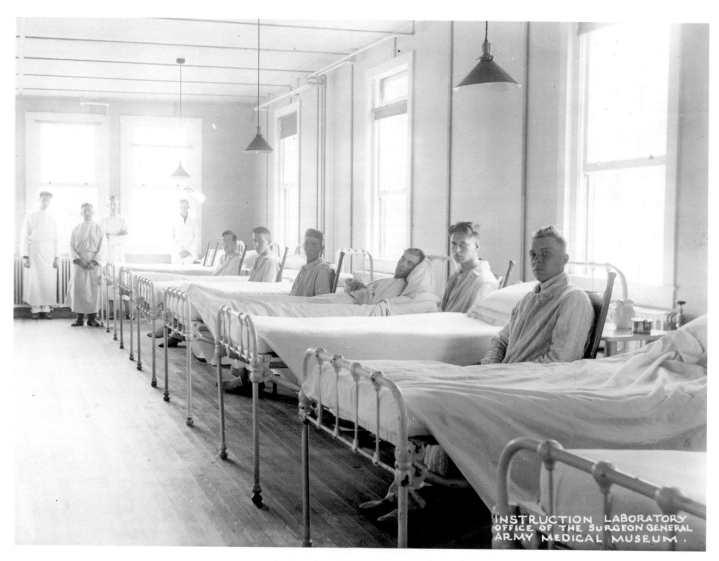

INSTRUCTION LABORATORY
OFFICE OF THE SURGEON GENERAL
ARMY MEDICAL MUSEUM.

▲ A typical hospital ward at Walter Reed. Patients are here for observation.
Source: National Museum of Health and Medicine, AFIP, WRAMC History Collection. Reeve 605

▶ Rehabilitation aides (later called physical therapists) attending to their patients in one of the temporary building wards in August 1922.
Source: Walter Reed Army Medical Center History Office

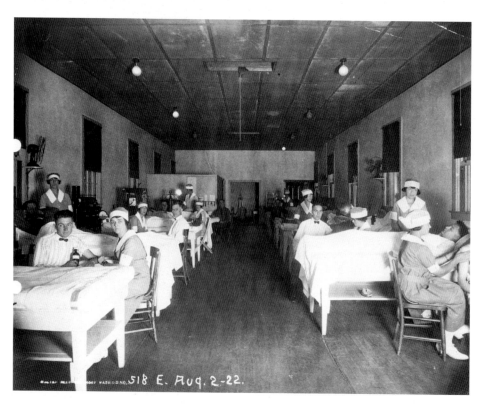

518 E. Aug. 2-22.

44

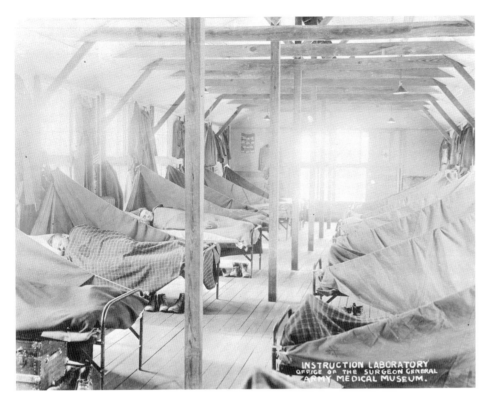

◄ Inside a hospital ward in a temporary building.
Source: National Museum of Health and Medicine, AFIP, Reeve 227

▼ Patients in Ward 72 on New Year's Day, 1920. This was one of the temporary wards built to accommodate the wounded from the Great War.
Source: National Museum of Health and Medicine, AFIP, WRAMC History Collection

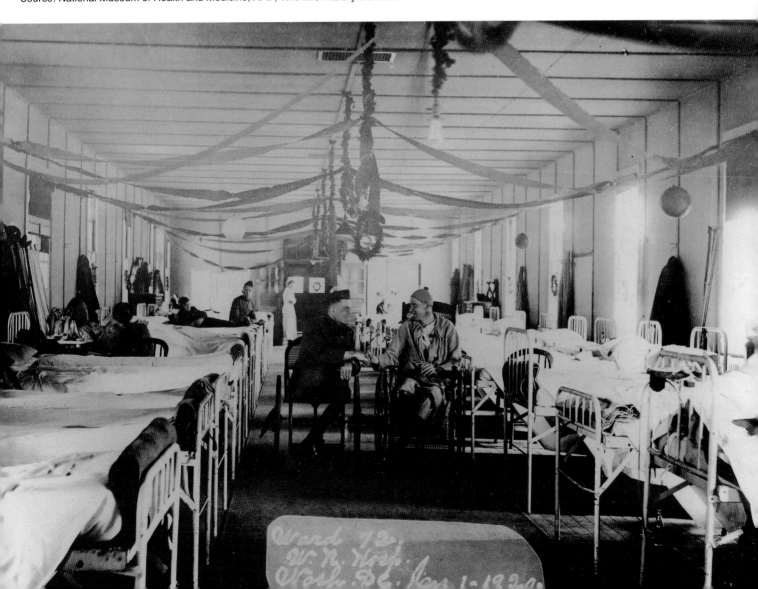

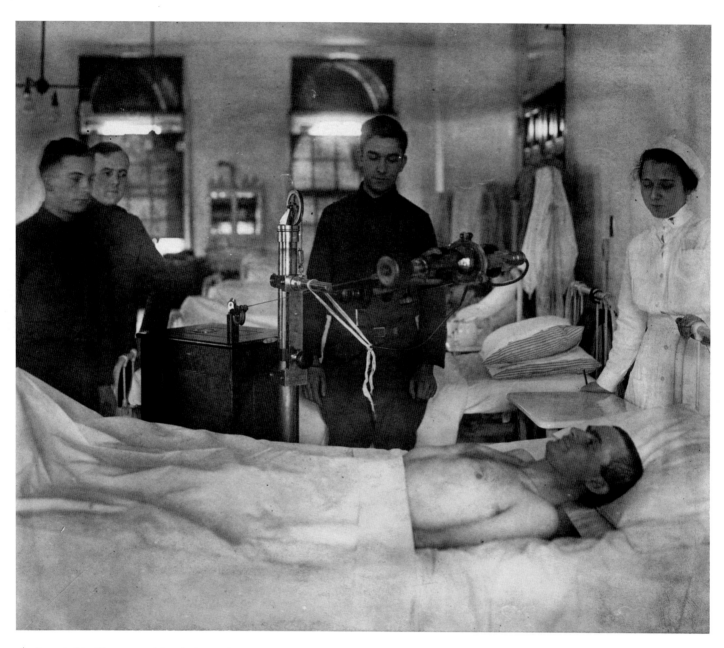

▲ A portable X-ray machine is brought to the patient on the ward. The practice at the time was not to use protective shielding.
Source: National Museum of Health and Medicine, AFIP, Reeve 2312

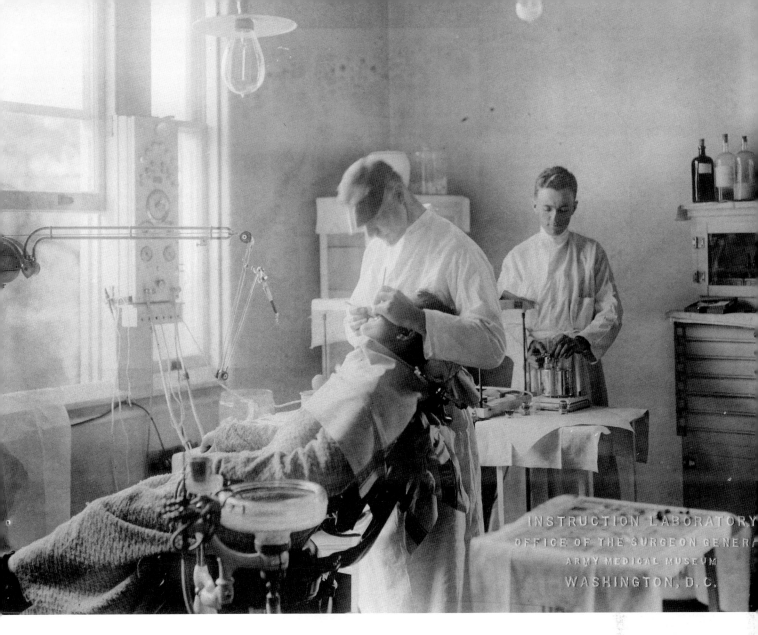

▲ Dental procedure using natural lighting.
Source: National Museum of Health and Medicine, AFIP, Reeve 225

▶ A Dental Technician positioning the X-ray machine for dental radiographs at Walter Reed General Hospital, 1922.
Source: National Museum of Health and Medicine, AFIP, NCP 2732

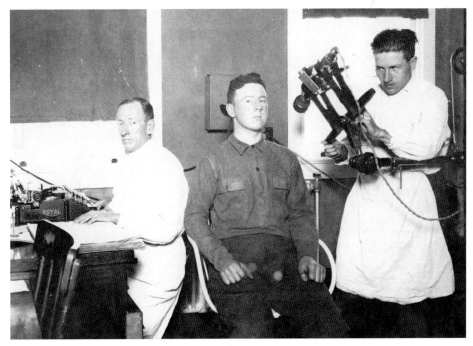

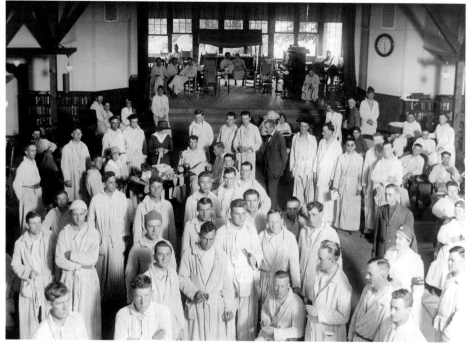

▶ Patients enjoyed a social event in the recreation center of the Red Cross Building.
Source: National Museum of Health and Medicine, AFIP, Reeve 740

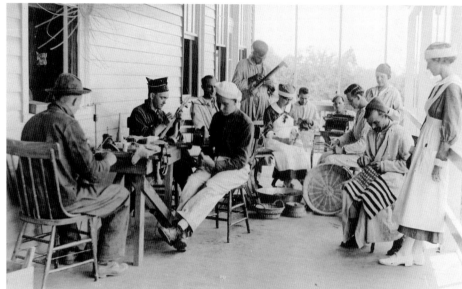

◀ Re-education in the form of occupational therapy is taking place on Ward X.
Source: National Museum of Health and Medicine, AFIP, Reeve 773

▶ A war veteran wearing temporary pilons, which precede permanent prosthetic limbs.
Source: National Museum of Health and Medicine, AFIP, WRAMC History Collection, Reeve 282

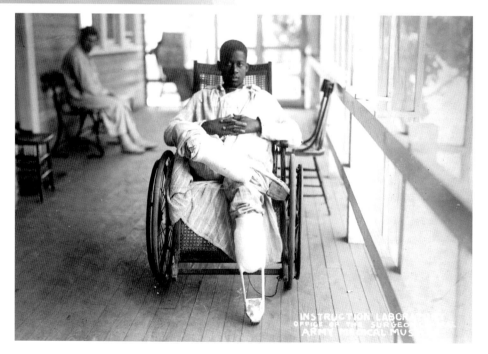

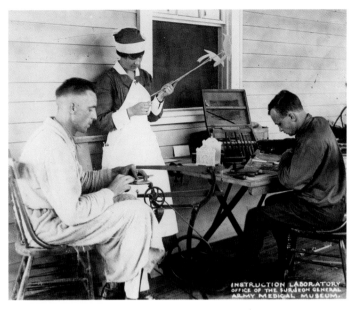

▶ Wounded soldiers being taught scroll work by a vocational aide at Walter Reed Hospital.
Source: National Museum of Health and Medicine, AFIP, Reeve 644

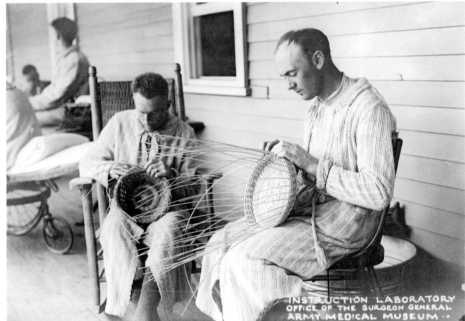

◀ Veterans recovering from wounds are taught basketry. The skills learned here will improve hand dexterity and eye-hand coordination.
Source: National Museum of Health and Medicine, AFIP, Reeve 286

▶ The process of making prosthetics is an essential part of training the patients to return to their normal lives. Here, technicians are shown creating the limbs lost in battle.
Source: National Museum of Health and Medicine, AFIP, Reeves 271

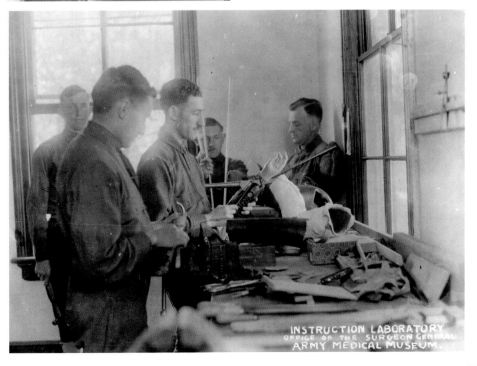

▶ Weaving is not only a creative way to pass time in the hospital, it also teaches eye-hand coordination, teaches injured muscles to work again, and gives the patient a sense of accomplishment when the project is completed.
Source: National Museum of Health and Medicine, AFIP, Reeve 645

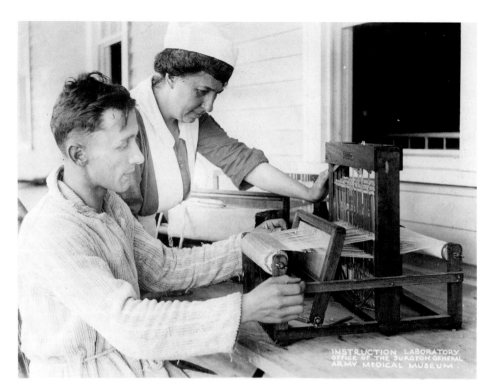

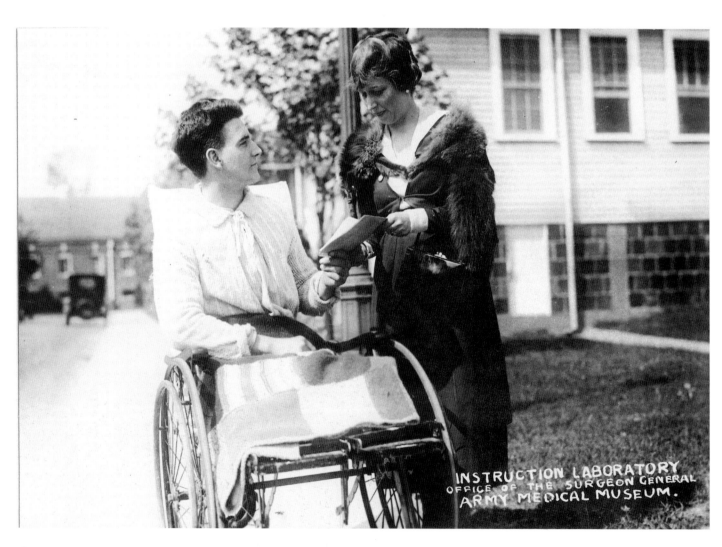

▲ World War I veteran enjoys a spring day on campus.
Source: National Museum of Health and Medicine, AFIP, Reeve 170

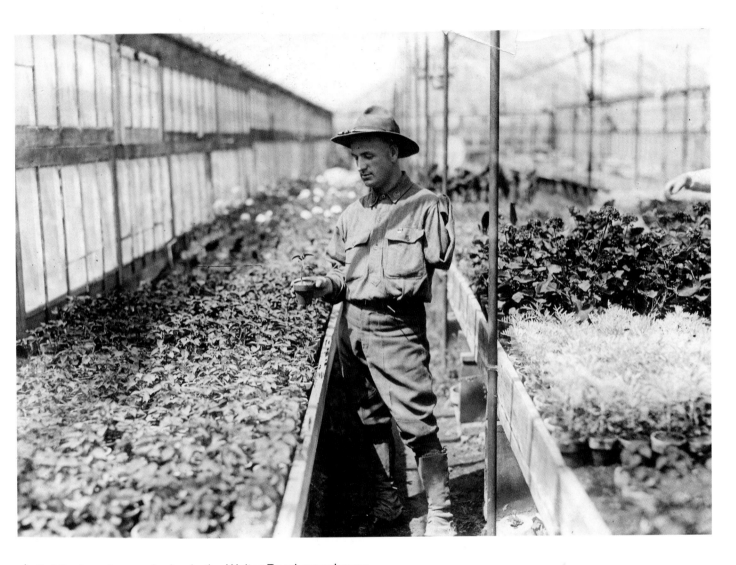

▲ Soldier learning gardening in the Walter Reed greenhouse.
Source: National Museum of Health and Medicine, AFIP, Reeve 280

▶ The World War I veteran received a practical course. Farming, gardening, chicken-raising, and carpentry were taught, as well as stenography, printing, and the crafts. (Original caption)
Source: National Museum of Health and Medicine, AFIP, Reeve 281

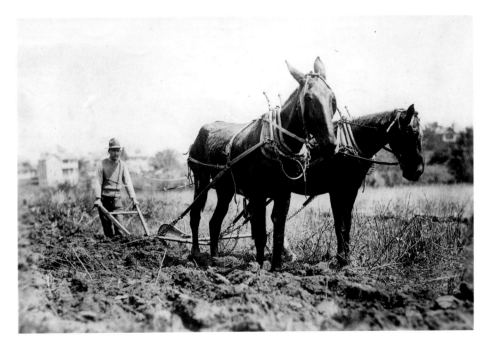

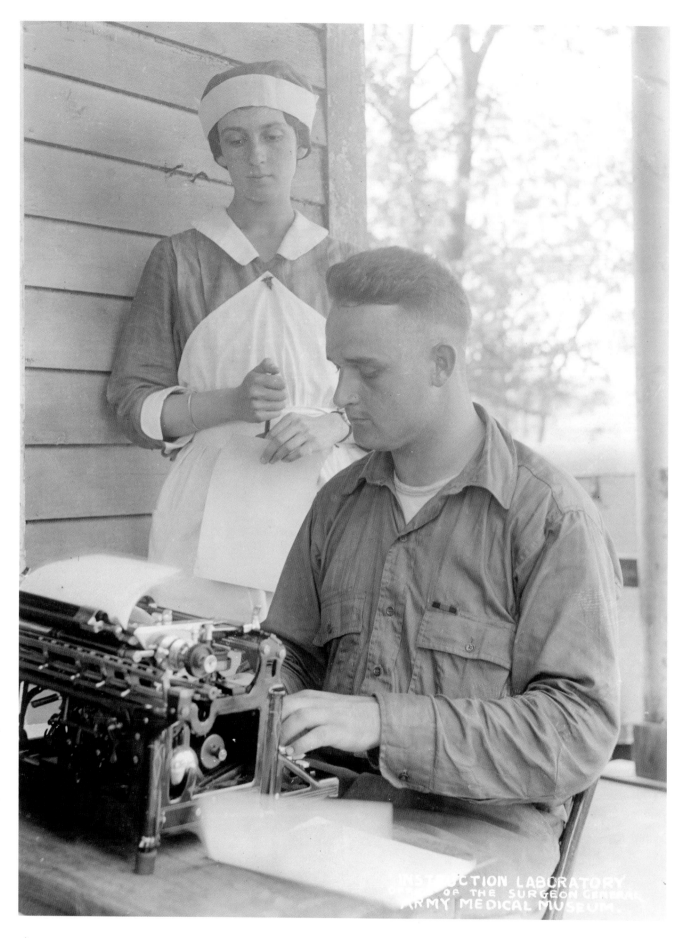

▲ Typewriting is another skill useful both in physical therapy to regain coordination and muscle strength, and also a useful tool for employment after release from the hospital. The patient is being observed by a Physiotherapy Aide.
Source: National Museum of Health and Medicine, AFIP, Reeve 646

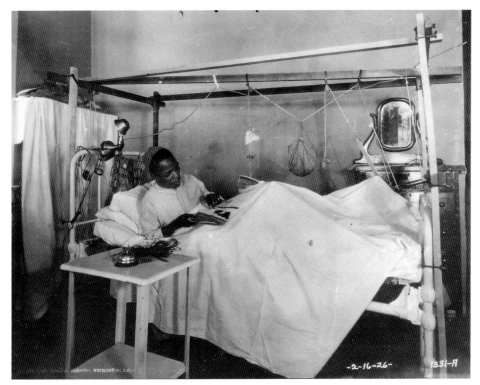

◀ A patient learning hand weaving in his hospital bed, February 16, 1926.
Source: National Archives and Records Administration, SC 560344

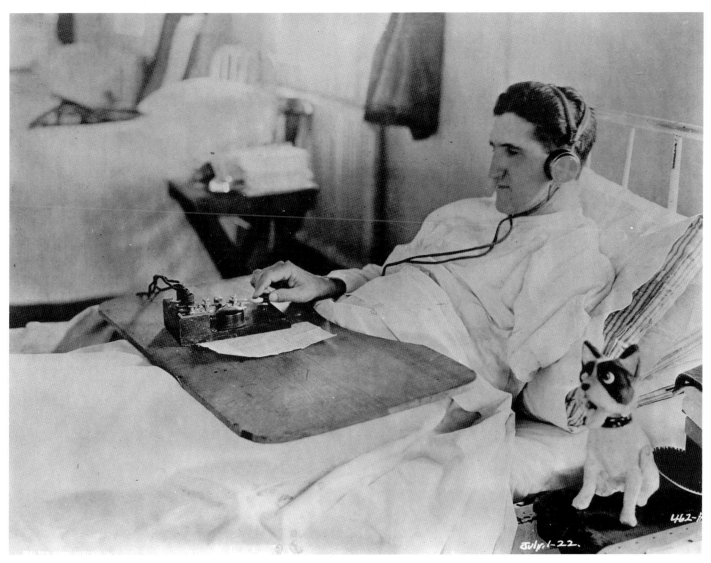

▲ Patient learning telegraphy, July 1922.
Source: National Museum of Health and Medicine, AFIP, Reeve 41849

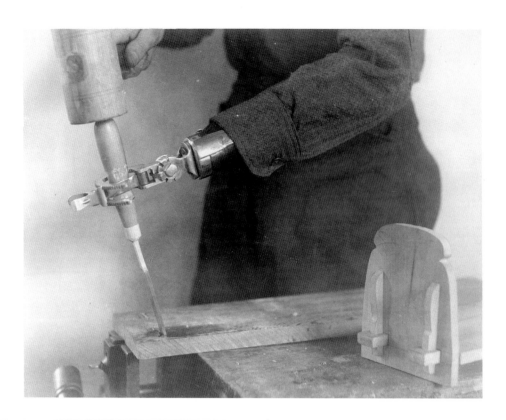

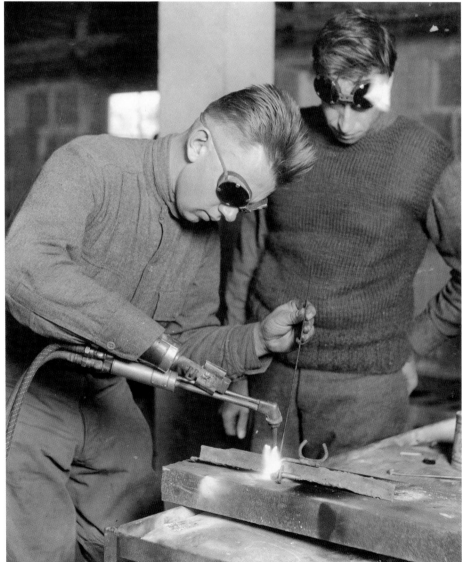

Learning to use prosthetics is critical to the patients' recovery. In this series of photographs, patients are learning dexterity as well as skills for vocations after their release from the hospital.

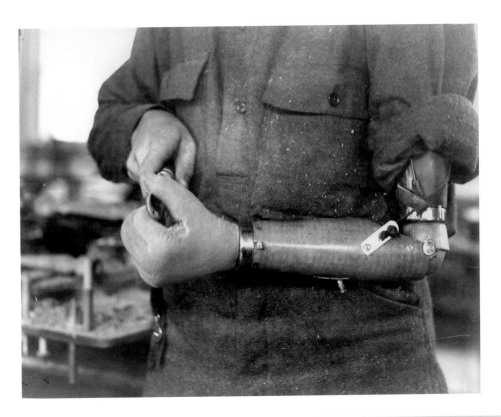

▲ Source: National Museum of Health and Medicine, AFIP, Reeve 4267

▶ Source: National Museum of Health and Medicine, AFIP, Reeve 4269

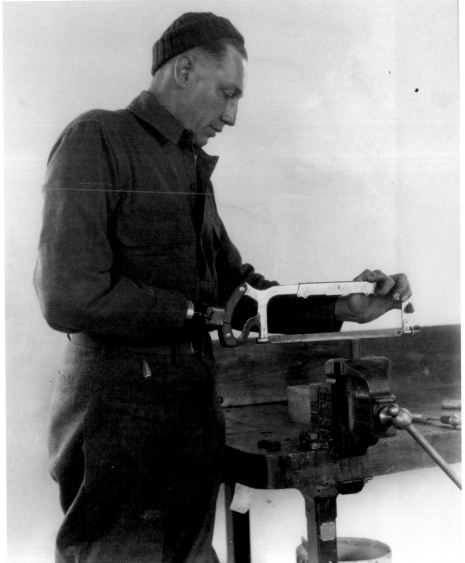

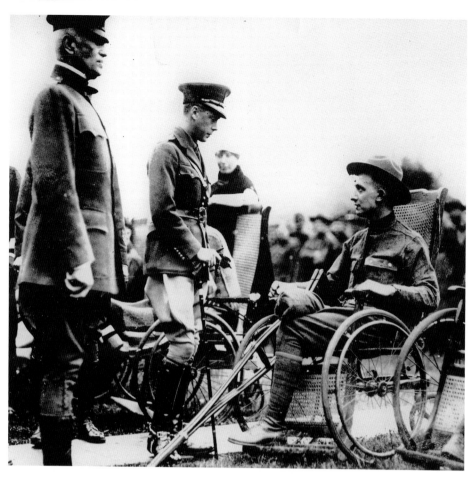

◀ Col. Glennan with the Duke of Windsor visiting with patients in 1920.
Source: National Museum of Health and Medicine, AFIP, WRAMC History Collection

▼ President Warren G. Harding was the first President to visit Walter Reed General Hospital in 1922. Here, he meets patients during his visit.
Source: National Museum of Health and Medicine, AFIP, WRAMC History Collection

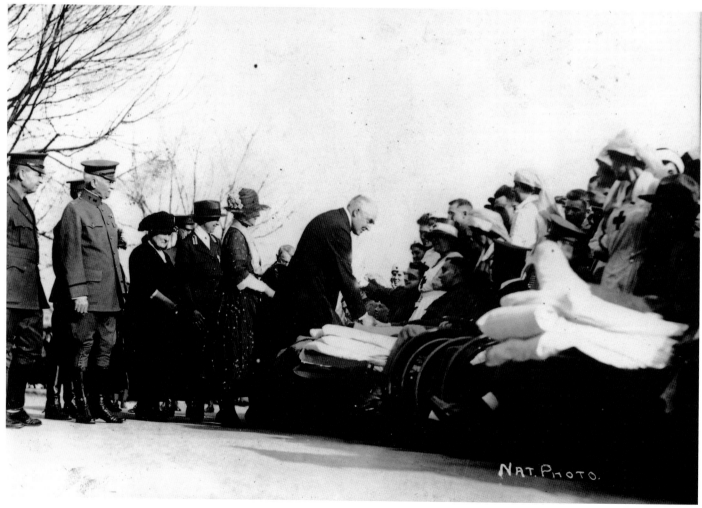

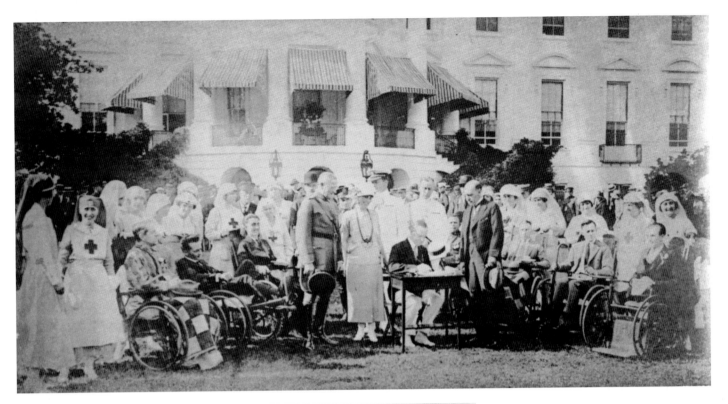

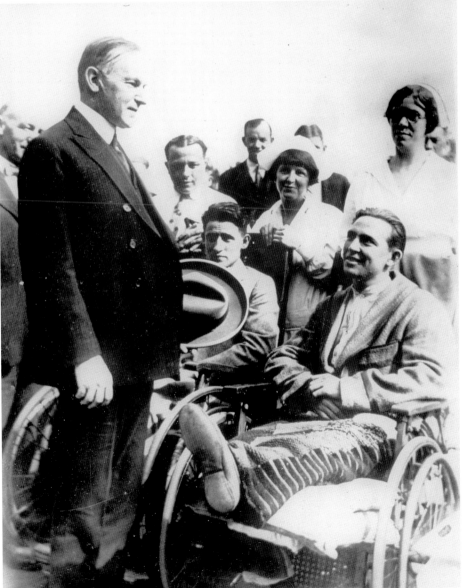

▲ Surrounded by Walter Reed patients and Red Cross Gray Ladies at the White House, President Calvin Coolidge signed a bill for veterans relief pay, June 5, 1924. Looking on is General of the Armies, John J. Pershing.
Source: National Museum of Health and Medicine, AFIP, WRAMC History Collection

◄ President Calvin Coolidge visiting with Walter Reed Hospital patients, 1926.
Source: National Museum of Health and Medicine, AFIP

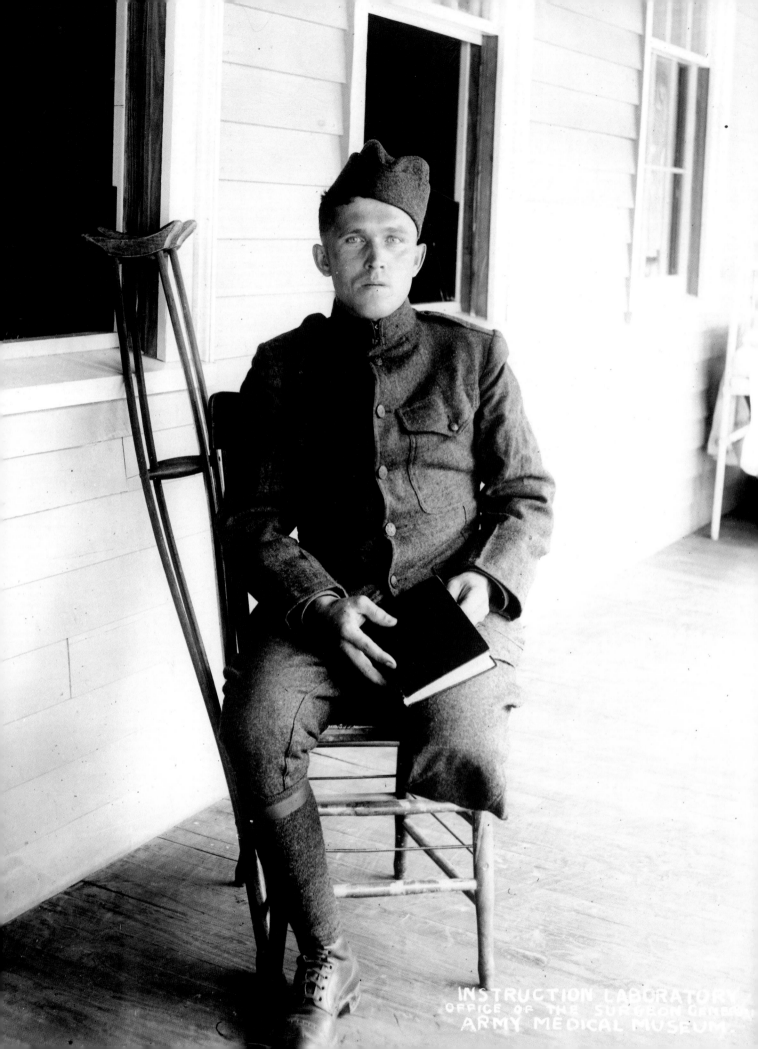

A determined and resolute Pvt. Maleskie poses for a picture in uniform at Walter Reed.
Source: National Museum of Health and Medicine, AFIP, Reeve 1299

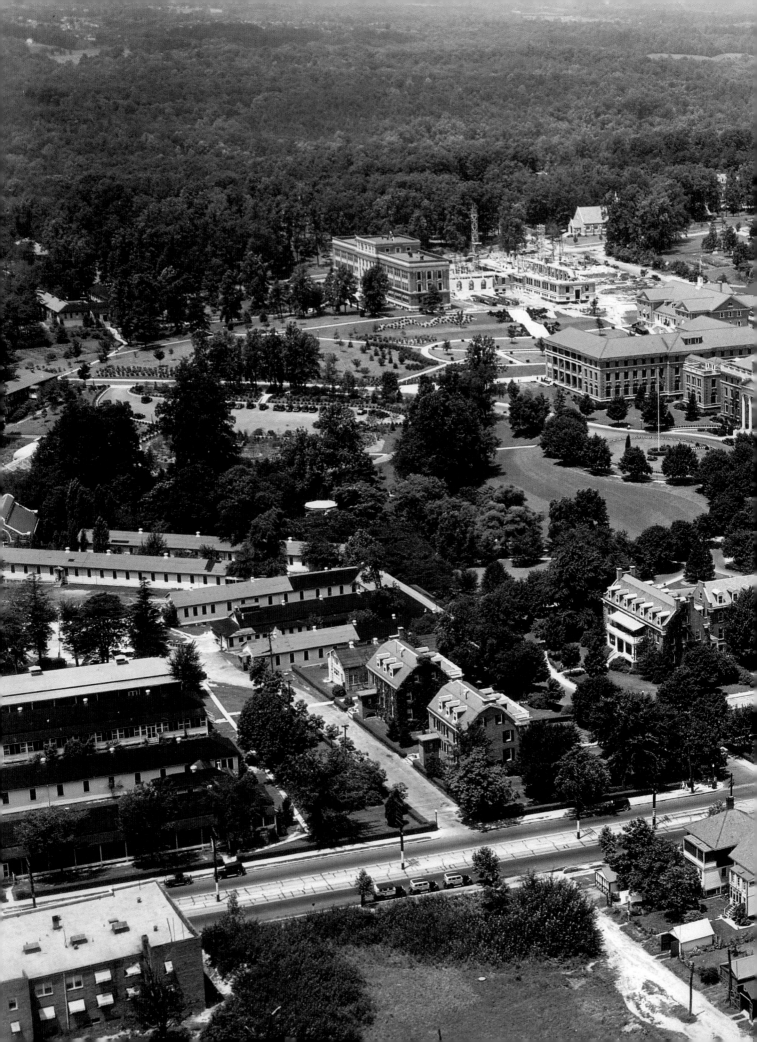

1930–1939

Title page - In comparison to the disorganized, chaotic photo taken in 1921 that opened the previous chapter, this northwest looking photo taken 10 years later shows an extraordinary transformation to an organized, orderly campus of uniform, symmetrical, and permanent buildings. During the 1920s, major additions to the campus had been massive east and west wings onto Building 1, permanent ward buildings north of Building 1, the initial Army Medical School (Building 40, upper left with additions being added), Red Cross Hall (Building 41), and Memorial Chapel. Some of the more orderly temporary buildings remain to the southeast of Building 1 and south of the General Officer's quarters. The flagpole remains in the traffic circle in front of Building 1.
Source: National Archives and Records Administration, 17128AC and 17132AC

▶ This view of an addition to the Army Medical School was taken in April 1931. It shows the massive amount of construction happening on the grounds.
Source: National Museum of Health and Medicine, AFIP, WRAMC History Collection

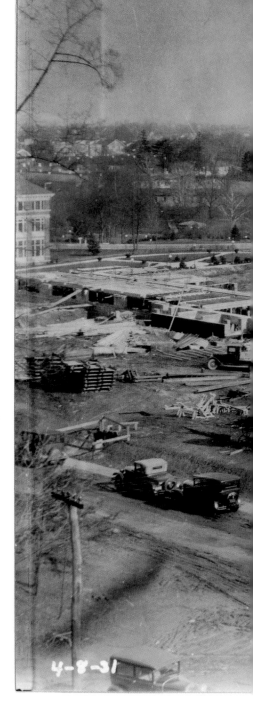

As the demands to care for and rehabilitate the war wounded declined, dependents made up a higher percentage of patients at Walter Reed. In addition, establishment of the Veterans Administration health care system took veteran patients away from all Army hospitals, including Walter Reed. However, Executive Order #6101 of April 5, 1933, authorized treatment of Civilian Conservation Corps members, which helped fill the bed space lost with the exodus of VA patients.

The 1930s brought together a trio of talented surgeons, all destined to leave their mark on Walter Reed and the Army Medical Department. The most senior was the already legendary William L. Keller, who had been Chief of the Surgery Service since returning from World War I. When he retired in 1935, he was the first person made a lifetime consultant by The Surgeon General. He was given an office at Walter Reed, where he returned twice weekly for 15 years until his health deteriorated and he was no longer able to do so. Keller died at Walter Reed in July 1959 at age 85. In August 1974, ground was broken for a new Army community hospital at West Point, NY, that was named for him.

Norman T. Kirk, a previous Chief of Orthopaedics at Walter Reed, returned from the Philippines to resume his old

position in 1930. He had previously served with the Punitive Expedition in Mexico with Pershing and Eisenhower, in Panama, and Texas. During World War I, when assigned to Walter Reed, Kirk had authored *Amputations, Operative Technique*, a book that became a classic in the field. Following World War I, he served in San Antonio, the Philippines, and San Francisco. He returned again to Walter Reed in 1941–1942. Before being promoted to General Officer, he commanded the Percy Jones General Hospital in Michigan. From June 1, 1943 until June 1, 1947, during the height of World War II, Dr. Kirk served as US Army Surgeon General. He died at Walter Reed in 1960 at age 72.

In 1930, James Claude Kimbrough, a veteran of World War I and recipient of the Purple Heart, became Chief of Urology at Walter Reed; he began a long and fruitful association for both. He had already served as Chief of Urology at the Station Hospital in San Antonio and at Letterman Army Hospital in San Francisco. Dr. Kimbrough became a legend in his own time and was known as the "Father of Army Urology." Following his retirement after 36 years of active duty, he was also made a lifetime consultant to Walter Reed. He died in 1956 at Walter Reed after a brief illness. The new Army Community Hospital at Fort Meade, MD, was named for him when it opened in June 1961.

Significant additions to the Army Medical School building (Building 40) were completed in 1932. With the additional administrative space, the Army Medical Center Commander moved out of Building 1 and into Building 40. With the Commander, the flagpole was moved from in front of Building 1 and placed at the east entrance of Building 40. In 1933, the Hoff Memorial Fountain was placed in the traffic circle in front of Building 1, where the flagpole had been.

Plans for a memorial chapel had begun as early as 1922, spurred by Miss Margaret Lower of the Red Cross and

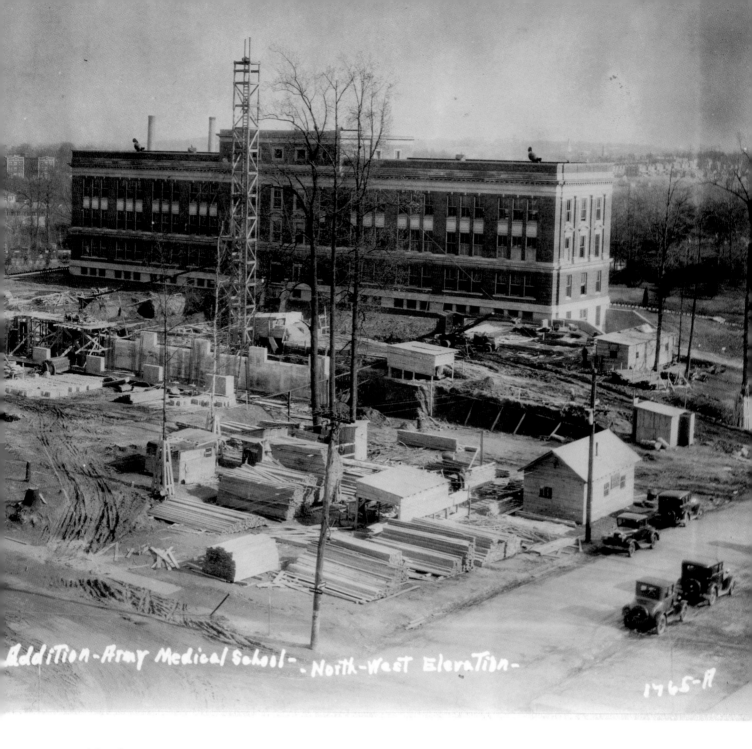

Addition-Army Medical School-. North-West Elevation-

1765-A

encouraged by the Commander, Gen. Glennan. At the time, chapels could not be built with government funds, so monies needed for the chapel were raised from donations. The nest egg was started with a $5 gift from a former vaudeville entertainer; gifts ranged from 25 cents to $32,000 from the ever benevolent Mrs. Rea. The groundbreaking took place on November 11, 1929 at 11 a.m., the eleventh hour of the eleventh day of the eleventh month, eleven years after the end of the "War to End All Wars." The cornerstone was laid May 28, 1930, and the dedication was on May 21, 1931. It was said that, "Ev-

erything in it is a memorial to someone much loved."

Built to house students of the Army School of Nursing and named for the second superintendent of the Army Nurse Corps, Jane Delano, the first section of Delano Hall was completed on November 29, 1930. Additional wings were added, and the entire building was completed in 1934. By that time, however, the Army School of Nursing had been closed since January 1933. The closure was due to the reduction in the number of nurses required, because many nurses were staying on

active duty due to the uncertain economic times, the cost of operation, and the lack of success in retention of those trained.

Most of the construction related to the clinical needs of patients occurred late in the previous decade and early in this one. It involved replacement of the temporary buildings constructed during World War I with permanent wards located north of Building 1. All but one of these was later razed to make way for the AFIP building in the 1950s and even later for the new hospital building in the 1970s.

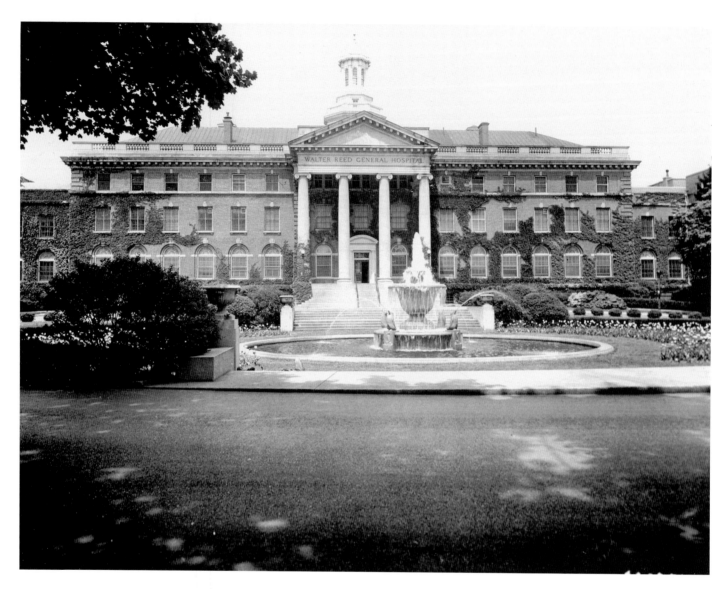

Dedicated October 25, 1935 in memoriam of Col. John Van Rensselaer Hoff. Mrs. Hoff was granted the permit to erect the memorial on January 19, 1931. She died, but the executor of her will, Mr. Van Rensselaer H. Green, carried out her wishes. Col. Hoff was one of the many noted surgeons whose untiring devotion to a cause raised the Medical Corps from a rather insignificant Army adjunct to an important branch of the service. He was born in 1848, entered the Army in 1874, and retired in 1912. He was recalled to active service during the World War and died in 1920. Col. Hoff was, above all, a military surgeon, and was the first officer to apply military drill and precision to the movements of corpsmen in handling wounded patients. During his 38 years of energetic duty, Col. Hoff saw service in the Philippine Islands, Puerto Rico, and Cuba. He was a military observer with the Russian army in the Russo-Japanese War and was Chief Surgeon of the American Expeditionary Force to China in 1900. Mr. James C. Mackenzie designed the fountain, and it was built under the direction of Capt. Kester L. Hastings, Post Engineer, U.S.A. Capt. Hastings' son is Brig. General James E. Hastings, US Army (ret), former Deputy Commander for Clinical Services at Walter Reed.
Source: National Archives and Records Administration, SC 320751

▶ The new nurses quarters, Delano Hall, under construction on April 8, 1931. The Hall had 196 bedrooms for nurses assigned to the hospital. It had sunporches, music rooms, reception rooms, and a ballroom. It was named for Jane Delano, the second superintendent of the Army Nurse Corps.
Source: National Archives and Records Administration, SC 590550

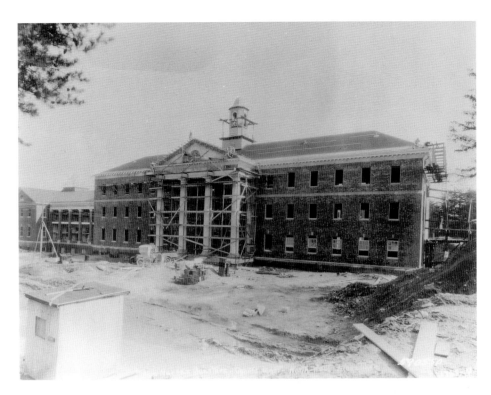

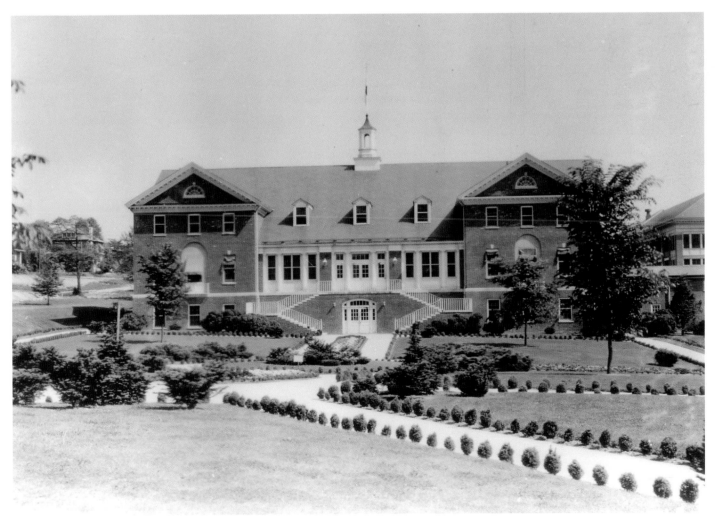

▲ The Red Cross Hall, South elevation, taken June 7, 1932. This new building, completed in 1928, replaced the original World War I period structure, and was paid for by the American Red Cross and donated to Walter Reed.
Source: National Archives and Records Administration, SC 59055

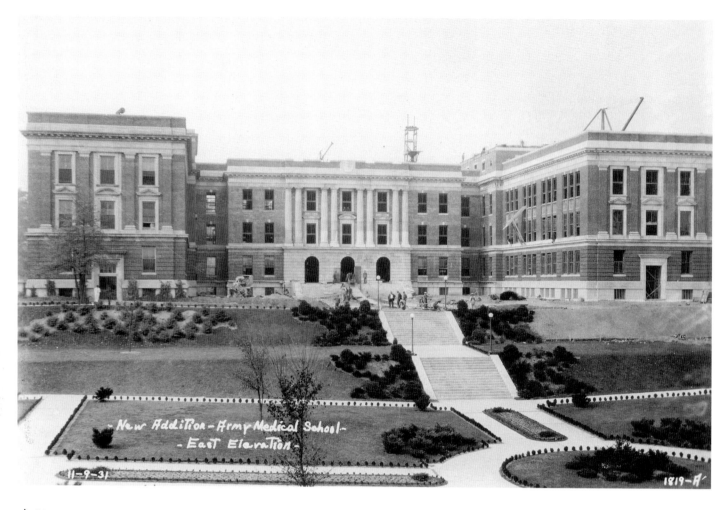

▲ New addition to the Army Medical School, East elevation. November 9, 1931.
Source: WRAMC Historians Office, PAO Historical Collection

▶ The new headquarters of the Army Medical Center in Building 40, September 13, 1935. The flag was moved from its previous location in front of the hospital when the headquarters moved to the new building.
Source: National Archives and Records Administration, SC 590700

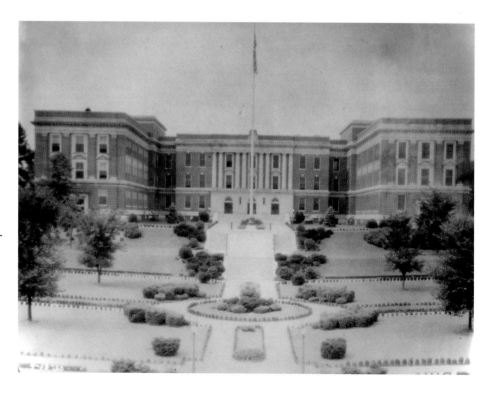

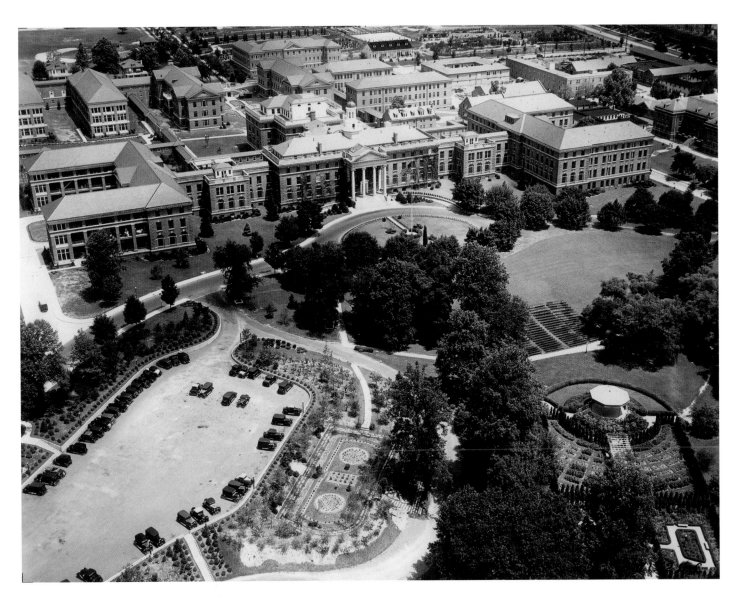

▲ This view of the front of the hospital was taken in early 1935. The pergola and rose garden can be seen in the foreground.
Source: National Archives and Records Administration, SC 320751

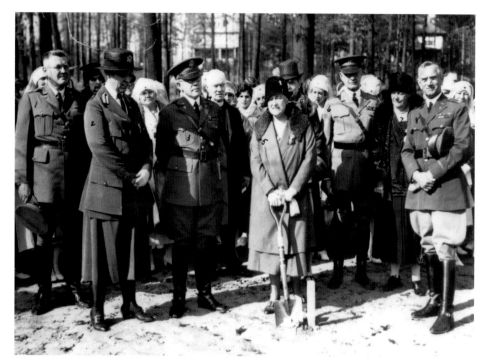

◄ The groundbreaking for the new chapel. In attendance is Chaplain Oliver, Miss Margaret Lower, Gen. Darnall, Father McGeary, Mrs. Edith Oliver Rea, Miss Boardman, General Merritte Ireland, Mrs. Walter Reed (black dress and black hat), and Col. Easterbrook. 1929.
Source: WRAMC History Collection

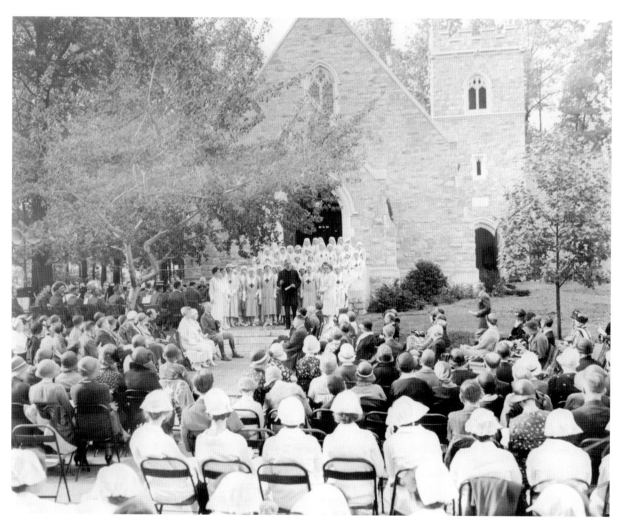

▲ Dedication services for the Memorial Chapel were held on May 21, 1931. Among the visitors were Mrs. Herbert Hoover, the Secretary of War, Mrs. Patrick J. Hurley, and Mrs. Woodrow Wilson.
Source: Pierce Collection

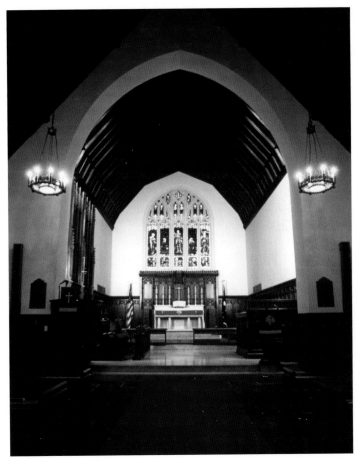 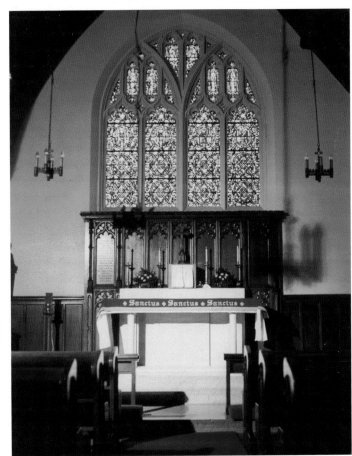

▲ These later interior views show the main altar in the Memorial chapel (left). The "Little Chapel" (right) equipped by the McCook family in memory of family members "who served their country in the war for the preservation of the Union." In time, this became a Roman Catholic sanctuary due to its frequent use.
Source: WRAMC History Office, PAO Historical Collection

The influenza epidemic of 1918 led to caskets filling every available space. In 1922, spurred by Miss Margaret Lower and supported by General James D. Glennan, Commander, the Gray Ladies began to plan for construction of a memorial chapel. By 1924, a site was identified and fund-raising efforts were begun. Donations ranged from twenty-five cents to $32,000. When construction bids were examined in October 1929, the estimate had increased to $84,900 without windows, an organ, the altar, a flagstone floor and foundation, or a Glennan memorial tower. When finally completed, the building cost $161,000. The costs were met by an impressive list of memorial gifts. The groundbreaking ceremony was held on the 11th hour of the 11th day of the 11th month on the 11th anniversary of the end of World War I.

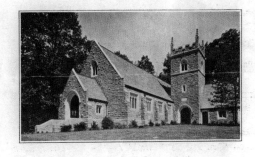

Services of Consecration
of the
Memorial Chapel

Walter Reed General Hospital

Army Medical Center
Washington, D. C.

June 7, 1931

▶ Cover of the Services of Consecration of the Memorial Chapel.
Source: National Museum of Health and Medicine, AFIP, Reid Collection

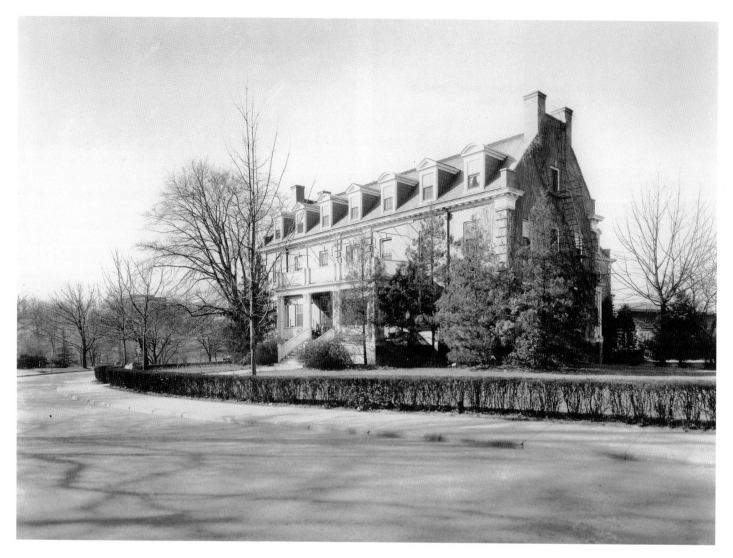

▲ Built in 1911 to house nurses, Building 12 was located near Georgia Avenue and the main entrance to the hospital. Jane Delano, the second superintendent of the Army Nurses Corps, insisted the barracks be located near the front of the property. When Delano Hall (Building 11) was completed in the 1930s the nurses quarters were moved there. Building 12 became officer's apartments. This photograph is from about 1931.
Source: National Museum of Health and Medicine, AFIP, WRAMC History Collection

▶ Brig. General Albert E. Truby, a contemporary of Walter Reed, was an advocate for the powers of healing from the enjoyment of nature. Here is a pergola with clinging roses in bloom as seen looking west through the Portal Garden about 1932.
Source: National Archives and Records Administration, SC 590597

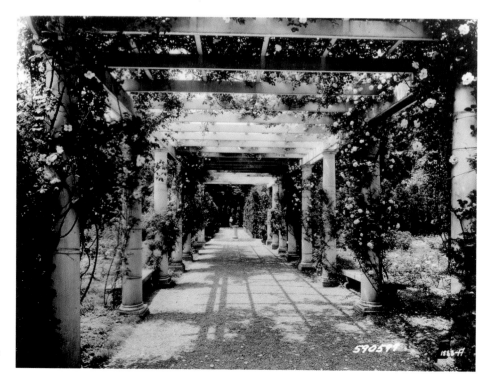

▶ Nurses relaxing in the reading and music room of the new Delano Hall. February 1, 1939.
Source: National Archives and Records Administration, SC 590777

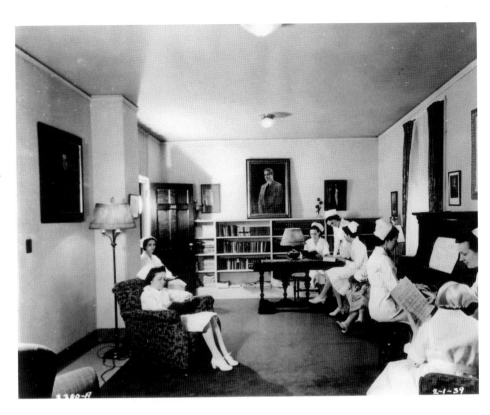

▼ A library was established to serve both the patients and the staff. The Library continues to serve the Walter Reed base.
Source: WRAMC Library

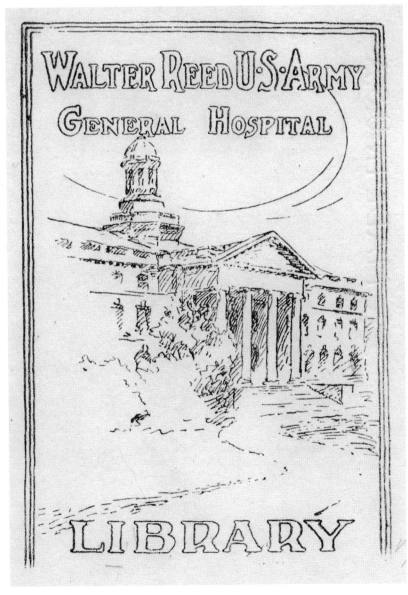

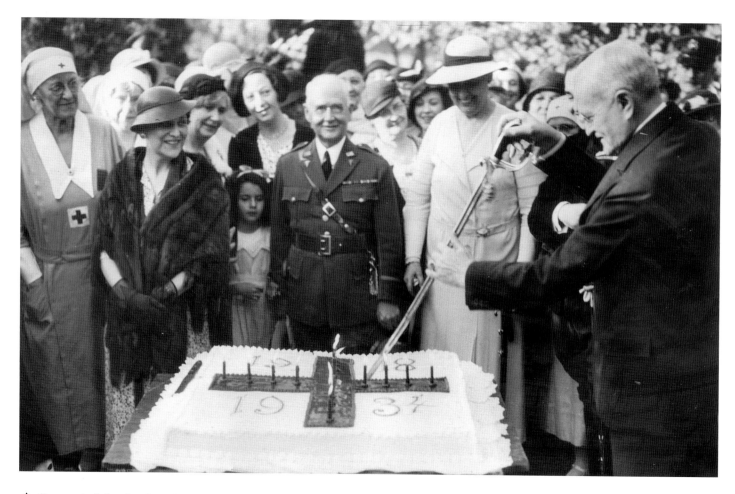

▲ General of the Armies, John J. Pershing, was an ardent supporter of the hospital and the medical care of the soldiers who served under him in World War I. He made numerous visits to the hospital, participating in many activities. Here, he is cutting the cake to celebrate the 16th Anniversary of the American Red Cross at Walter Reed in 1934. Also pictured are Brig. General Albert Truby, CG, and Miss Margaret Lower, Field Director, ARC.
Source: National Archives and Records Administration, SC 590677

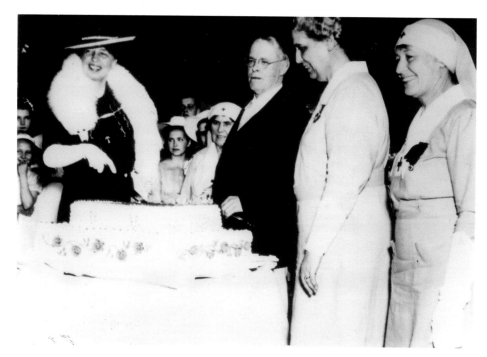

◀ In 1938, Mrs. Eleanor Roosevelt, wife of the President, cut the cake at an American Red Cross party at the hospital. Brig. General Wallace DeWitt and Miss Lower stand in the foreground.
Source: National Archives and Records Administration, SC 590763

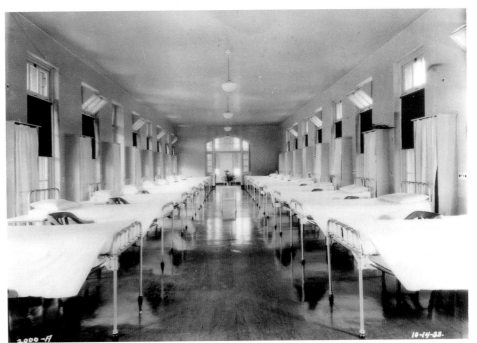

► Interior view of Ward 9A waiting for patients. October 14, 1933.
Source: National Archives and Records Administration, SC 590631

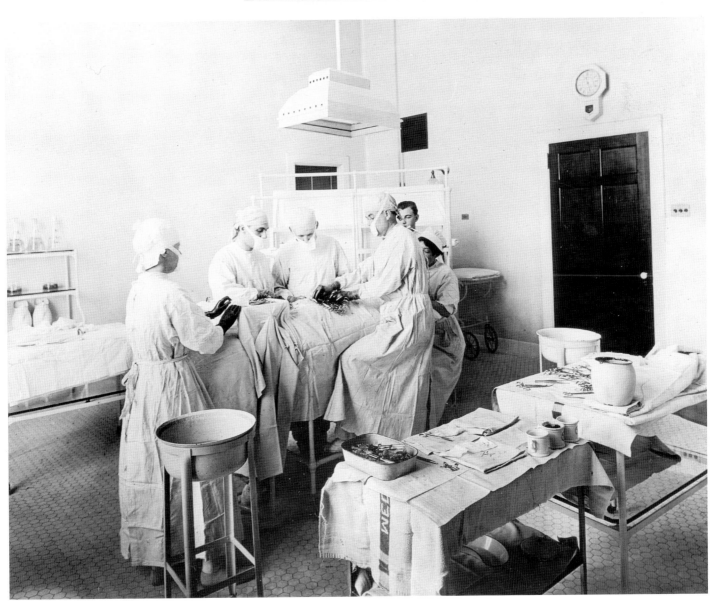

▲ Surgical Operating Room at Walter Reed Hospital about 1935.
Source: Walter Reed Army Medical Center History Office

WARD 21

G UR-R-RL, you're wonderful!" There is just one question we want answered before we leave: "What is 21 going to be when Major Lehman has gone?" The class of 1930 was the first entire class to have its Obstetrics at Walter Reed, and thank goodness we all got through before Major Lehman was transferred!

Twenty-one is many things beside the Obstetrical Service. For one thing, it is the water-tight excuse,—"on call to 21"—and that "call" lasts three months. Anything and everything can be sidestepped for the evenings of that time,—not only can, but must.

It is also the happiest, most informal service on the Post, and no one concerned is really sick. We learned a lot,—or thought we did,—about the psychology of early parenthood. Some of it comes under "Grandiose Delusions", and a lot of it under "Situation Psychoses." But the complete non-repression of our resistive little charges in the Nursery was the real revelation,—that and their individuality. Don't ever believe that a Mother doesn't know her child from all the rest,—its been tried.

Whole days we spent making supplies, down in the Utility Room, days when we talked sixteen to the dozen all our time on duty, with never a long breath. And who could forget Duffy's doll? It was made of a suture pad, a sponge, and a 4x4, with a face painted in mercurochrome! Yet the covers vanished into the big bag, filled, in spite of all the sociable hours.

Before we leave the subject of 21, we want to give special mention to the young lady on night duty at the time, who, on going upstairs with a tray of nourishments, fell up with twenty-four glasses of chocolate malted milk be-showering her. She broke every glass but one. We want to congratulate her on that one glass, but in the same breath hope that life won't always give her such a deal.

But take heart, all you who are leaving your time in 21,—for Public Health awaits you in another year, with dozens more of little babies to care for, and loads of doting mothers.

Eighty-one

The nursing class of 1930 was the first entire class to train in obstetrics at Walter Reed.
Source: National Museum of Health and Medicine, AFIP, WRAMC History Collection (TAPS 1930)

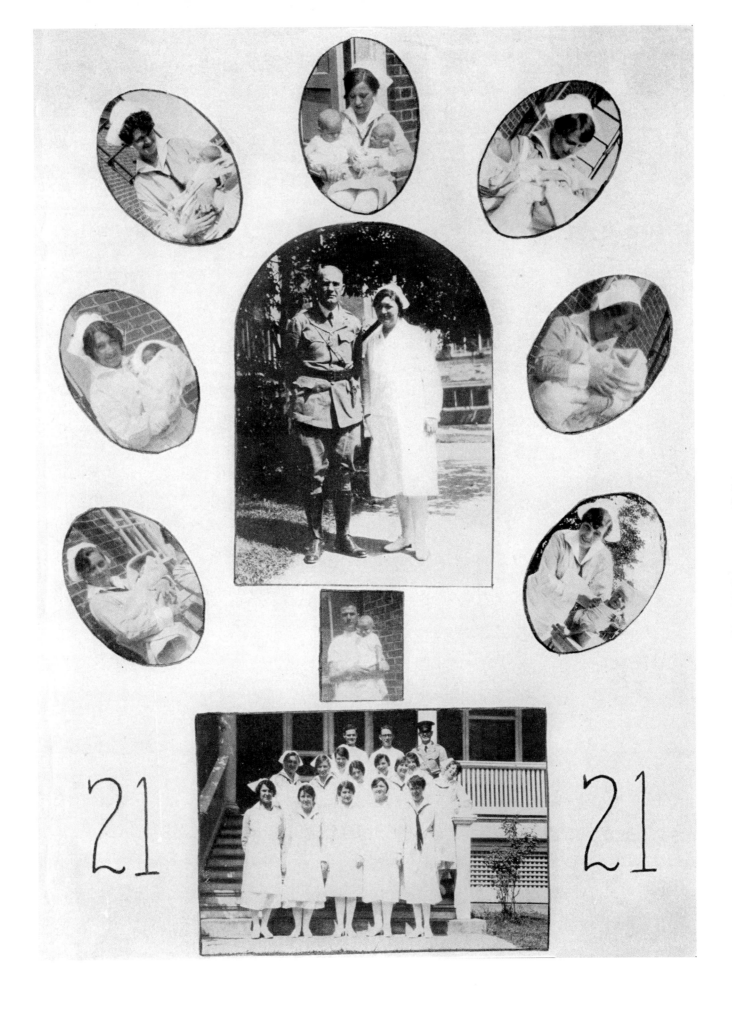

21 21

75

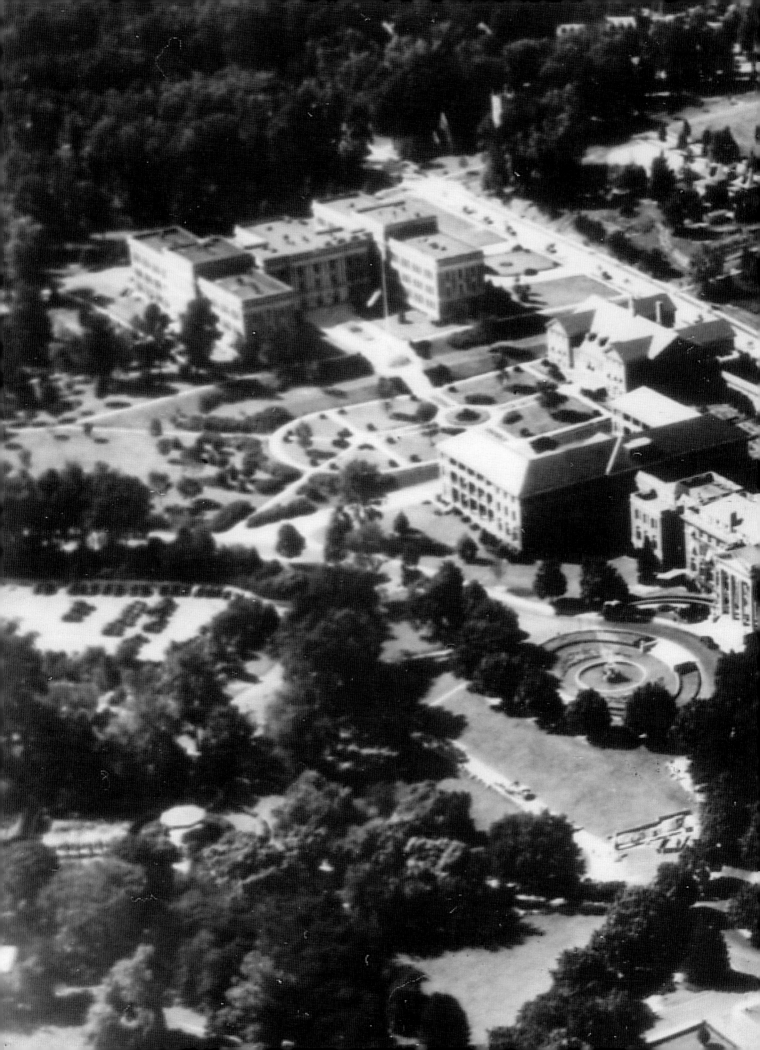

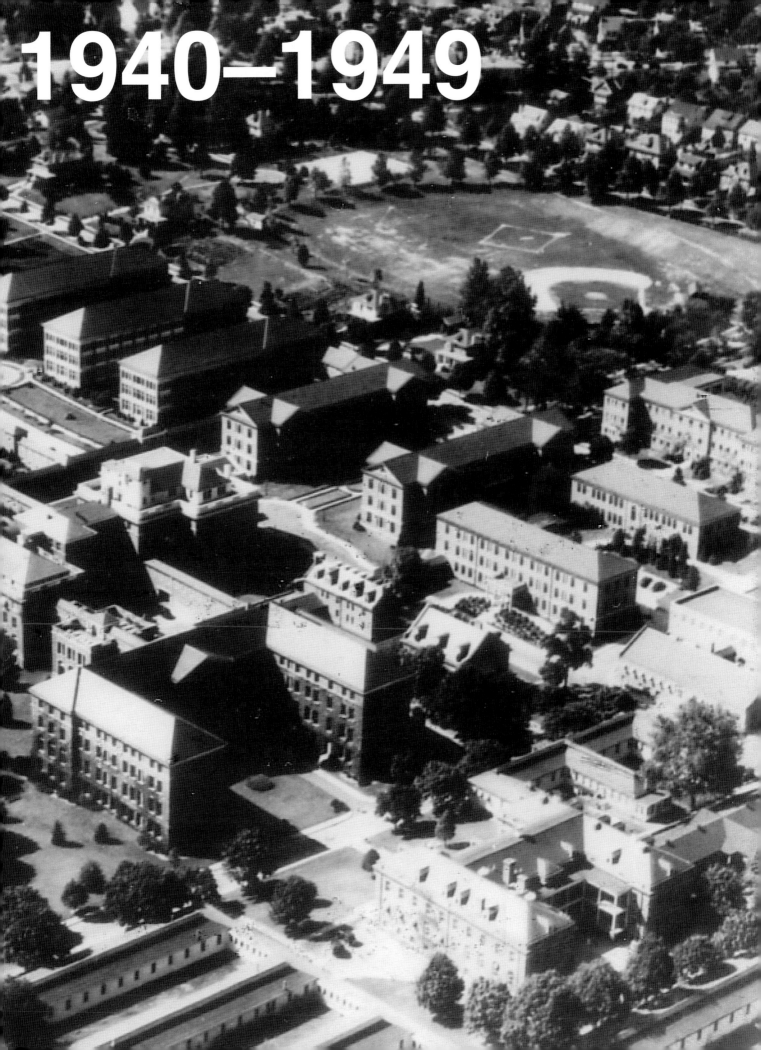

1940–1949

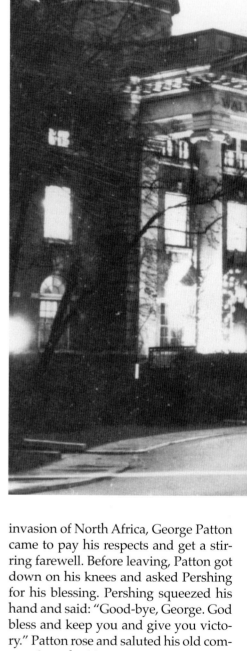

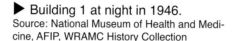

▶ Building 1 at night in 1946.
Source: National Museum of Health and Medicine, AFIP, WRAMC History Collection

World War II was by far the most extraordinary event of this decade, as well as the century for the United States and the world. The cataclysm that was the Second World War is hard to grasp. How do you come to grips with an estimated 50–60 million deaths worldwide during those war-riddled years? As in World War I, the United States was not involved in all the years of the war, entering after Pearl Harbor on December 7, 1941 and continuing through the Japanese surrender on September 2, 1945. United States involvement in World War I (4.7 million mobilized, with 116,000 deaths and 204,000 wounded) paled in comparison to World War II (16 million mobilized, with 400,000 deaths and 670,000 wounded). The worldwide loss of human life and property simply has no comparison in human history.

At Walter Reed, even the significant building expansion that took place along with and after World War I could not accommodate the patients generated by the Second World War. The busiest year for admissions in World War I was 1918, with 13,752 admissions of which about 1,800 were related to the influenza epidemic. The 18,046 admissions in 1943 easily topped that total. Walter Reed needed additional facilities; thus, in September 1942, the Army purchased the old National Park Seminary at Forest Glen. The 185-acre

property was initially called the New Section, then the Convalescent Section, and finally simply Forest Glen. As the second name implies, it was primarily used for convalescence. In addition, the Army temporarily took possession of a former Civilian Conservation Corps Camp at Beltsville, MD, about 7 miles from the main campus and 4 miles from Forest Glen. Camp Ord, as it became known, was an independent and self-sufficient station where soldiers wore fatigues rather than Class A or convalescent clothing. Rehabilitative work was mostly agricultural. Camp Ord was operated until March 7, 1945.

In May 1941, at age 81, General of the Armies, John J. Pershing, former Commanding General of the American Expeditionary Forces during World War I and former Army Chief of Staff, left the Carlton Hotel in Washington, DC, where he lived and moved into Walter Reed General Hospital. A special suite was built for him on the third floor of what had been called Ward B of Building 1. While the suite was being finished, he stayed on Ward 4, the male officer's medical ward. Shocked by the Japanese attack on Pearl Harbor, he wrote President Roosevelt and offered to do whatever he could. However, he knew that this war was not his war, but belonged to the men who had earlier worked for him and to the sons of the Doughboys of World War I. Before sailing for the

invasion of North Africa, George Patton came to pay his respects and get a stirring farewell. Before leaving, Patton got down on his knees and asked Pershing for his blessing. Pershing squeezed his hand and said: "Good-bye, George. God bless and keep you and give you victory." Patton rose and saluted his old commander, who likewise rose and smartly returned the salute.

On Sunday April 22, 1945, the newly sworn-in President of the United States, Harry S. Truman, came to Walter Reed to pay his respects to General Pershing, his World War I commander. President Truman had taken the oath of office just ten days before following the unexpect-

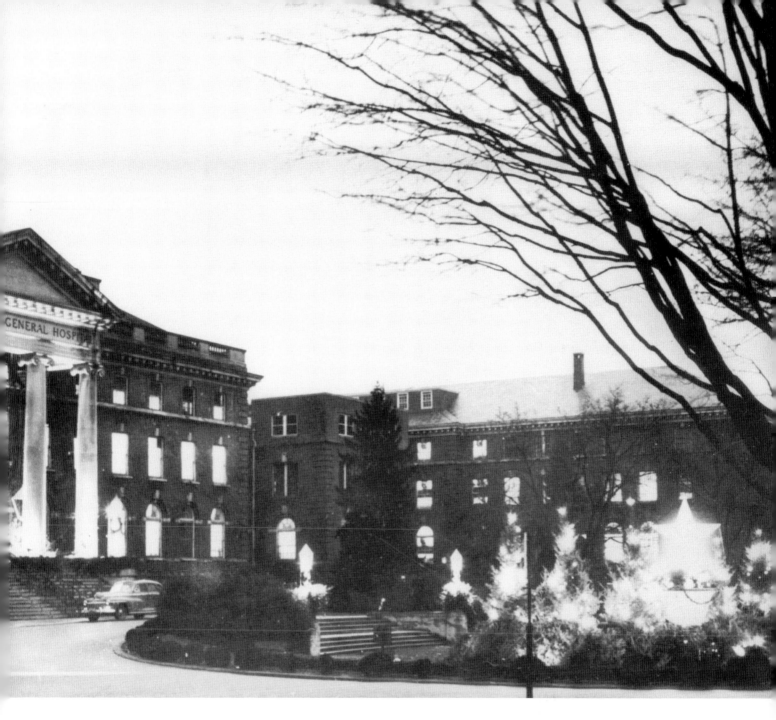

ed death of Franklin Delano Roosevelt. Prior to visiting General Pershing, President Truman wanted to attend church and did so at Walter Reed's Memorial Chapel.

General Pershing lived in the "penthouse" until his death on July 15, 1948 at age 88. The penthouse became known as the Pershing Suite; subsequently, other famous officers were hospitalized in the Pershing Suite, including General Peyton C. March, Chief of Staff of the Army during World War I. He was hospitalized at Walter Reed General Hospital circa 1954 and died there on April 3, 1955. At times, the suite was used as overflow for the labor and delivery service. President

Eisenhower was a patient in the Pershing Suite for approximately one month during his eleven-month stay at Walter Reed between May 1968 and March 1969. He used the Pershing Suite while the Presidential Suite on Ward 8 was being redecorated. The area was closed after clinical care moved to the new hospital facility in 1978; but, when space got tight, it was used off and on for administrative space. In the late 1980s, it was used by The Surgeon General's Consultant for Academic Medicine as office and conference space. From the late 1990s until today, it has been used by the Walter Reed Society.

Following the end of World War II,

many physicians were interested in specialty medical and surgical training. Across the Army Medical Department, physician residency training began in earnest and Walter Reed was no exception. In the past 60 years, Graduate Medical Education (internships, residencies, and fellowships) has become an integral part, if not the engine, that has driven expansion and excellence of clinical services at Walter Reed. While these individual specialty and subspecialty programs have numbered in the 50s to 60s, trained thousands of physicians, and contributed immeasurably to the stature of Walter Reed, it is simply not possible to even begin to address them in this volume.

▶ The Memorial Chapel saw heavy use not only for memorial services, but also for many weddings. This photograph is from May 1948.
Source: National Museum of Health and Medicine, AFIP, WRAMC History Collection

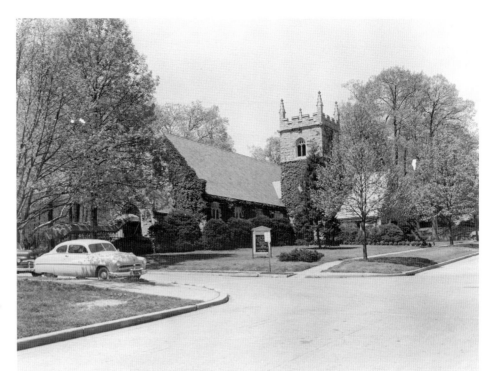

▼ The entrance used by the Army Medical Department Research and Graduate School is also the headquarters of the Army Medical Center. On the right is the solarium wing of the Red Cross Building. May 1948.
Source: National Museum of Health and Medicine, AFIP, SC 320757

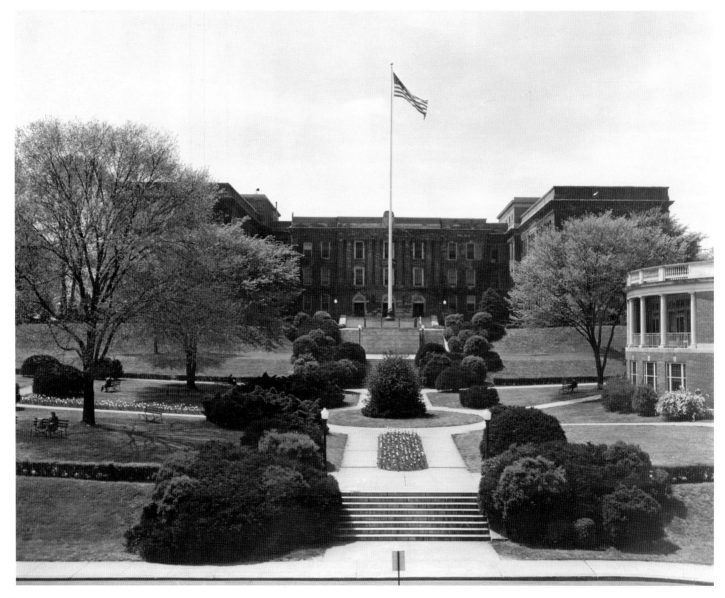

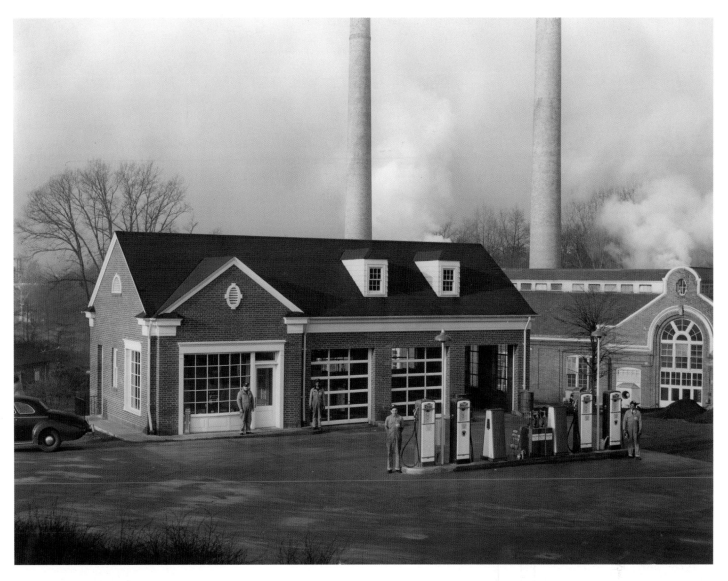

▲ Gas station on Walter Reed General Hospital grounds in 1942.
Source: National Museum of Health and Medicine, AFIP, WRAMC History Collection

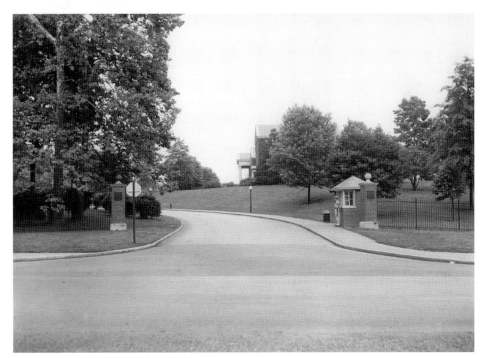

◄ 16th Street Entrance to Walter Reed on May 19, 1949. Delano Hall is seen in the background.
Source: National Museum of Health and Medicine, AFIP, WRAMC History Collection

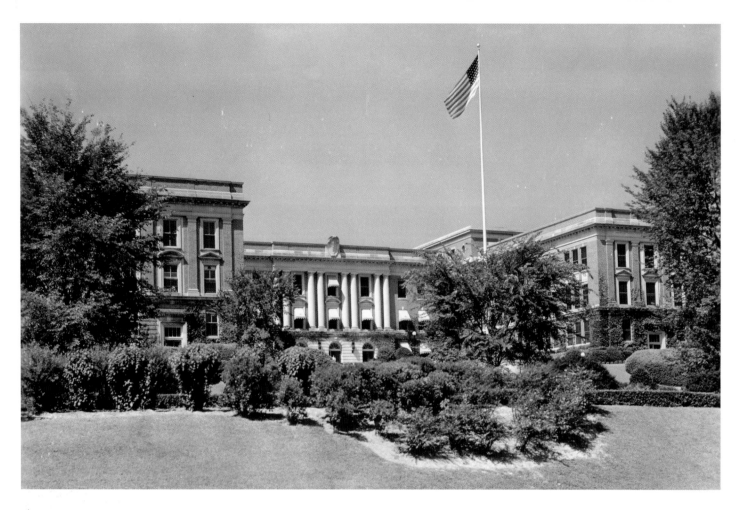

▲ East elevation of Building 40, formerly the Army Medical School.
Source: Walter Reed Army Medical Center, Directorate of Public Works Archives

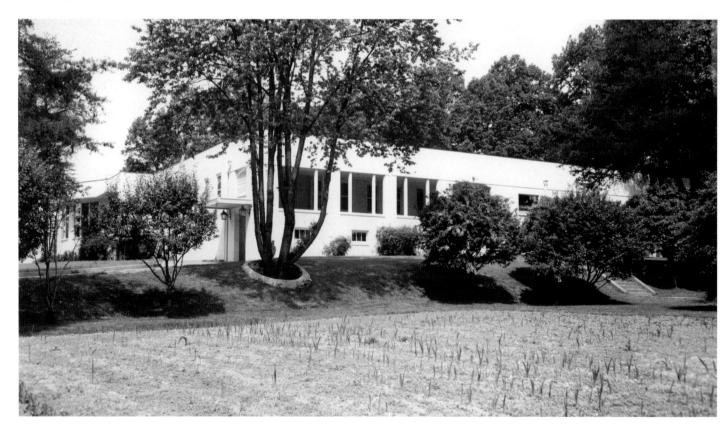

▲ The Officer's Club at the Army Medical Center, Walter Reed General Hospital, Washington, D.C., May 29, 1949.
Source: Walter Reed Army Medical Center, Directorate of Public Works Archives

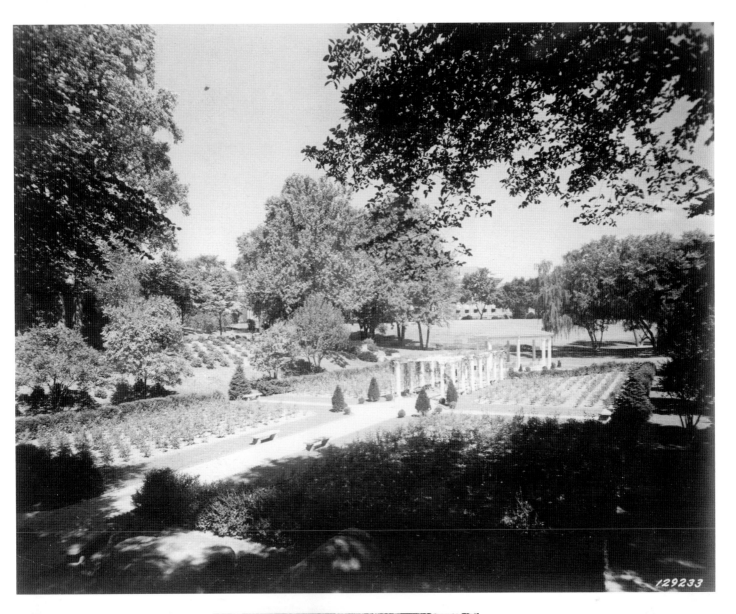

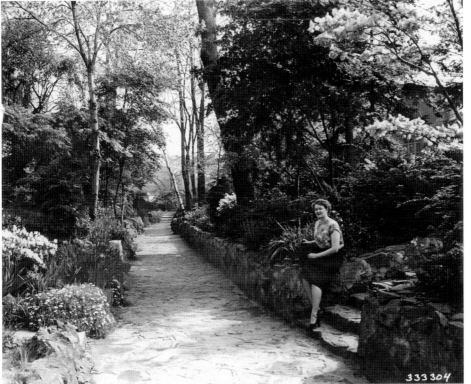

▲ The formal garden of Walter Reed Hospital, September 8, 1941.
Source: National Museum of Health and Medicine, AFIP, WRAMC History Collection

◀ Woman on garden path, April 21, 1948.
Source: National Museum of Health and Medicine, AFIP, WRAMC History Collection

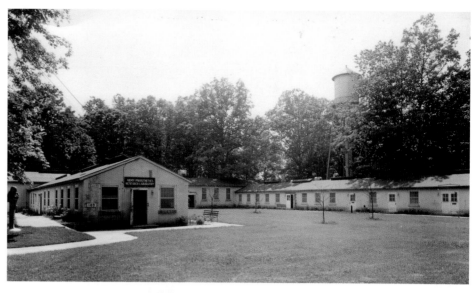

▶ The Army Prosthetics Research Laboratory at Army Medical Center, Forest Glen, MD. May 19, 1949.
Source: National Archives and Records Administration, SC 321908

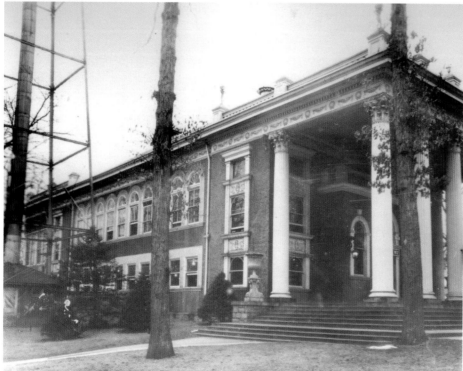

◀ Post Theater at Forest Glen, MD. 1946.
Source: National Archives and Records Administration, SC 321816

▶ The Aural Rehabilitation Center. Forest Glen, MD. 1946.
Source: National Archives and Records Administration, SC 321815

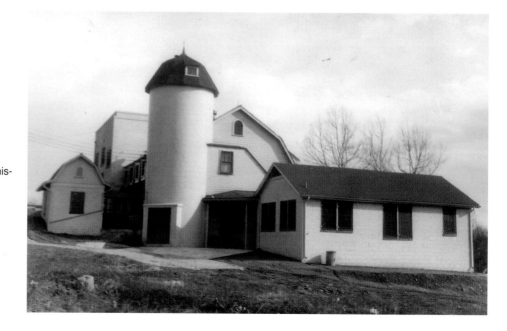

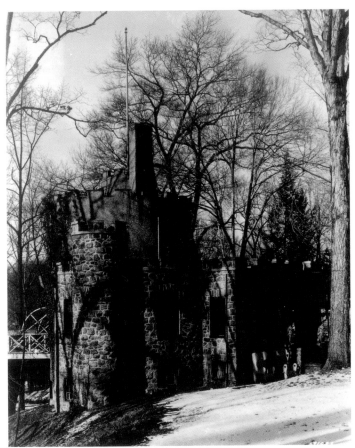

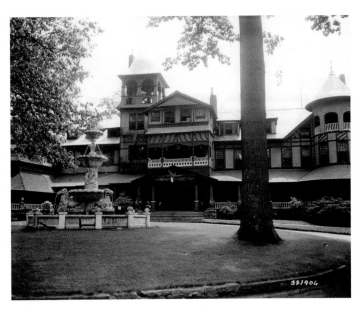

▲ Administration Building of the Forest Glen Annex.
May 19, 1949.
Source: National Archives and Records Administration, SC 321906

▲ Castle at Forest Glen, January 18, 1945.
Source: National Archives and Records Administration, SC 591022

The Army purchased a 188-acre site from National Park College, a private school for young women that had occupied the site since 1894. For its 1943 opening, it transformed the 70 college buildings of varied architecture into the nucleus of a convalescent branch for Walter Reed Army Hospital's ambulatory patients, thus freeing much needed bed space at the main Washington campus for patients needing constant medical attention.

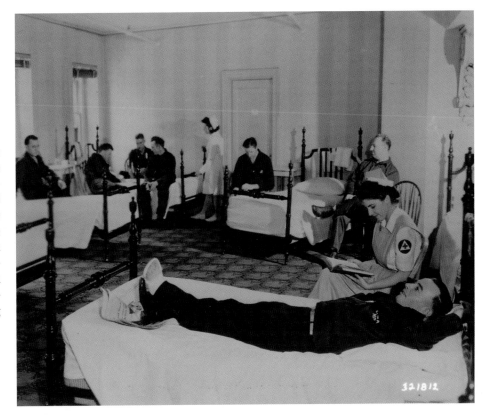

▲ Ward Room in the Forest Glen Section, Walter Reed General Hospital. Most of the original furnishings of the National Park College were retained after it was taken over as an annex to Walter Reed Hospital. 1944.
Source: National Archives and Records Administration, SC 321812

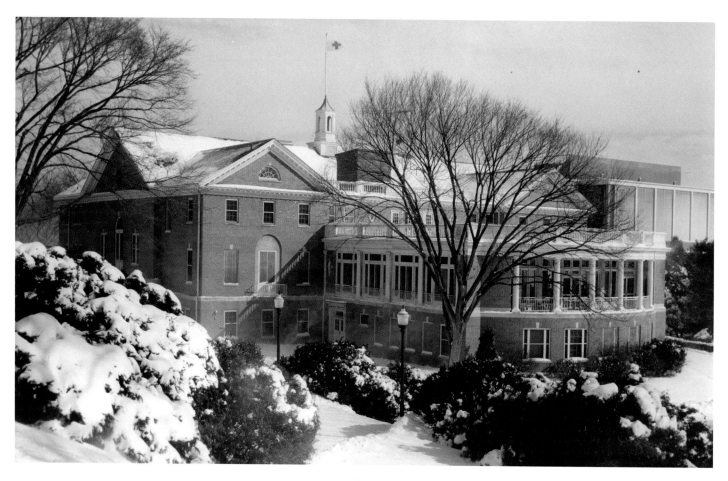

▲ A solarium was added to Red Cross Hall in 1948.
Source: Walter Reed Army Medical Center, Directorate of Public Works Archives

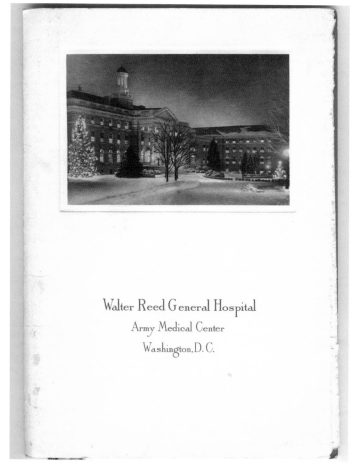

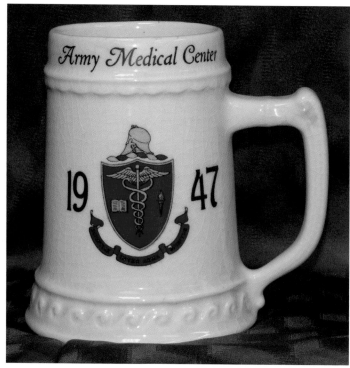

Christmas dinner brochure and mug from 1947.
Source: Pierce Collection

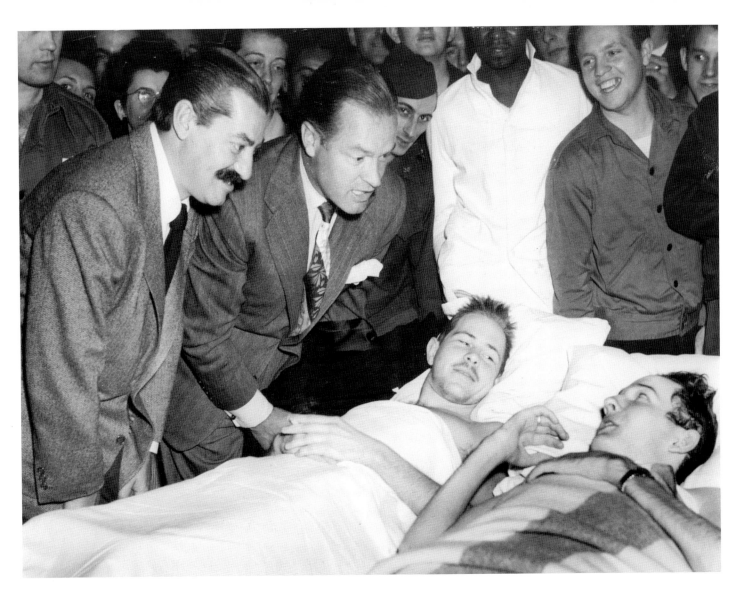

▲ Jerry Colonna and Bob Hope greeting patients after a show at the Red Cross Hall on February 10, 1948.
Source: National Museum of Health and Medicine, AFIP, WRAMC History Collection

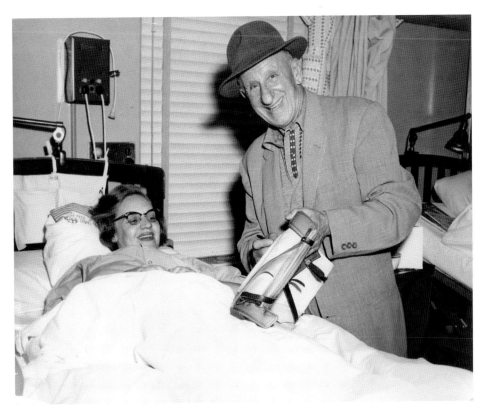

▶ Jimmy Durante, star of radio and television, performed for patients at Walter Reed. After, he toured some of the wards. Here, he pens an autograph for a fan.
Source: WRAMC History Office, PAO Historical Collection, Celebrity 2

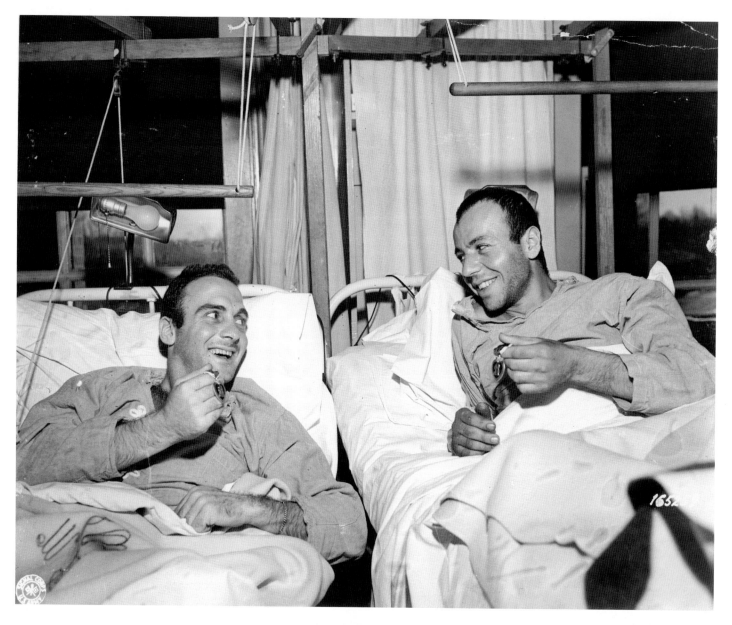

▲ Sgt. Ernest H. Robson, Orange, NJ, and Pvt. Rocco R. Parrotti, Orange, NJ, show each other the Purple Hearts they were awarded after being wounded in the engagement in North Africa. They were wounded in the same action at Safi, Morocco, and brought back to the transport and occupied adjoining beds at Walter Reed Hospital, Washington, D.C., where they are in high spirits and recovering from their wounds. (Original caption)
Source: National Museum of Health and Medicine, AFIP, SC 165259

▶ A Gray Lady writes a letter for a GI patient, 1944.
Source: National Archives and Records Administration, SC 333302

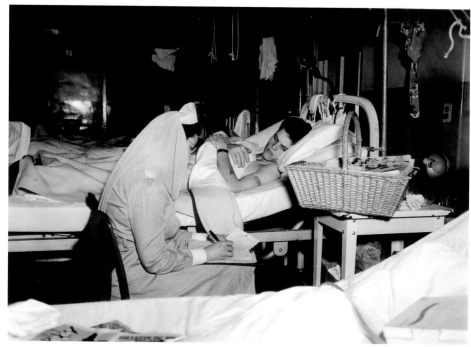

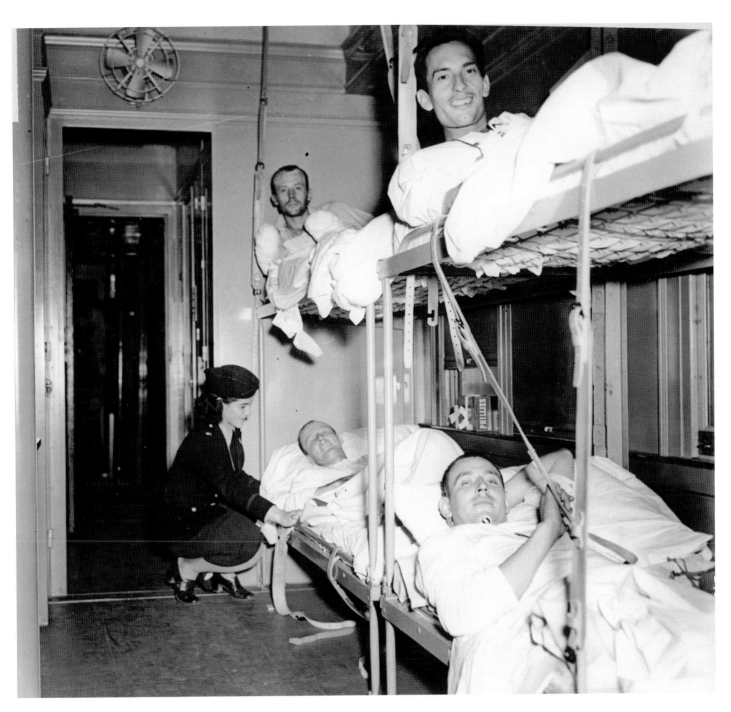

▲ United States Army officers and enlisted men, home after service in the North African campaign, were brought to Walter Reed Hospital in Washington, D.C., after arriving at an East Coast port. They were cheerful despite wounds suffered during the successful military operations. The accompanying picture was taken as the wounded were being removed from the special hospital train for transport to the hospital. An Army nurse prepares a wounded soldier for transfer from the train to the hospital. (Adapted from original caption)
Source: National Museum of Health and Medicine, AFIP, SC 139698

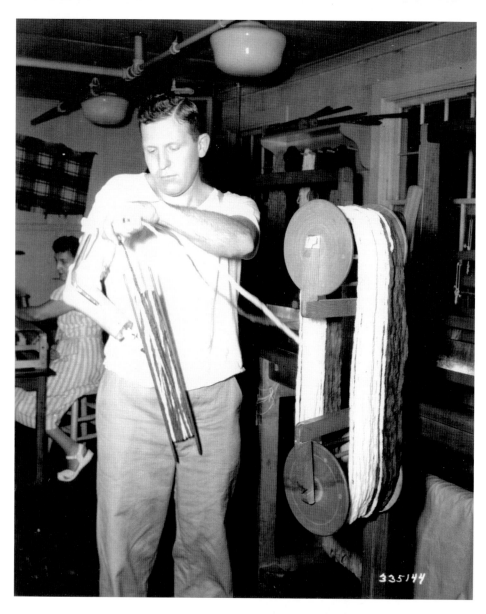

◄ An arm amputee veteran winding rug yarn on a reel in the Occupational Therapy Shop at Walter Reed Hospital, 1946.
Source: National Archives and Records Administration, SC 335144

▶ Rehabilitation continues to be a critical part of patient care at the Hospital. Here, patients are taught the visual methods of piano on August 20, 1945.
Source: National Archives and Records Administration, SC 335161

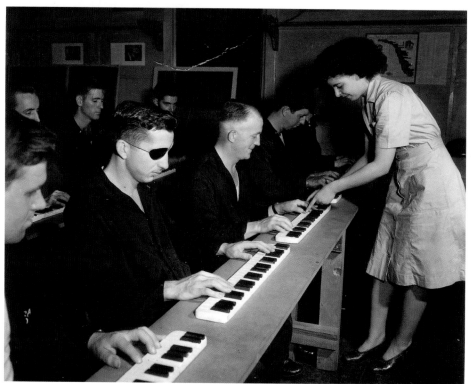

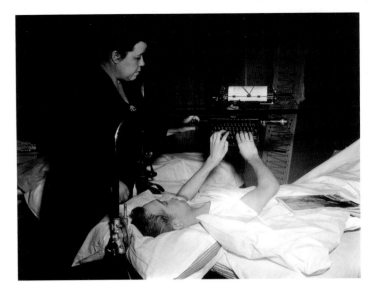

▲ An instructor teaching typing to a patient in the supine position, 1946.
Source: National Archives and Records Administration, SC 335158

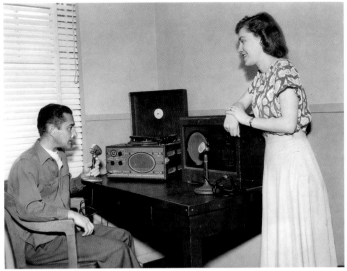

▲ Ms. Lois Senft, a speech correctionist, plays a recording of a patient's voice on voice recording and playback equipment. May 5, 1949.
Source: National Archives and Records Administration, SC 335757

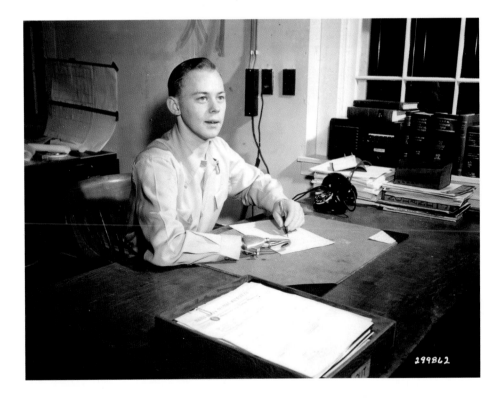

▲ After nearly three years of research and experimentation the Army's prosthetics research laboratory, Forest Glen, Maryland has developed a cosmetic hand that is Life-Like in appearance and may be adapted to many tasks normally allotted its human counterpart. The primary improvements of the hand over the hook are its appearance and facility of articulation. In addition to veterans, civilian amputees have volunteered for the experiments which have led to the development of the cosmetic prosthesis in its present stage. Mr. Jerry Leavy, Los Angeles, California a civilian amputee who has volunteered for the Army's prosthetic research program demonstrates the use of the cosmetic hand. The hook offers a marked contrast to the neat life-like hand. May 7, 1948. (Original caption)
Source: National Archives and Records Administration, SC 299862

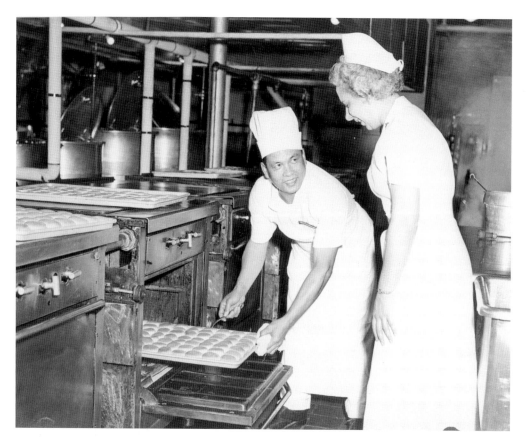

▲ Hot biscuits from the oven.
Source: Walter Reed Army Medical Center History Office, PAO Historical Collection

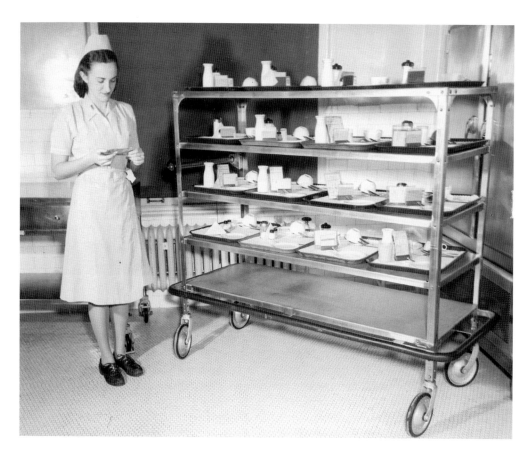

▲ 2nd Lt. Lorraine Shandolmier, a dietician, checks the contents of a tray cart.
Source: Walter Reed Army Medical Center History Office, PAO Historical Collection

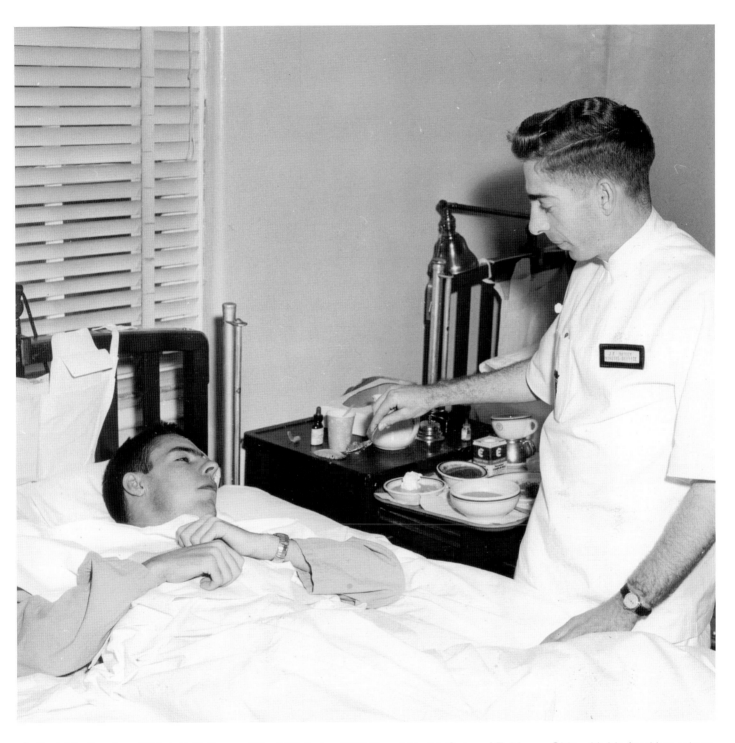

▲ Bedside Service. SP4 J. F. Bailey on Ward 39, helps PFC Ronald L. McGuire of Fairborn, Ohio with his food brought to the ward via the Centralized Tray Service Cart, one of the 30 such carriers recently purchased by the Food Service Division. (Adapted from original caption)
Source: Walter Reed Army Medical Center History Office, PAO Historical Collection

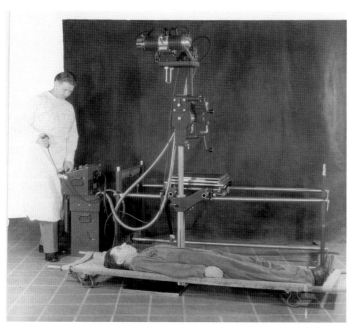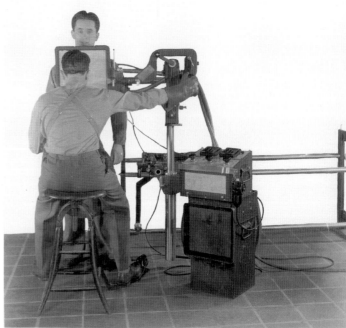

▲ (Left and Right) Demonstrations of a portable X-ray apparatus as used in the field, Army Medical School, 1941.
Source: Walter Reed Army Medical Center History Office, PAO Historical Collection

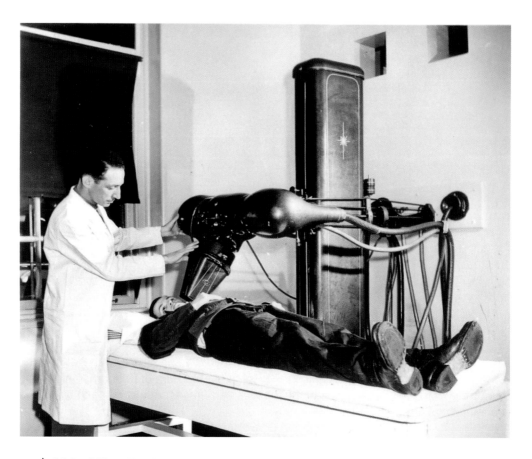

▲ Major Milton Friedman of the Roentgenology Department gives a high-voltage X-ray treatment to a soldier-patient at Walter Reed General Hospital. 1944.
Source: National Archives and Records Administration, SC 321749

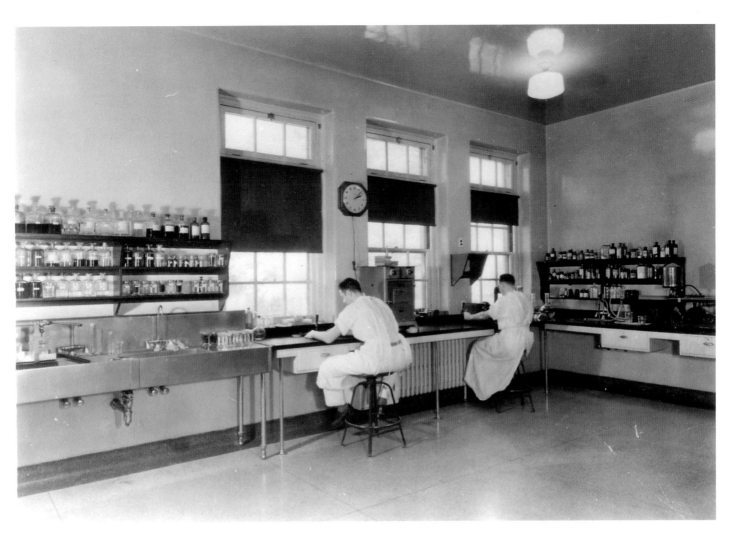

▲ Men at work in the clinical Laboratory Pathology Preparatory Room, October 4, 1940.
Source: National Archives and Records Administration, SC 590849

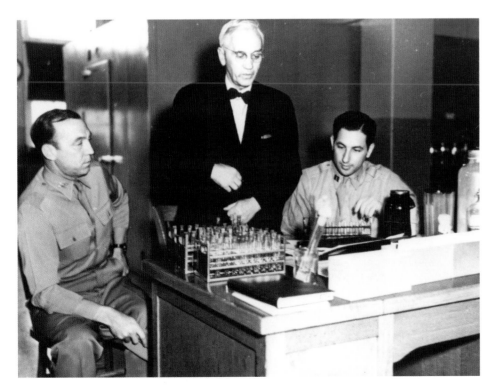

▲ Sir Alexander Fleming, discoverer of penicillin, visits Capt. Monroe Romansky (right) in the Penicillin Laboratory. Capt. Romansky developed a beeswax and peanut oil carrier, called Romansky's Formula, that extended Sir Fleming's penicillin shot from every 3 hours to single daily injections. 1945.
Source: Walter Reed Army Medical Center, Directorate of Public Works Archives

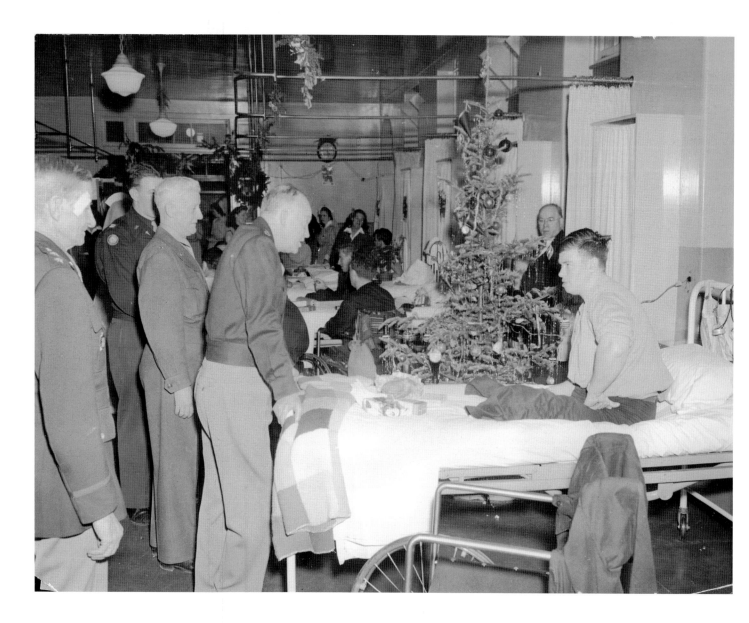

▲ Where Heroes Meet. General Dwight D. Eisenhower visits PFC Ray E. Stevenson of Fayetteville, TN, on Ward 36 of the Hospital. 1945.
Source: National Museum of Health and Medicine, AFIP, WRAMC History Collection

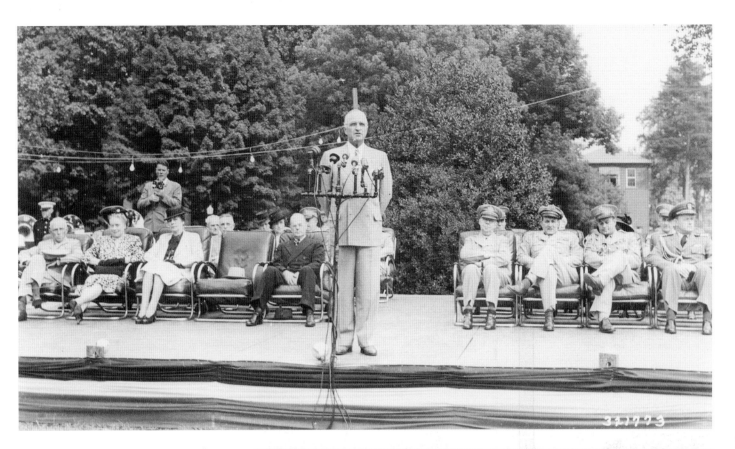

▲ President Harry S. Truman officially opened the country fair for benefit of the Nurses' National Memorial at Walter Reed General Hospital on September 11, 1946. Truman attended his first church service after becoming President at Memorial Chapel at Walter Reed. He had come to Walter Reed to visit General Pershing, his commander during World War I who resided in the Pershing Suite.
Source: National Archives and Records Administration, SC 321773

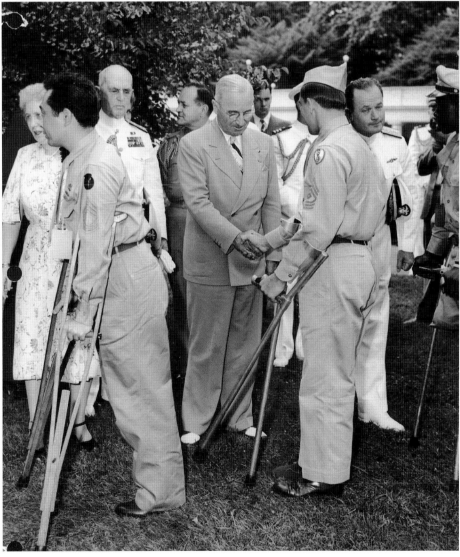

▶ President Truman greeting soldier-patients at a White House reception.
Source: National Museum of Health and Medicine, AFIP, WRAMC History Collection

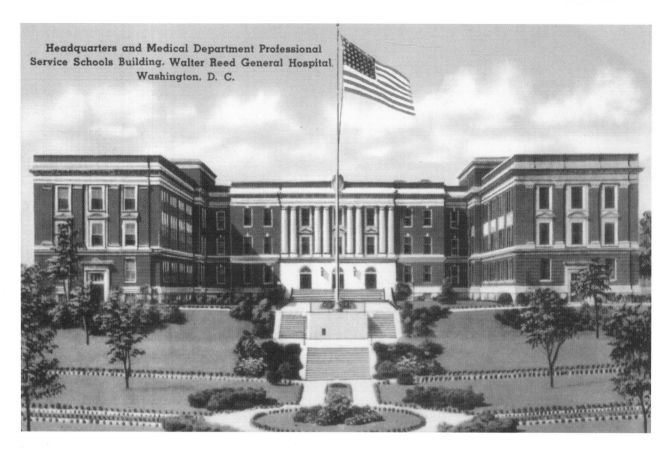

Headquarters and Medical Department Professional Service Schools Building, Walter Reed General Hospital. Washington. D. C.

The back of this postcard reads: The Headquarters Army Medical Center and Army Medical Department Professional Service Schools Building is located at Alaska Avenue and 16th Street, Washington D.C.
Source: Pierce Collection

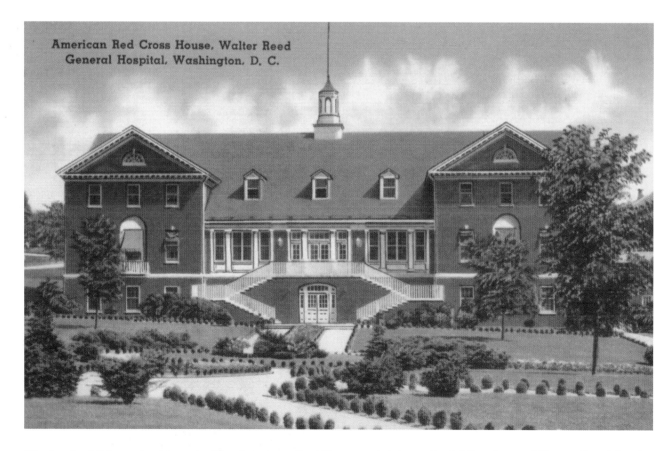

American Red Cross House. Walter Reed General Hospital. Washington. D. C.

The back of this postcard reads: The American Red Cross maintains a Social Service and Recreational Center for patients in Walter Reed General Hospital.
Source: Pierce Collection

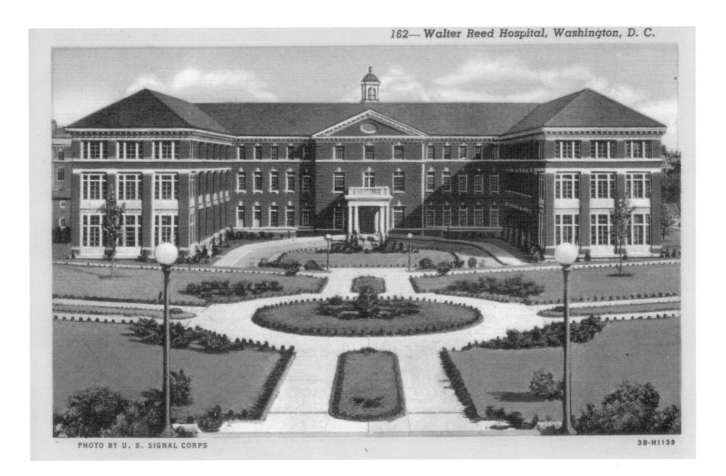

162— Walter Reed Hospital, Washington, D. C.

PHOTO BY U. S. SIGNAL CORPS

3B-H1139

Source: Pierce Collection

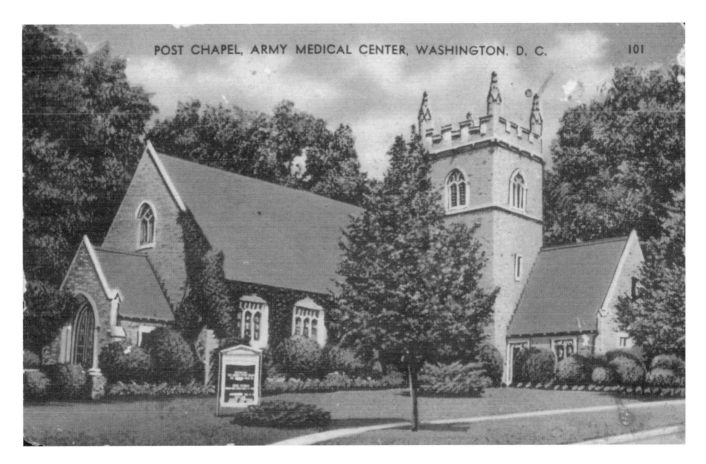

POST CHAPEL, ARMY MEDICAL CENTER, WASHINGTON. D. C.

101

Source: Pierce Collection

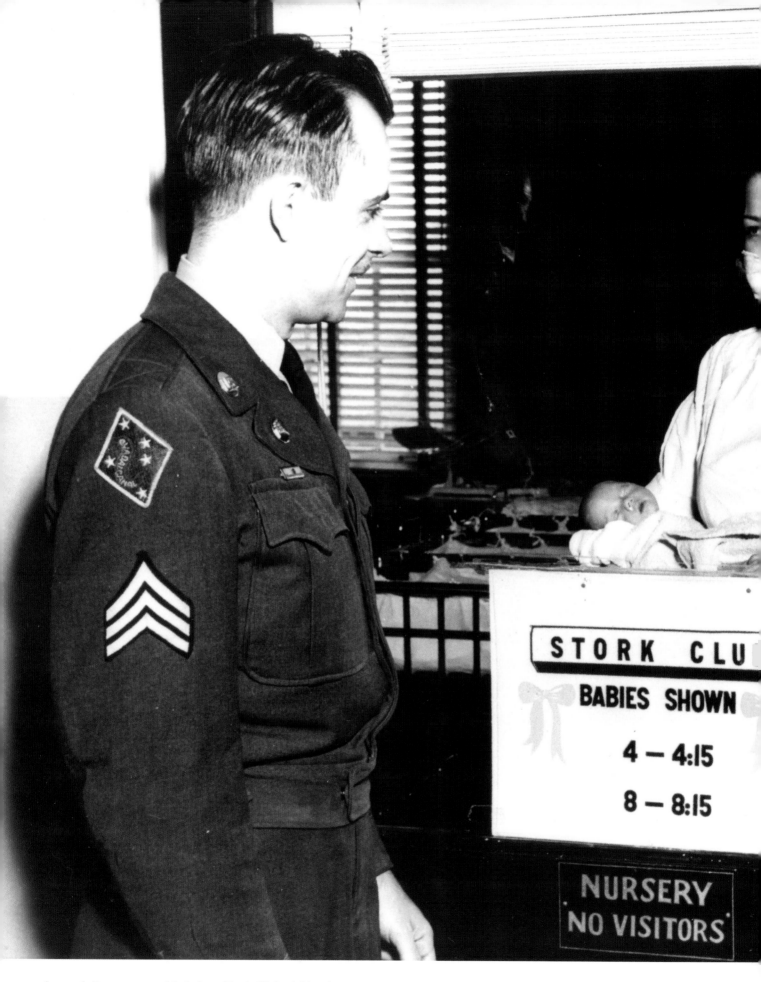

A new father surveys his twins. Stork Club visiting hours as posted.
Source: Walter Reed Army Medical Center, Directorate of Public Works Archives

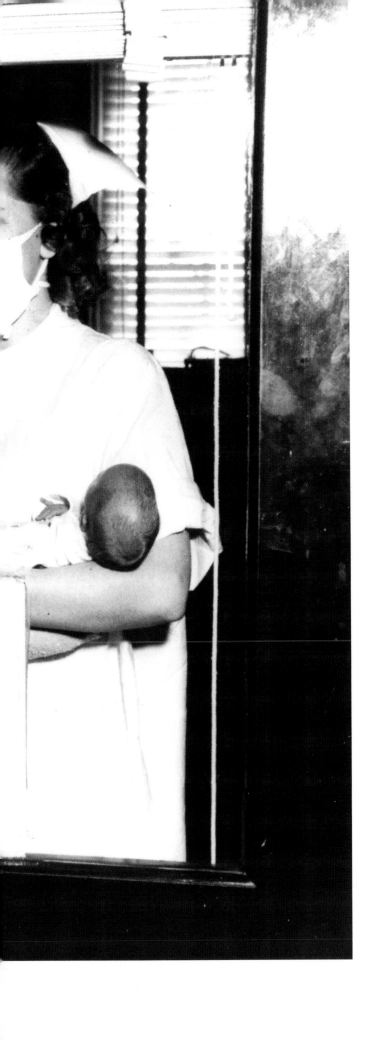

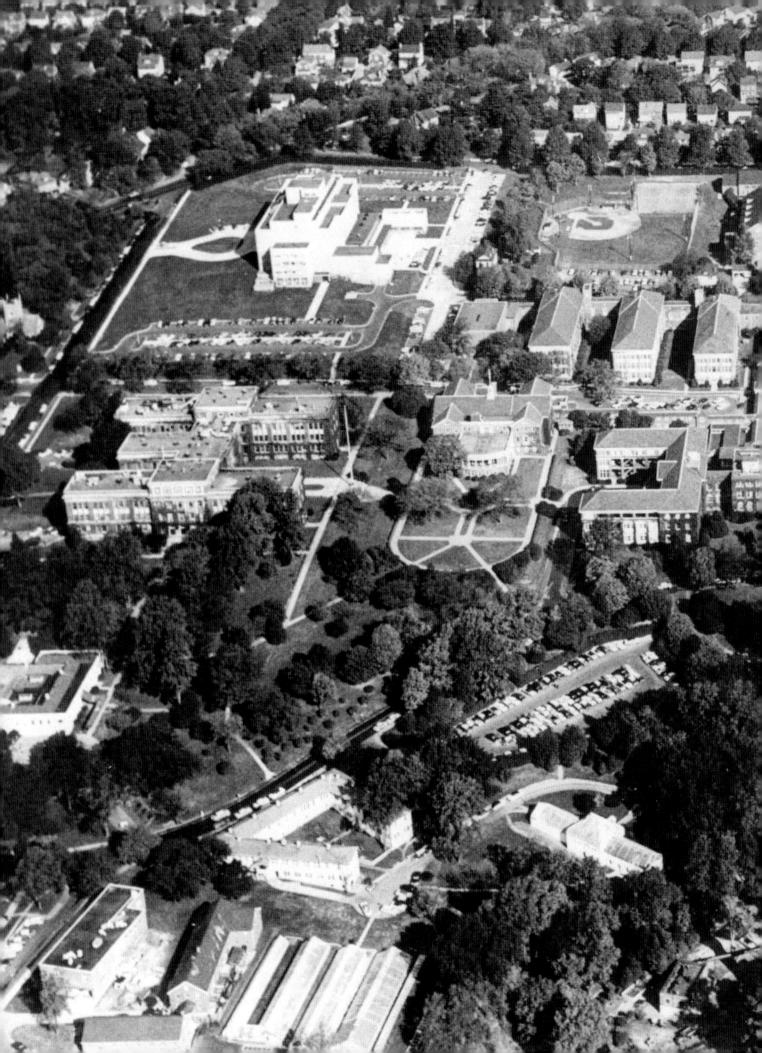

1950–1959

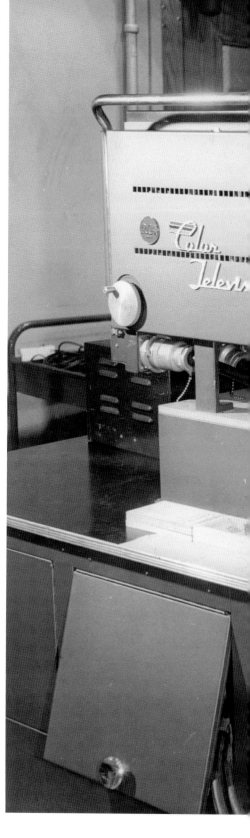

Title page - The aerial view looking north shows the biggest addition to the campus during the 1950s in the upper left of the photo: the Armed Forces Institute of Pathology (AFIP) building. The ball field in the upper center of the photo has been reoriented and appears to have been downsized, probably to softball size. A solarium has been added to the south elevation of the Red Cross Hall intruding into the landscaped garden area. To the far left of the photo, below Building 40, is the Officer's Club. In the 1940s, the Pershing Suite was added as the third floor to B wing of Building 1; A wing was triple decked for symmetry.
Source: National Museum of Health and Medicine, AFIP, SC 526813

▶ Lt. Colonel Helmuth Sprinz, Surgical Pathologist, Walter Reed Army Hospital, operates the completely new color TV microscope, designed by Walter Reed and RCA technicians. Light passes through the microscope and engages a beam splitter which directs a sufficient amount of light to the microscopist's eye permitting him to examine suspect tissue just as though television was not involved. The remaining amount of light passes directly through the beam splitter and is reflected through a prism into a three-vidicon color television of special design. The whole assembly is mounted on an instrumentation table which may be easily wheeled into many different laboratories, classrooms and conference rooms. With this system it is possible for the microscopist to see a parallax corrected field with any number of students in as many different locations as can be reached by the Television Division's distribution system. 14 November 1957. (Original caption)
Source: National Museum of Health and Medicine, AFIP, SC 521401

In 1951, to coincide with the 100th anniversary of the birth of its namesake Major Walter Reed, the name of this now world-famous medical institution was changed from the Army Medical Center and Walter Reed General Hospital to Walter Reed Army Medical Center. A member of the campus family since 1923, the Army Medical School had undergone name changes over the years, from Army Medical School to Medical Department Professional Services School in 1934, to Army Medical Department Research and Graduate School in 1947, to Army Medical Service Graduate School in 1950, and finally to Walter Reed Army Institute of Research (WRAIR) in 1955.

The Armed Forces Institute of Pathology (AFIP), formerly the Army Medical Museum, moved to the Walter Reed campus in the 1950s, bringing together three of the four institutions needed to complete Borden's Dream. The majority of the fourth institution, The Surgeon General's Library, would become the National Library of Medicine, be

transferred to the Public Health Service, and moved to the National Institutes of Health campus in Bethesda, MD. The Army Medical Museum, established in 1862, had maintained that name until 1946, when it was renamed the Army Institute of Pathology. With the addition of the Navy and Air Force, it became the Armed Forces Institute of Pathology in 1949.

AFIP's unique mausoleum-style building, started in 1951 and completed in 1955, was windowless with thick concrete walls and considered atomic bomb proof. Fortunately, that unique characteristic has never been tested. During construction of the AFIP building, a number of civilian houses that had existed as part of the 16th Street Heights subdivision that was purchased for expansion of the Post in the early 1920s were moved to create a cul-de-sac of officers housing on 15th Street off of Dahlia Street. President Eisenhower dedicated the AFIP building on May 26, 1955.

The following year, healthwise, would be very difficult on the 65-year-old President. He suffered a heart attack in September 1955, recovering at Fitzsimons Army Medical Center in Denver. In June 1956, he was hospitalized at Walter Reed for abdominal surgery that would place in question his run for a second term that

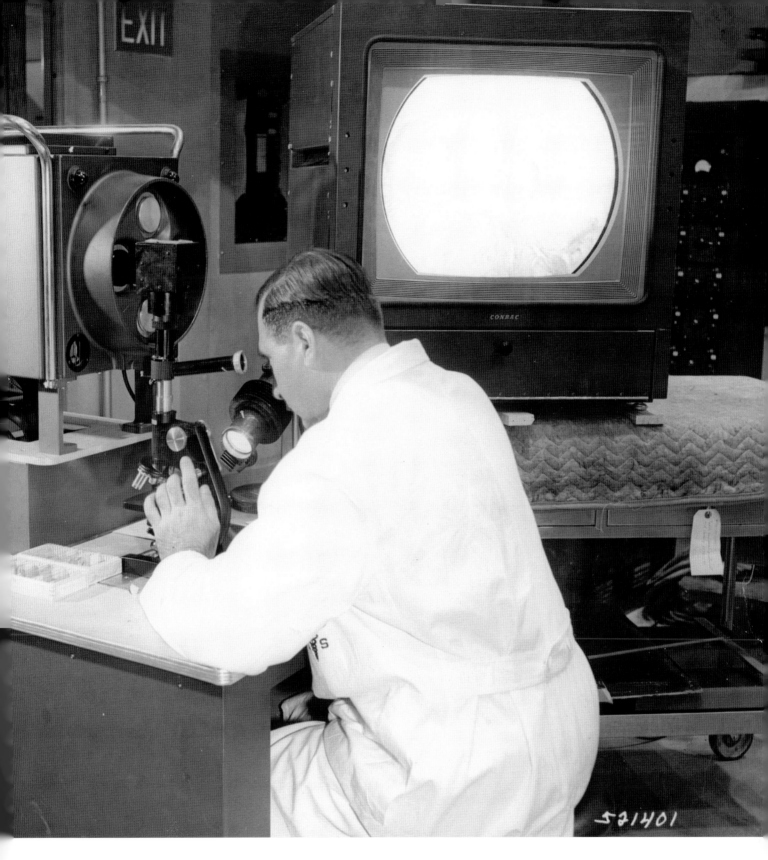

coming fall. Operated on by the Walter Reed Commanding General, Maj. General Leonard Heaton, Eisenhower would make a full recovery, and run and win a second term. Eisenhower and Heaton became lifelong friends. Heaton followed his six-year command at WRAMC with promotion to Surgeon General, a position he held for ten years, and a three-star rank—the first physician to hold that rank.

The 1950s brought many international visitors to Walter Reed; some for care and others to visit patients. With President Eisenhower as escort, Sir Winston Churchill visited General of the Army, former Secretary of Defense and Secretary of State George C. Marshall, on Ward 8 in May 1959. They also paid respects to John Foster Dulles, Eisenhower's former Secretary of State, a patient on Ward 8. During the visit, Eisenhower presented a portrait he had painted of Churchill to the hospital to be hung in the sitting room on Ward 8.

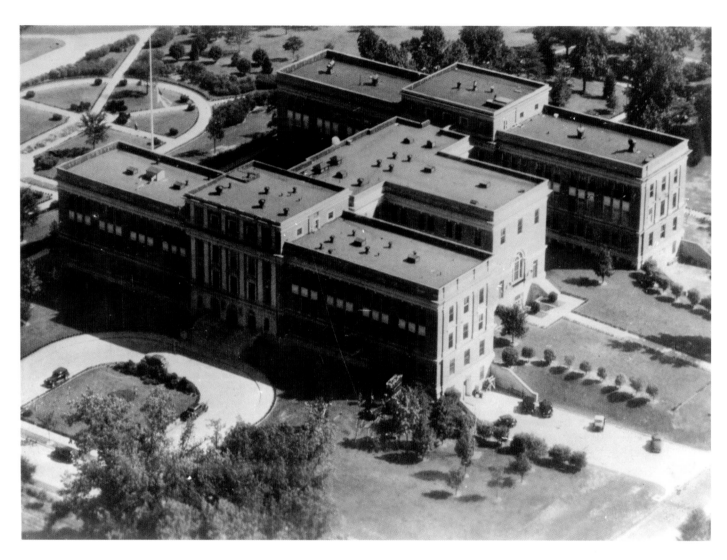

Building 40, the original Army Medical School building (upper portion) was opened in 1923. The center and lower portions were added in the early 1930s about the time the name was changed to Medical Department Professional Services School. The name changed again in 1947 to AMEDD Research and Graduate School, in 1950 to Army Medical Graduate School, and finally in 1955 to Walter Reed Army Institute of Research.
Source: Walter Reed Army Medical Center History Office, PAO Historical Collection

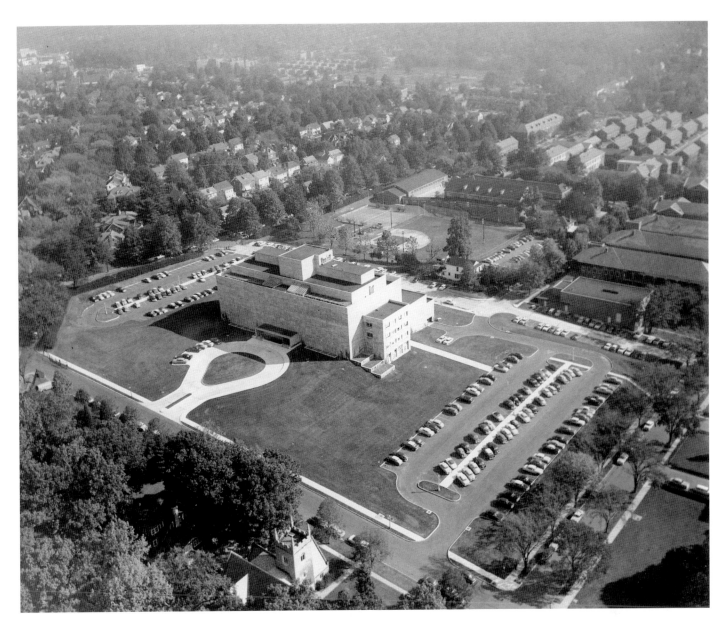

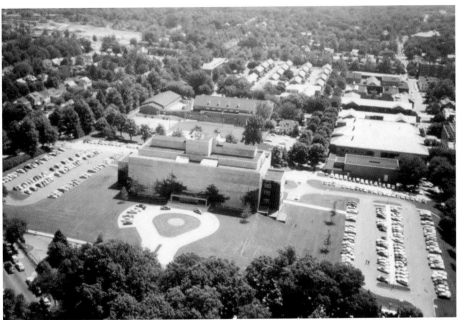

The Armed Forces Institute of Pathology moved from downtown Washington, DC to this impressive new building on the grounds of Walter Reed Army Medical Center and dedicated by President Eisenhower on May 26, 1955. It had four major departments, the Department of Pathology, American Registry of Pathology, Medical Illustration Service and the Medical Museum. The eight story bomb proof building was designed to provide working space for the central consultative, research and teaching center for pathology, serving the needs of all the military services as well as other government agencies. (Original caption)
Source: (top) National Museum of Health and Medicine, AFIP, WRAMC History Collection, (bottom) Directorate of Public Works

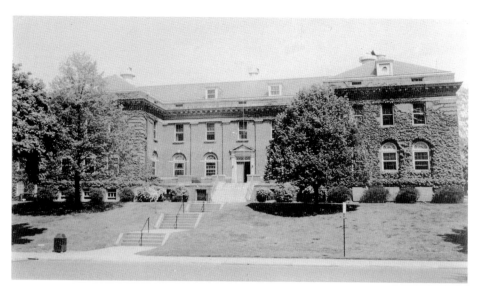

◀ The Outpatient Clinic, Walter Reed Army Hospital. This building — now completely modern and air conditioned — was originally constructed in 1911 for the purpose of housing enlisted personnel stationed at the Hospital during those first years of its operation. After undergoing extensive renovation, it opened again in May 1950 to offer, for the first time since outpatient service was begun at the Center in 1939, adequate facilities for the treatment of some 900 military personnel and dependents living in this area who visit the clinic daily — a most important milestone in the four-year history of a greatly expanded Out Patient Service at Walter Reed Army Medical Center. (Original caption)
Source: National Museum of Health and Medicine, AFIP, WRAMC History Collection

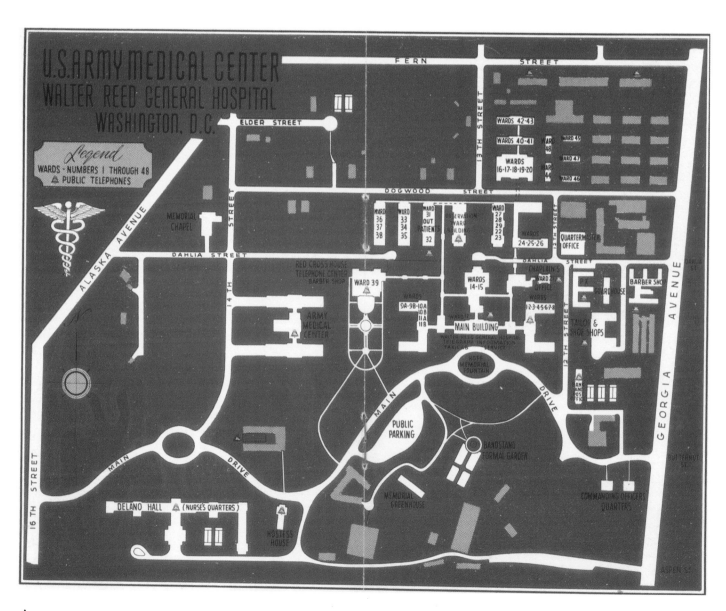

▲ Source: Pierce Collection

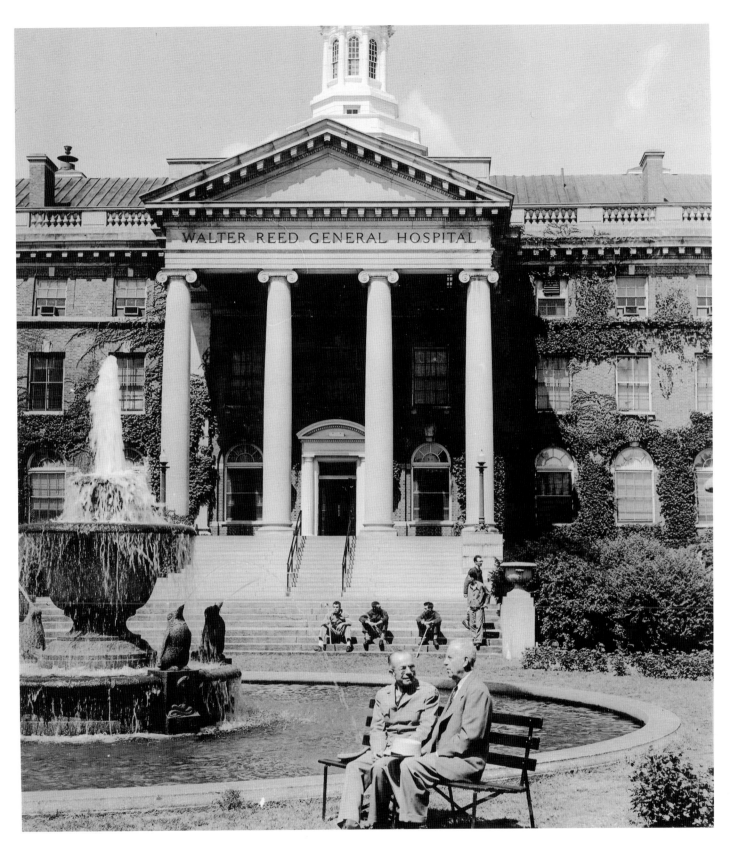

▲ Maj. General Walter Reed [seated right] visits September 11, 1951 the Hospital named for his father, Maj. Walter Reed. He is reliving his boyhood memories of the famed conqueror of yellow fever for Korean war patients [pictured in the background] and for Maj. General Paul H. Streit, the 19th Commanding Officer of these portals of healing. Maj. General Reed was the Inspector General of the Army at the time of his retirement in 1940. General Reed was recalled to active duty as a member of the War Department Personnel Board. He retired again on June 25, 1946. He died at Walter Reed Hospital May 1, 1956. (Adapted from original caption)
Source: WRAMC History Office, PAO Historical Collection

▶ New Central Dental Laboratory opened at Walter Reed. Maj. General George E. Armstrong, The Army Surgeon General (left) cuts the ribbon across the main entrance to the new Central Dental Laboratory building at Walter Reed Army Medical Center during a ceremony. Col. Lynn C. Dirksen, Commanding Officer of the laboratory (right) assists the general. February 23, 1954.
Source: WRAMC History Office, PAO Historical Collection

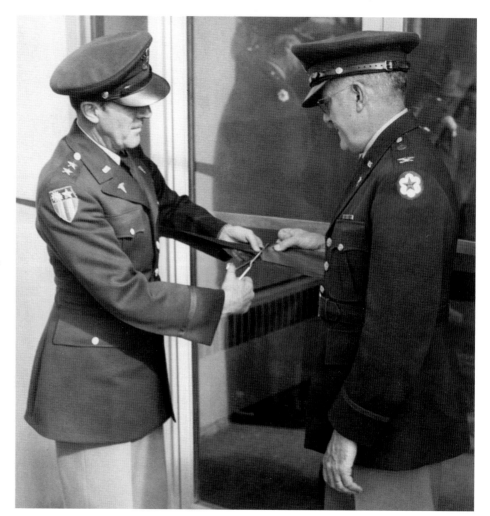

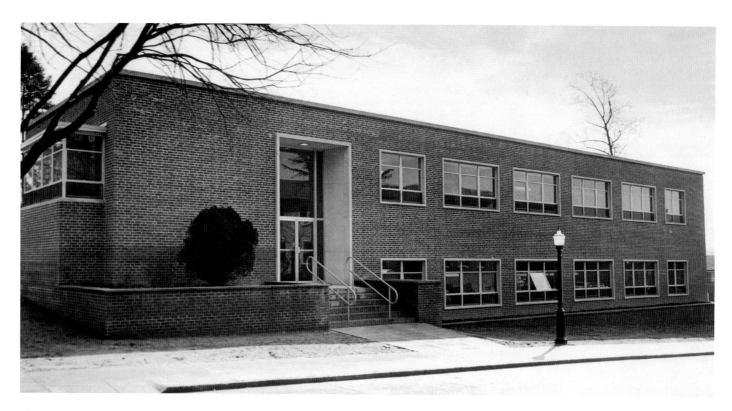

▲ The Central Dental Laboratory moved out of the Walter Reed Army Institute of Research and into its own 9,500 square foot building on February 23, 1954. Founded in 1927, the Laboratory mission is to provide military patients with the best prosthodontic therapy.
Source: WRAMC History Office, PAO Historical Collection

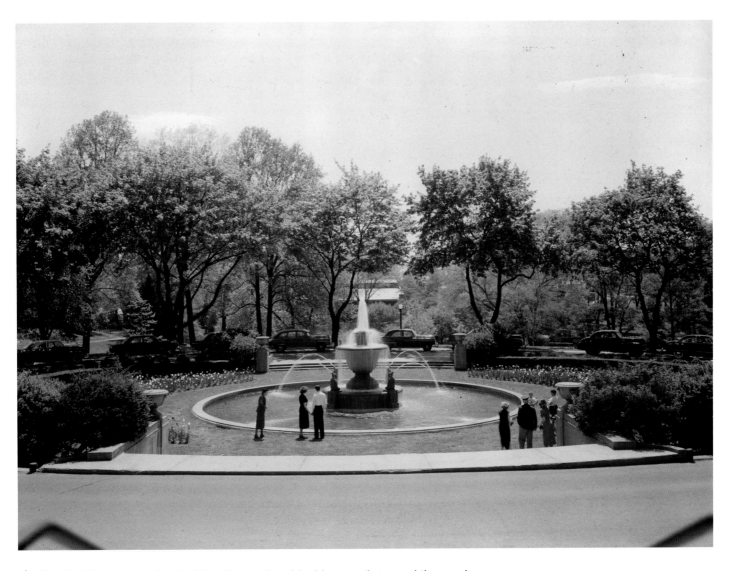

▲ The Hoff Fountain in front of the Hospital and looking south toward the garden.
Source: National Museum of Health and Medicine, AFIP, WRAMC History Collection

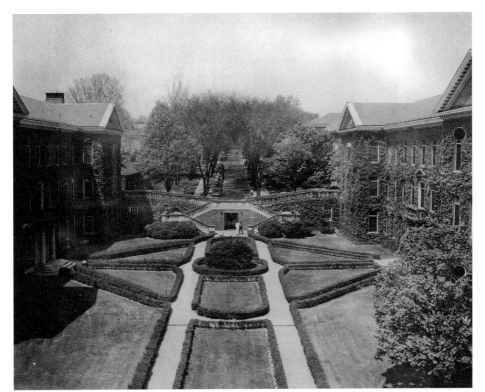

◀ The beauty of the grounds of the Hospital was definitely part of the healing process for patients. The garden was on the North side of Building 1 and between two wards.
Source: National Museum of Health and Medicine, AFIP, WRAMC History Collection

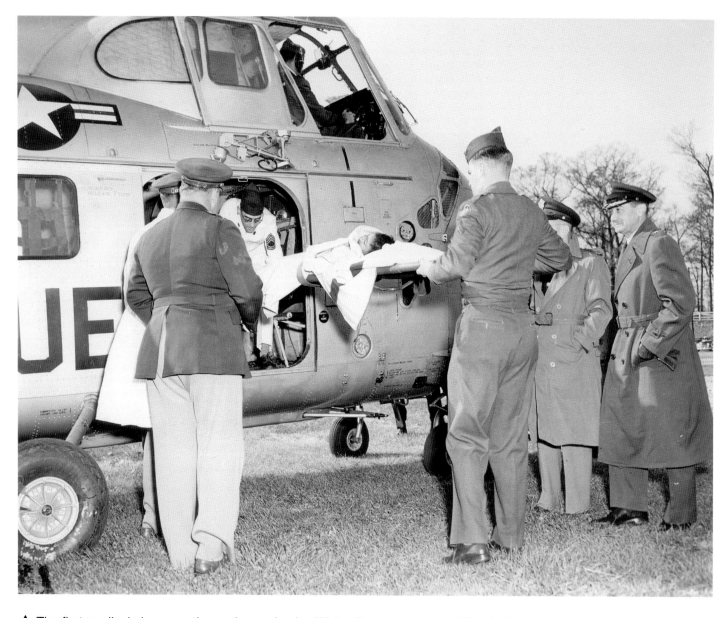

▲ The first medical air evacuation patient arrived at Walter Reed on board a Sikorsky H-19 in 1952.
Source: WRAMC History Office. PAO Historical Collection

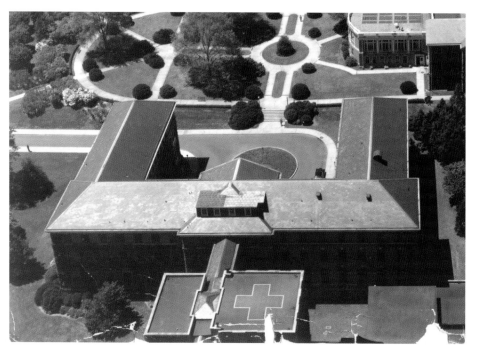

◄ A large red cross on the roof of Building 1 indicated to passing aircraft that this is a hospital. The actual landing site was nearby on the grass.
Source: Walter Reed Army Medical Center, Directorate of Public Works Archives

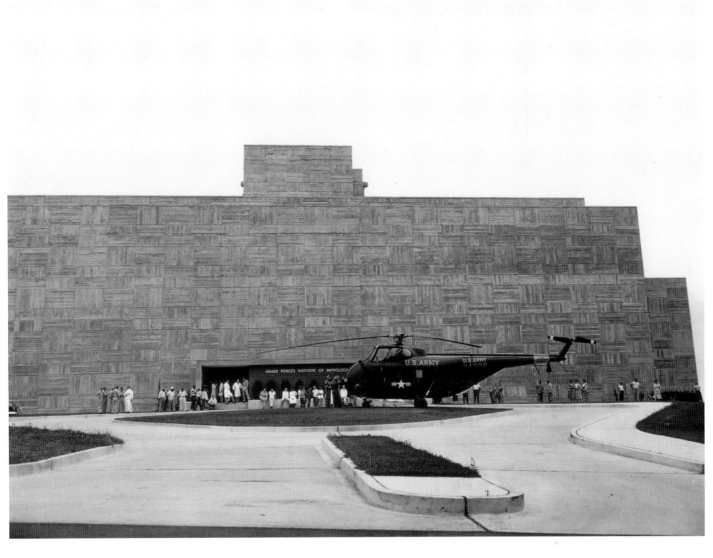

This Sikorsky H-19 helicopter ran low on fuel and made an emergency landing in front of the Armed Forces Institute of Pathology en route to Forest Glen with three soldiers involved in a car accident outside of Petersburg, VA. Source: National Archives and Records Administration (top) SC 521913 and (right) SC 521914

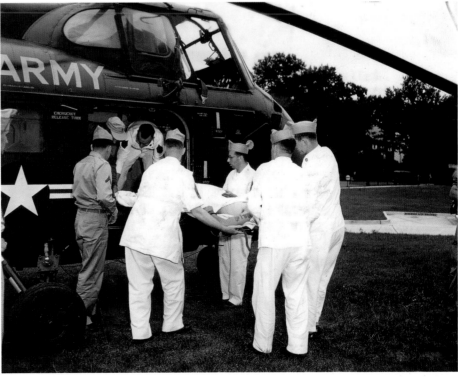

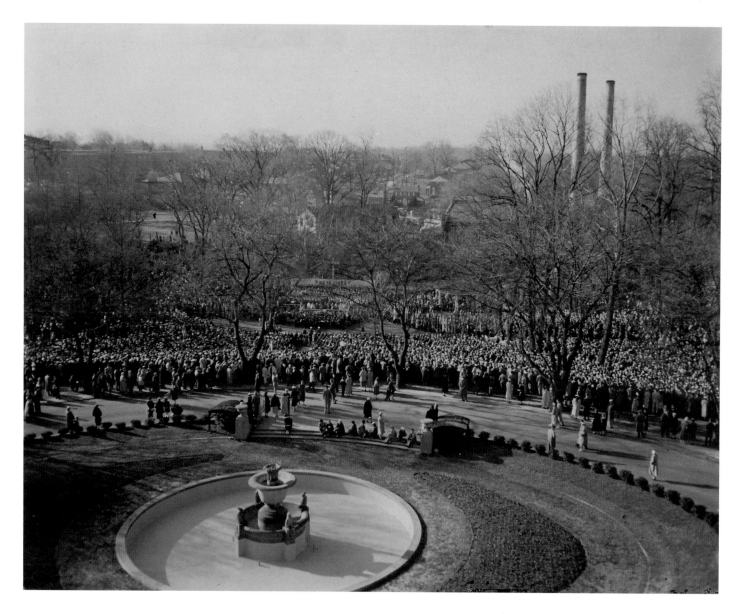

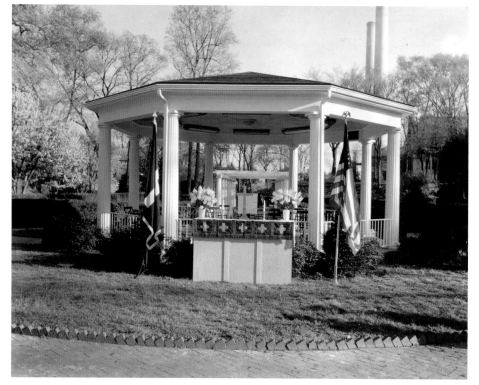

▲ The Easter Sunrise Service, April 1, 1956. Estimated attendance was 30,000–40,000, the largest attendance in history.
Source: WRAMC History Office, PAO Historical Collection

◄ The bandstand in the garden setup for Easter Sunrise Service.
Source: National Museum of Health and Medicine, AFIP, WRAMC History Collection

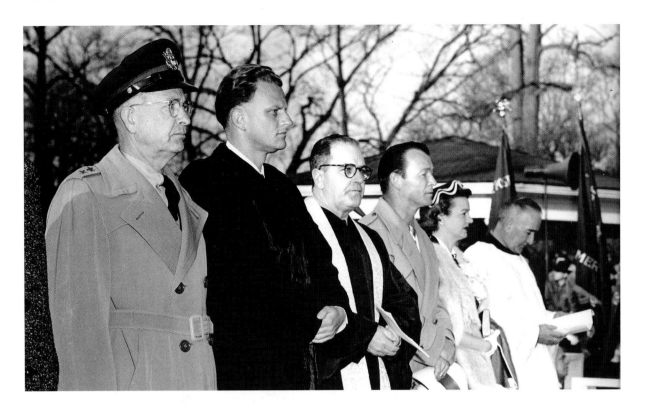

▲ Rev. Billy Graham led the ceremony at the 1956 Easter Sunrise Service. Maj. General Heaton is to Graham's left and Chaplain (Lt. Colonel) Alford V. Bradley is to the right.
Source: WRAMC History Office, PAO Historical Collection

▼ Actors and singers, Roy Rogers and Dale Evans also appeared at the 1956 Easter Sunrise Service.
Source: WRAMC History Office, PAO Historical Collection

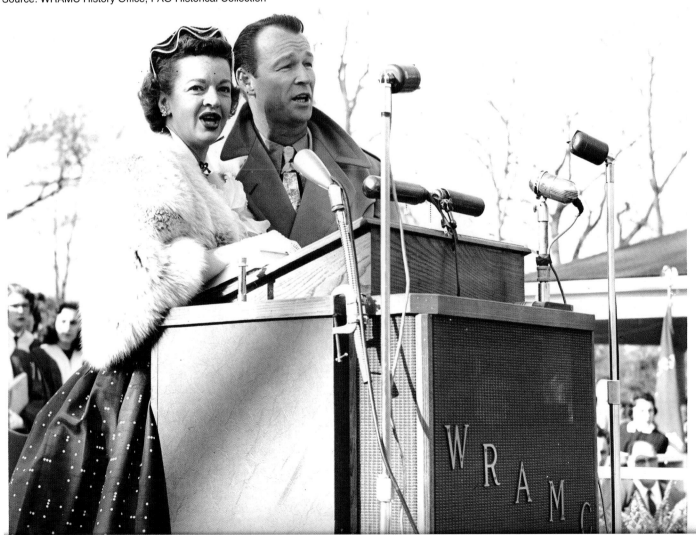

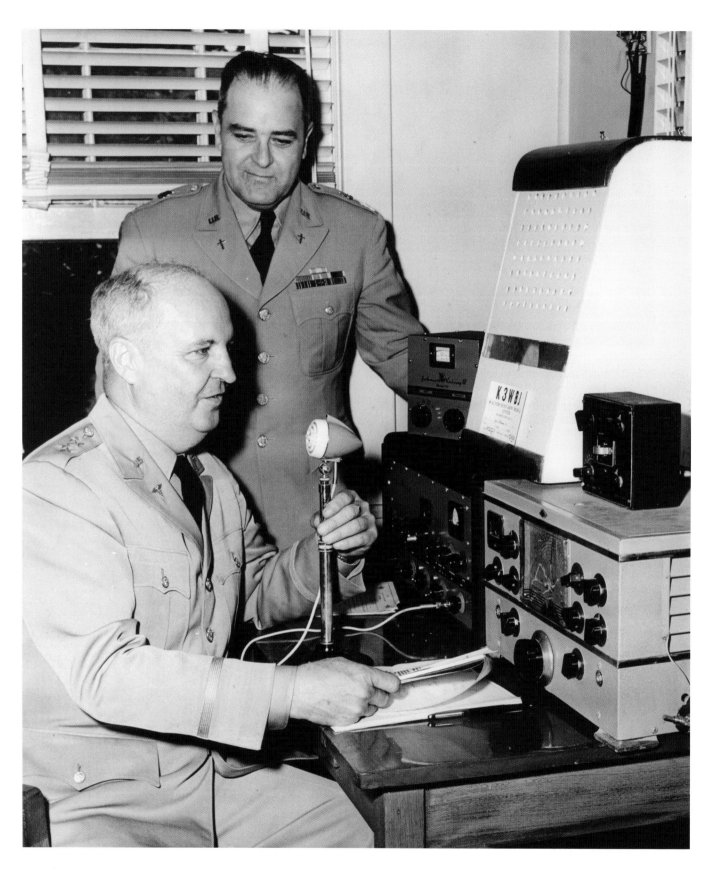

Maj. General Alvin L. Gorby sends the first message over Walter Reed's new Military Affiliate Radio Station (MARS), K3WBJ, during ceremonies. Looking on is Lt. Colonel Alford V. Bradley, Post Chaplain for the Center, who is a "ham" radio operator and was responsible for the unit being set up. The station will permit patients and duty personnel to send free messages all over the world. (Adapted from original caption)
Source: Walter Reed Army Medical Center, Directorate of Public Works Archives

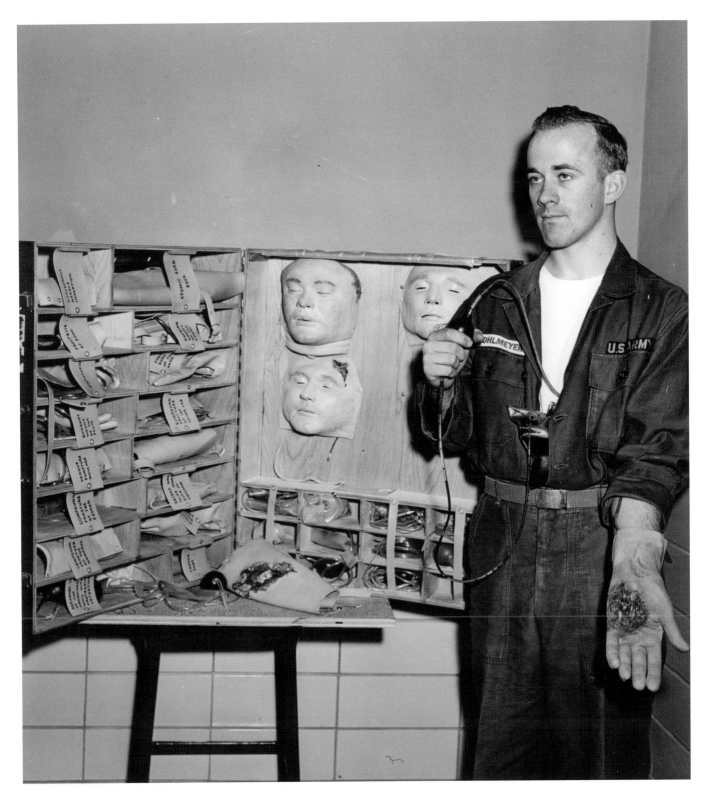

Mass casualties course completed at Walter Reed — A highlight of the week-long course in Management of Mass Casualties completed Saturday, May 17, at Walter Reed Army Institute of Research was a demonstration of wound moulages as a training aid in first aid treatment of wounds. The moulages realistically duplicate almost any type of wound that may occur in armed combat or as a result of a nuclear explosion. As is demonstrated above by PFC Carl W. Bohlmeyer, a flow of "blood" to the wound is controlled by pressure on a bulb which spurts the blood through a system of tubes concealed in the clothing of the "victim". Either venal or arterial bleeding can be simulated by the rapidity with which the blood is pumped, and the tubes are placed so that the bleeding can be stopped by normal first aid measures. In major wound moulages, the tubes can be "tied off" in the same manner that a normal artery would be. The moulage kit shown above contains twenty of the simulated wounds, including duplications of radiation burns. [The] course was attended by military and civilian defense officials from throughout the United States. (Original caption)
Source: Walter Reed Army Medical Center, Directorate of Public Works Archives

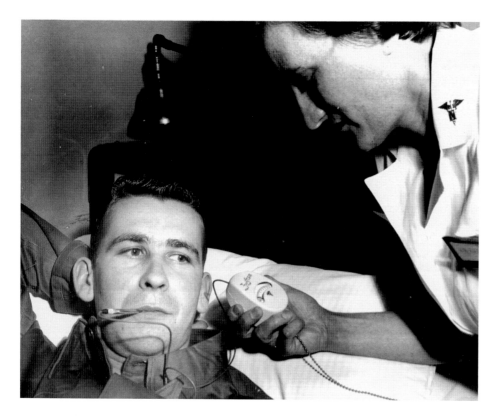

▲ Capt. Mary Rukesvine, U.S. Army
Nurse, takes the temperature of
Thomas L. Darby Remersburg, PA
with a new electronic thermometer at
Walter Reed Army Medical Center.
The device, the first change in a clinical thermometer since the introduction
of the mercury column type in 1867,
was developed by Colonel George T.
Perkin, Army Dentist. 1954. (Original
caption)
Source: National Archives and Records Administration, SC 54-7759

▶ Pediatric radiology.
Source: WRAMC History Office, PAO Historical
Collection

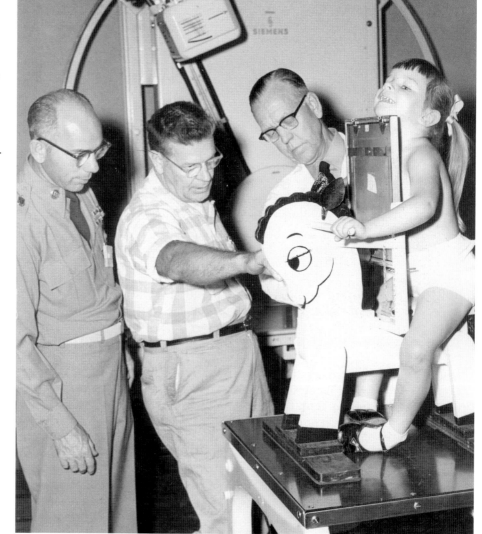

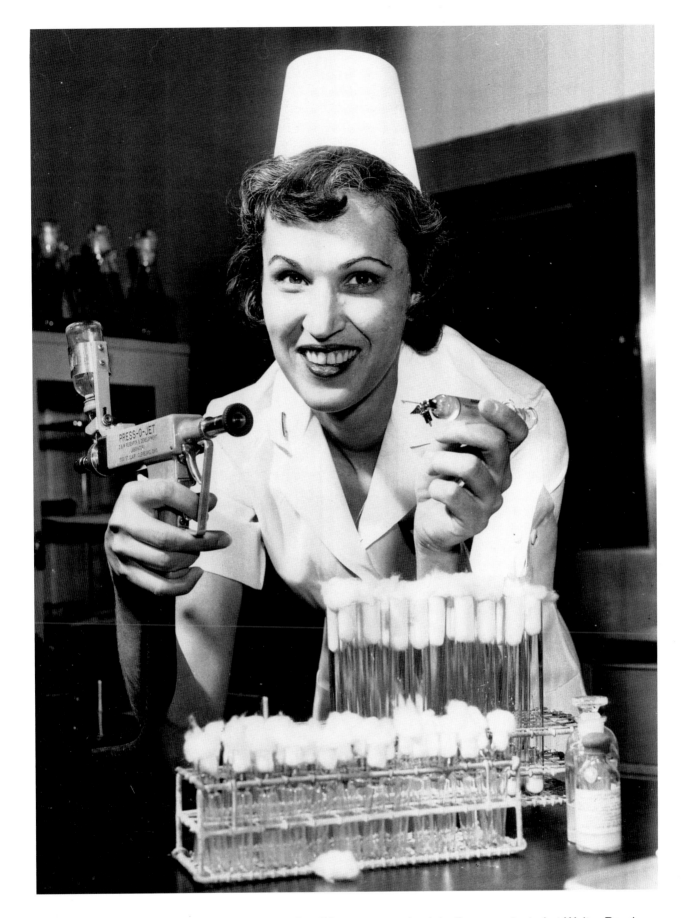

▲ A needleless, automatic, multiple nose jet "gun" for mass vaccine injections was tested at Walter Reed Army Medical Center in 1955. The new inoculation mechanism gives promise that someday the Army's soldiers may receive quick and practically painless inoculation. Here a nurse holds an old-style needle in her left hand and the new inoculator in her right. (Original caption)
Source: National Archives and Records Administration, SC 553312

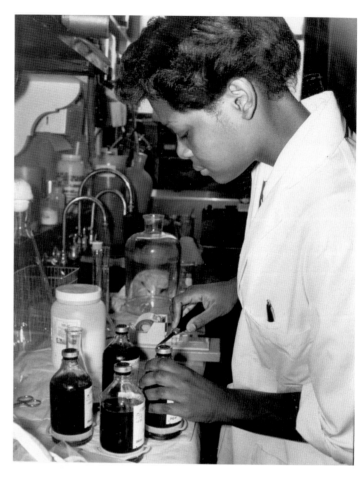

► SP4 Renee Poreey, Department of Gastroenterology separating blood for use in testing antibodies for vaccine studies.
Source: WRAMC History Office, PAO Historical Collection

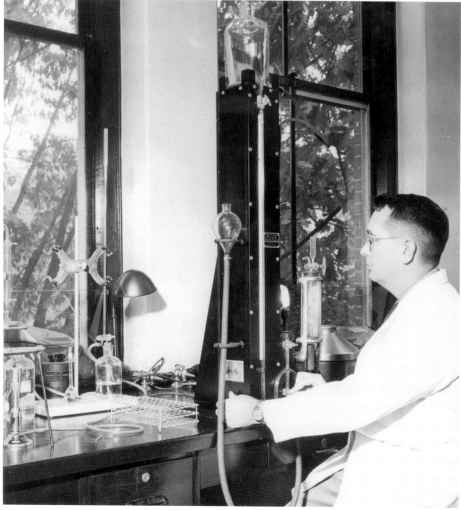

◄ Lt. Colonel George W. Burnett, Chief of Dental Research Department, Dental Division, Army Medical Service Graduate School, is shown using Van Slyke apparatus to analyze effect of fluorides upon tooth tissue. He is shown here measuring rate of removal of gasses from fluoride-treated tooth tissues during their destruction by acids in an attempt to find a treatment for prevention of dental caries. September 1, 1954. (Original caption)
Source: WRAMC History Office, PAO Historical Collection

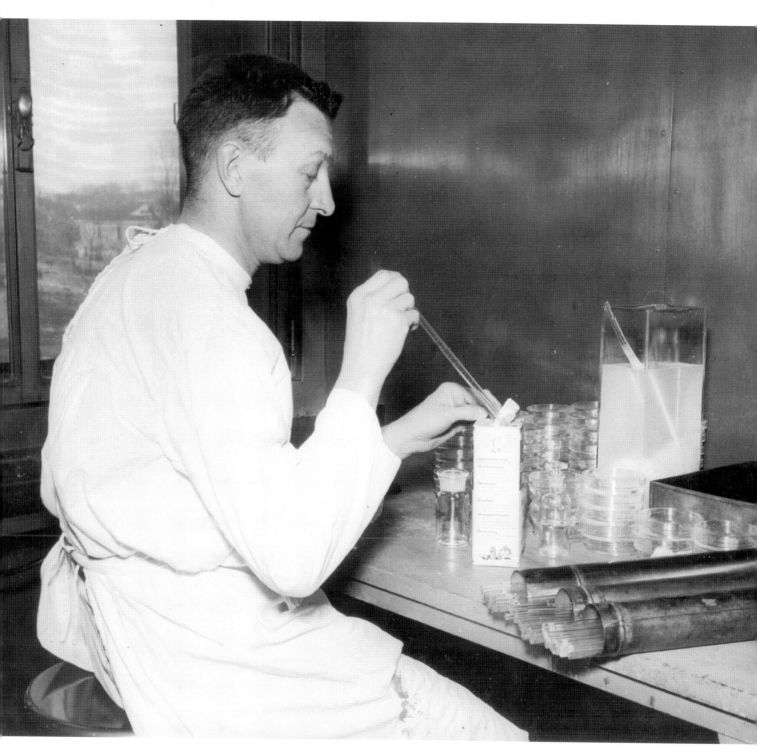

▲ Phillip Sidmore of the School's Veterinary Bacteriology Department is testing bacterial count in milk served to patients and duty personnel at Walter Reed. September 1, 1954.
Source: WRAMC History Office, PAO Historical Collection

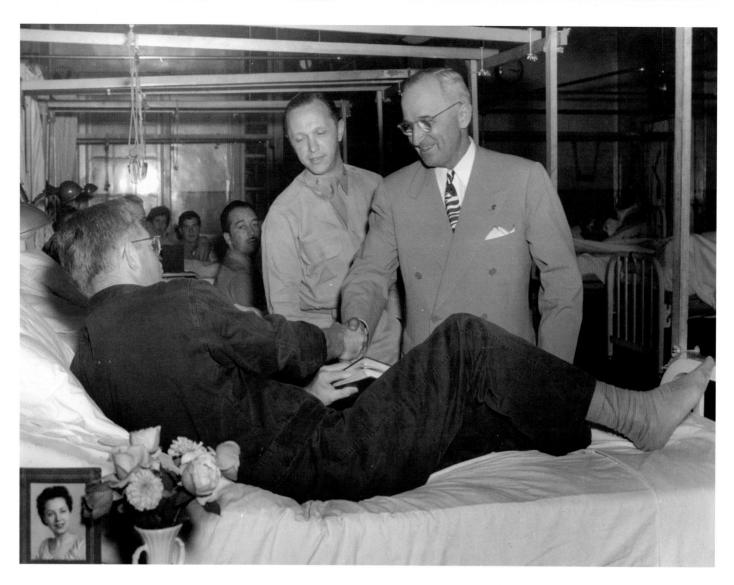

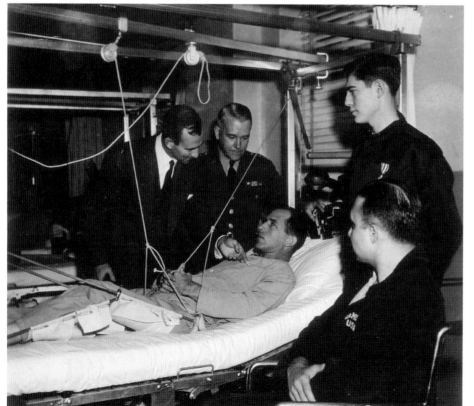

▲ President Harry S. Truman visits with a veteran of the Korean conflict whose leg amputation necessitated hospitalization at Walter Reed. (Original caption)
Source: Walter Reed Army Medical Center, Directorate of Public Works Archives

◀ First Korean Service Ribbons awarded by Secretary of the Army Frank Pace, Jr. (left) and Gen. J. Lawton Collins, Chief of Staff, US Army, to three wounded veterans - 1st Lieutenant Howard W. Cardoza, Jr. (seated right), PFC Francis Phillips (standing), and Master Sergeant Andy Partin (recumbent) - of the Korean Conflict in a ceremony at Walter Reed Hospital. February 6,1951. (Original caption)
Source: National Archives and Records Administration, SC 355362-S

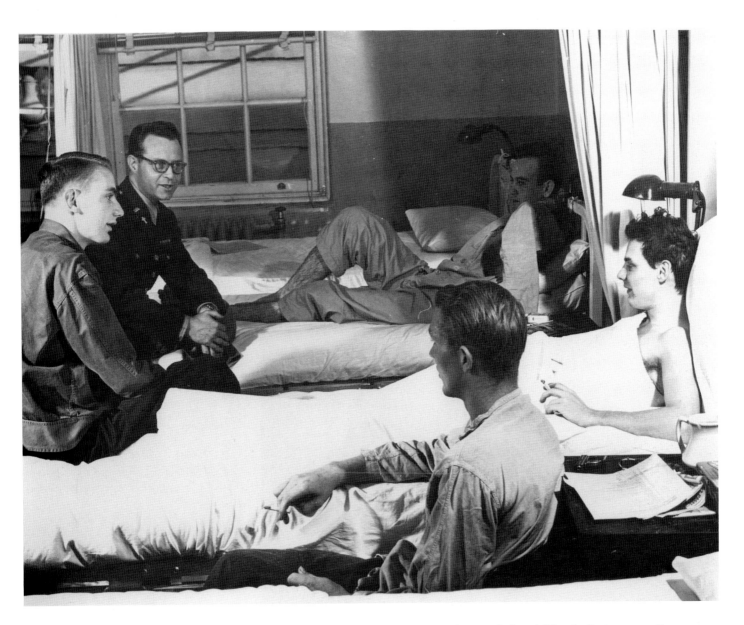

▲ Chaplains of all faiths are stationed at Walter Reed Hospital. They tour the wards in addition to their many other religious activities. Shown here are Capt Lowell G. McCoy (second from left) of Cincinnati, Ohio, holding a bedside chat with (from left to right): PFC Karl Lynn of Sandusky, Ohio; Captain McCoy; Corporal Leo D. Wallace of Savannah, Georgia; PFC Daniel Shoffstall of Lancaster, Pennsylvania; and PFC Carl H. Rice of Chester, South Carolina. (Adapted from original caption) 1951.
Source: Pierce Collection

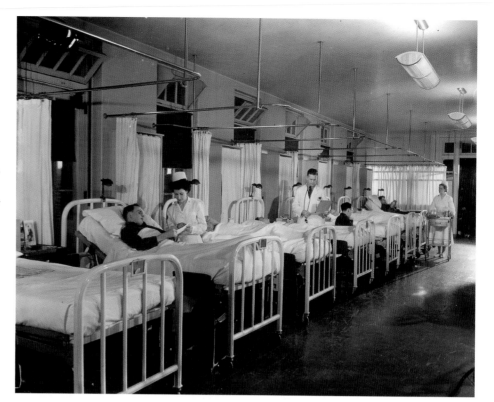

▶ View of a ward at Walter Reed Hospital, January 3, 1951.
Source: National Archives and Records Administration, SC 389632

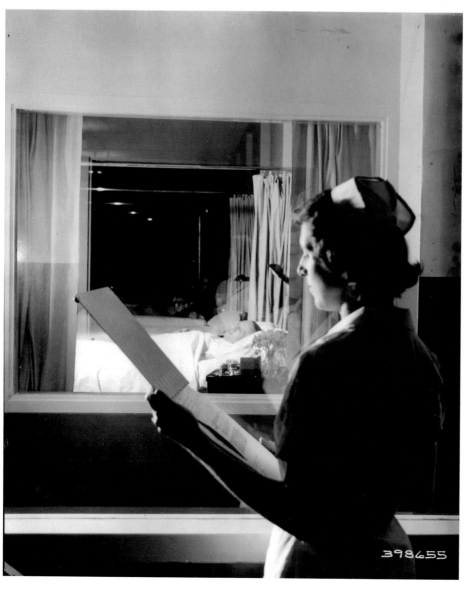

◀ An Army nurse prepares her ward report as she keeps vigil at Walter Reed General Hospital. July 9, 1952.
Source: National Archives and Records Administration, SC 398655-S

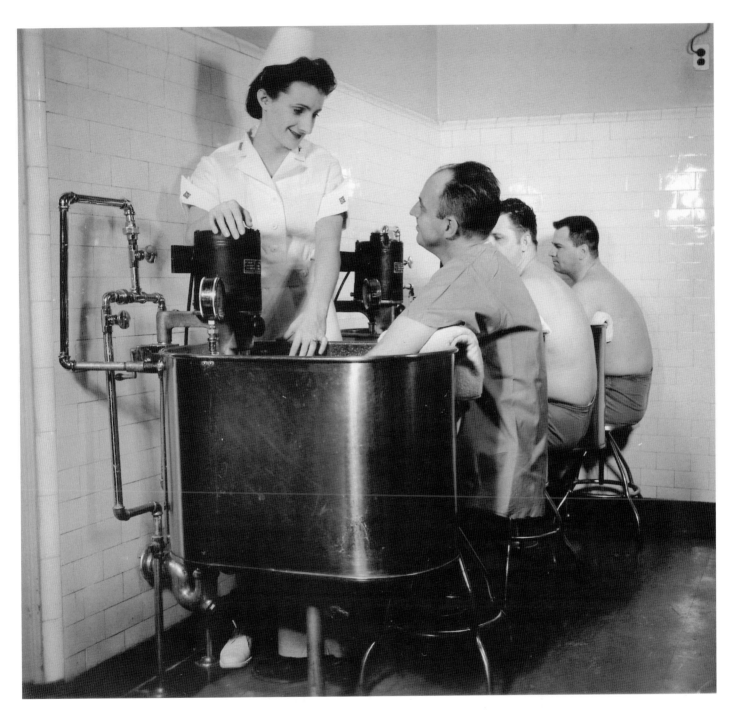

▲ Physical therapists at Walter Reed Army Hospital have some of the best equipment available to any hospital in the world. Here, Lt. Jean Brady (Boone, NC) assists Capt. R. E. Staaes (Loveland, CO) in daily water treatment in a hand whirlpool. (Original caption)
Source: National Museum of Health and Medicine, AFIP, SC 548658

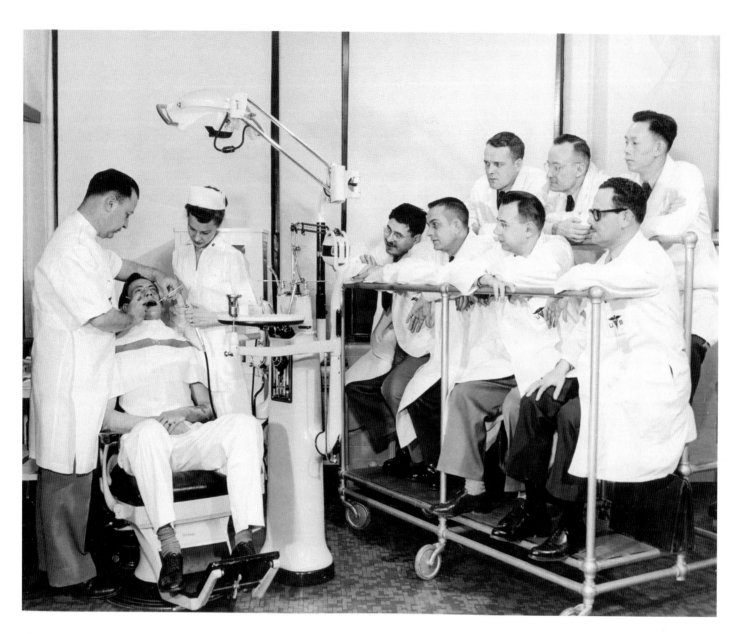

▲ Dental interns in the Central Dental Lab. April 12, 1957.
Source: WRAMC History Office, PAO Historical Collection, DIP-1

▶ The new color television camera in Operating Room #6 Walter Reed Army Hospital is equipped with a number of lenses of varying focal length. The camera looks at the surface of a mirror that is suspended at an angle above the operation. The center of the operating light is always focused on the operating field. November 14, 1957. (Original caption)
Source: National Archives and Records Administration, SC 521403

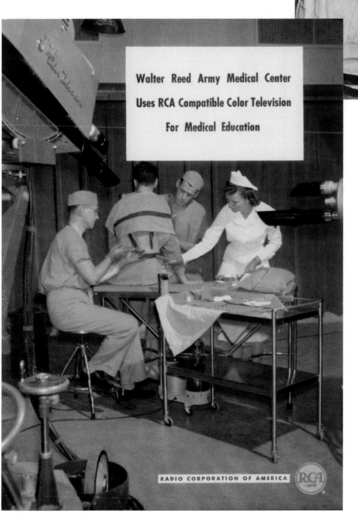

Walter Reed Army Medical Center
Uses RCA Compatible Color Television
For Medical Education

RADIO CORPORATION OF AMERICA RCA

◀ Cover from the brochure for the new color TV camera used in teaching to demonstrate surgical procedures.
Source: National Museum of Health and Medicine, AFIP, AFIP History Collection

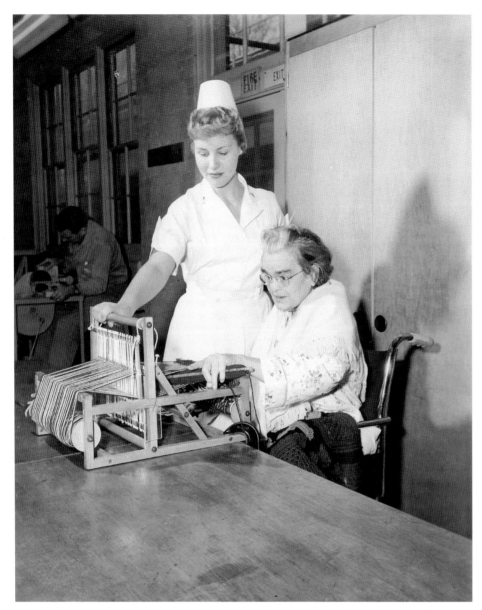

◀ Occupational therapists work with a wide variety of patients while serving their clinical affiliation at Walter Reed Army Hospital. Here, 2nd Lt. Mary E. Mueller works with an elderly patient who is weaving to promote use of her left arm.
Source: National Museum of Health and Medicine, AFIP, SC 548656

▶ Teaching amputees and patients who have lost the use of a limb how to perform routine functions is an important part of the daily activity of an occupational therapy clinical affiliate at Walter Reed Army Hospital. Here, 2nd Lt. Mary E. Mueller shows an Army Officer patient how to tie a Windsor knot with one hand.
Source: National Museum of Health and Medicine, AFIP, SC 548655

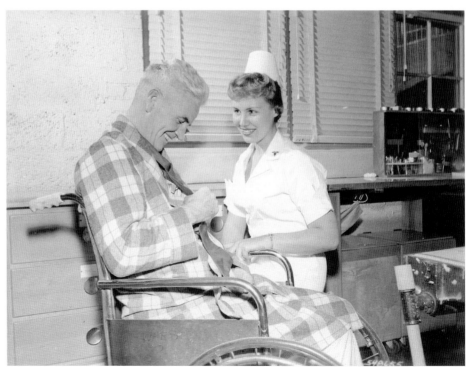

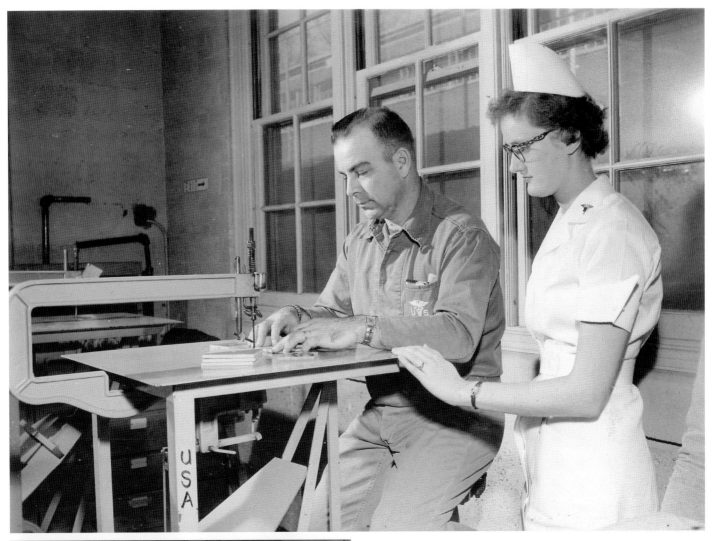

▲ Many kinds of tools and other equipment are available in the Occupational Therapy Section of Walter Reed Army Hospital to help patients in their rehabilitation. Here, OT clinical affiliate 2nd Lt. Joyce F. Jana works with a patient at a bicycle saw to increase tolerance and coordination.
Source: National Museum of Health and Medicine, AFIP, SC 548657

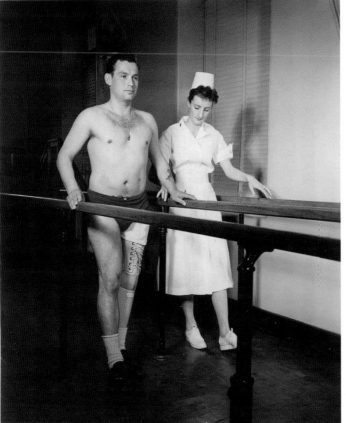

◀ Learning to walk again, 1959.
Source: National Museum of Health and Medicine, AFIP, SC 548660

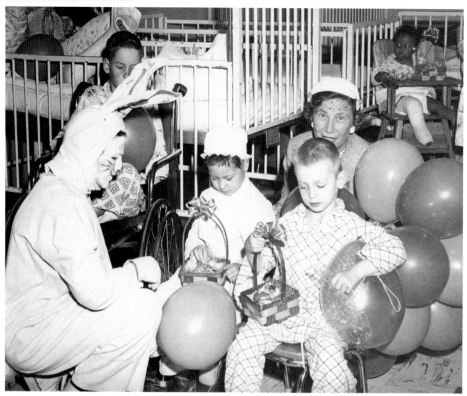

◀ A soldier's family also needs medical care and Walter Reed General Hospital served many dependents. Here, the Easter Bunny is paying a visit to some of the younger patients.
Source: WRAMC History Office, PAO Historical Collection

▼ SFC Alphonso Spencer, assigned to the Army Prosthetic Research Laboratory, Walter Reed Army Medical Center, meets Diana Beckett, a fellow amputee. Diane wears the new polyvinylchloride mitten, which was fitted on her by Mr. Chester Shelton. November 1, 1956.
Source: National Archives and Records Administration, SC 485317

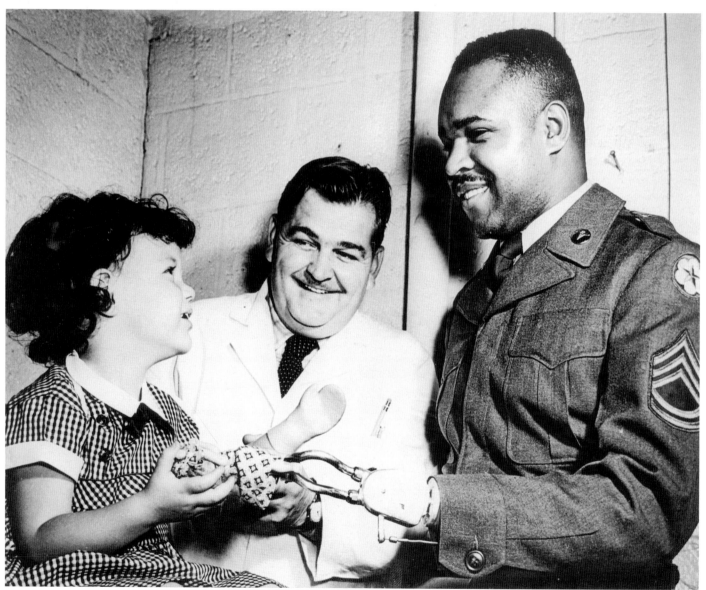

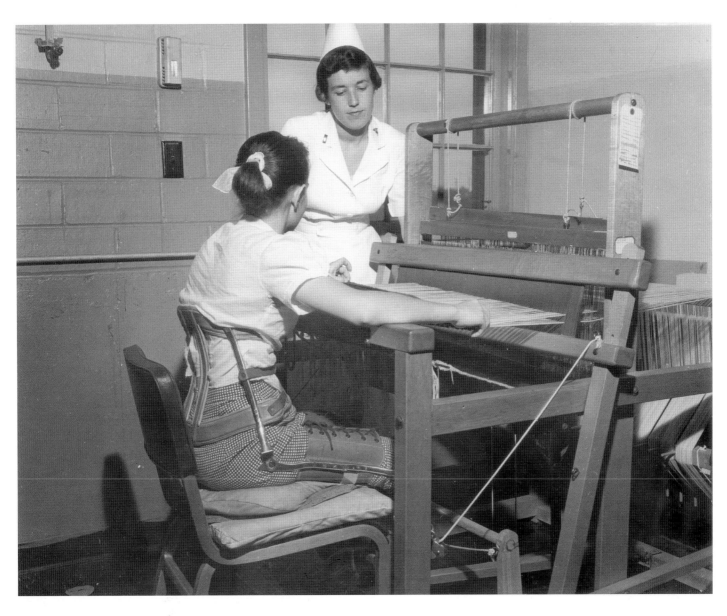

▲ Polio patient working with an occupational therapist at a handloom.
Source: National Museum of Health and Medicine, AFIP, NCP 2747

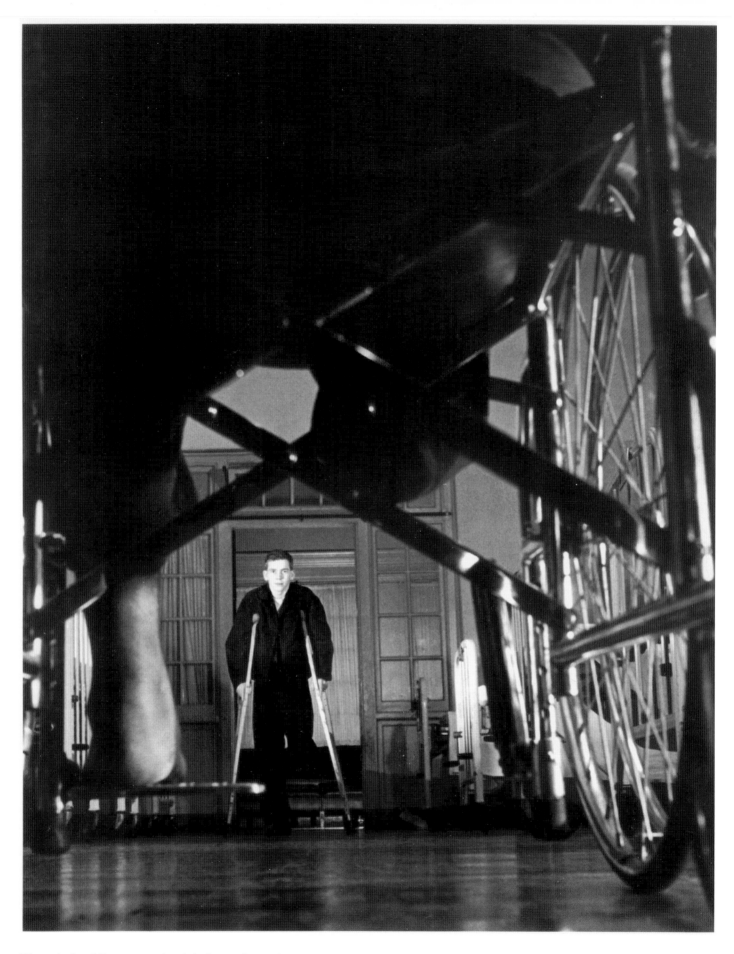

Wounded soldiers use wheelchairs and crutches until they learn how to walk with a synthetic limb. PFC Charles Woody, injured near Taegu, Korea, walks on crutches.
Source: National Archives and Records Administration, 306-PS-50-16899

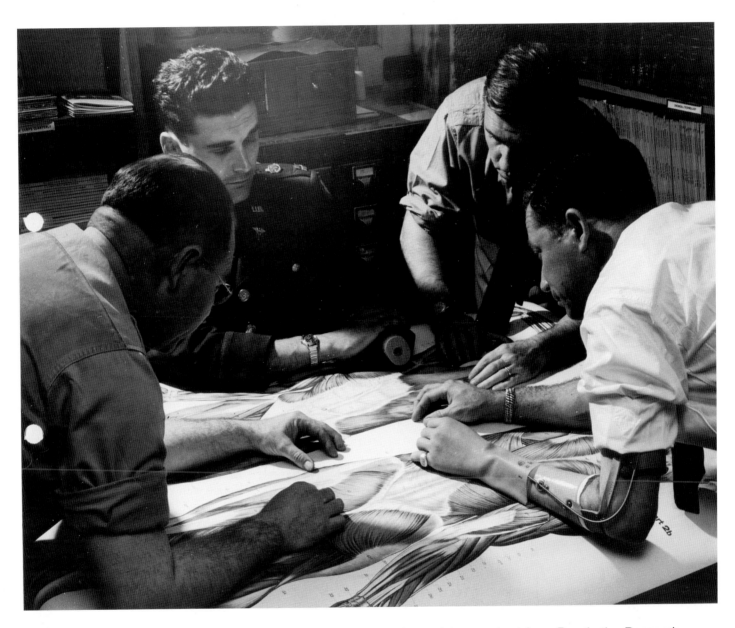

The amazing similarity of real and artificial hands is shown in the above picture made at Army Prosthetics Research Laboratory, Army Medical Center, Washington, D.C. Worn by CPO Joseph A. Phillips, Falls Church, Va. (right), the glove requires one further process before completion — the addition of hair to match that of the patient's own hand. Opposite Chief Phillips is Lt. Albert P. Clark, Portsmouth, N.H., whose artificial hand has been removed to show portions of the prosthesis to which it is normally attached. Others in the picture are (facing camera) Captain John Butchkosky, assistant director of the laboratory, Silver Spring, Md. and Sgt. Walter A. Stanley, Fort George Meade, Md. (wearing glasses) (Adapted from original caption)
Source: Walter Reed Army Medical Center, Directorate of Public Works Archives

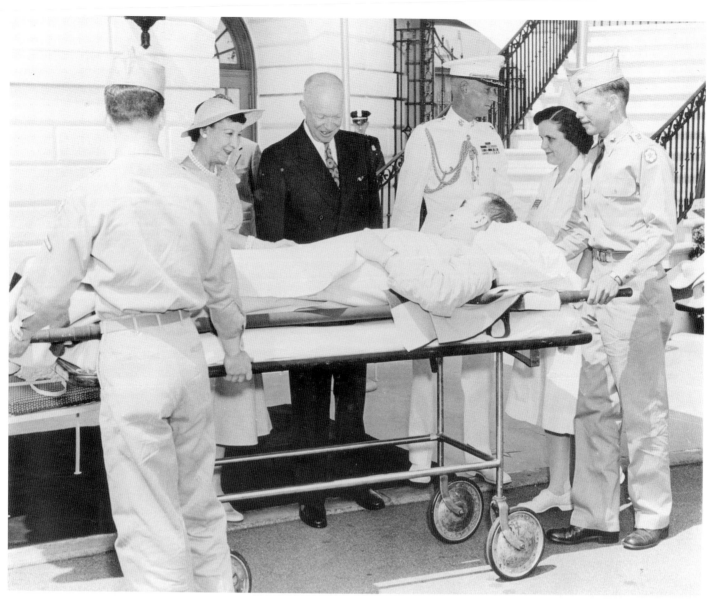

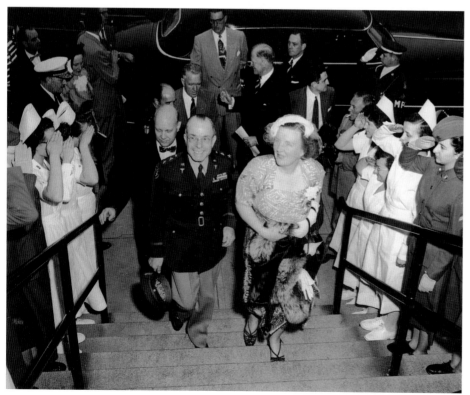

▲ President Eisenhower at White House with WRAMC patient and Captain Anna Mae McCabe. In 1967 Anna Mae (McCabe) Hays became Chief of the Army Nurse Corps and was later promoted to Brig. General.
Source: WRAMC History Collection

◄ Queen Juliana of the Netherlands, escorted by Maj. General Paul H. Streit, Commanding General, Walter Reed Army Medical Center, passes through saluting columns of Army medical and nurse officers, members of the Women's Medical Specialist Corps and the Women's Army Corps. Entering Walter Reed Army Hospital, Her Majesty visited many soldier-patients, casualties of the Korean conflict. April 9, 1952.
Source: National Museum of Health and Medicine, AFIP, WRAMC History Collection

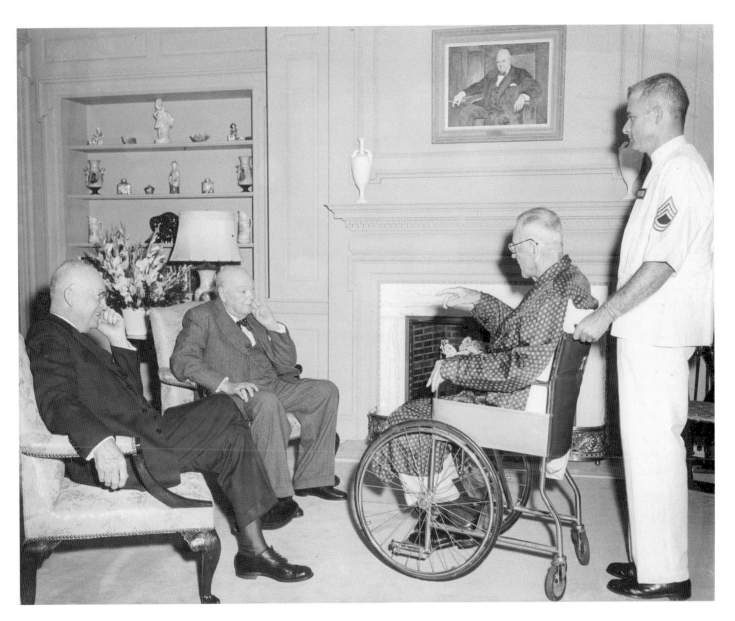

▲ Prime Minister Winston Churchill and President Dwight Eisenhower visit with John Foster Dulles in the sitting room on Ward 8. Above the fireplace is the portrait that President Eisenhower painted of his friend Winston Churchill. May 5, 1959.
Source: WRAMC History Collection

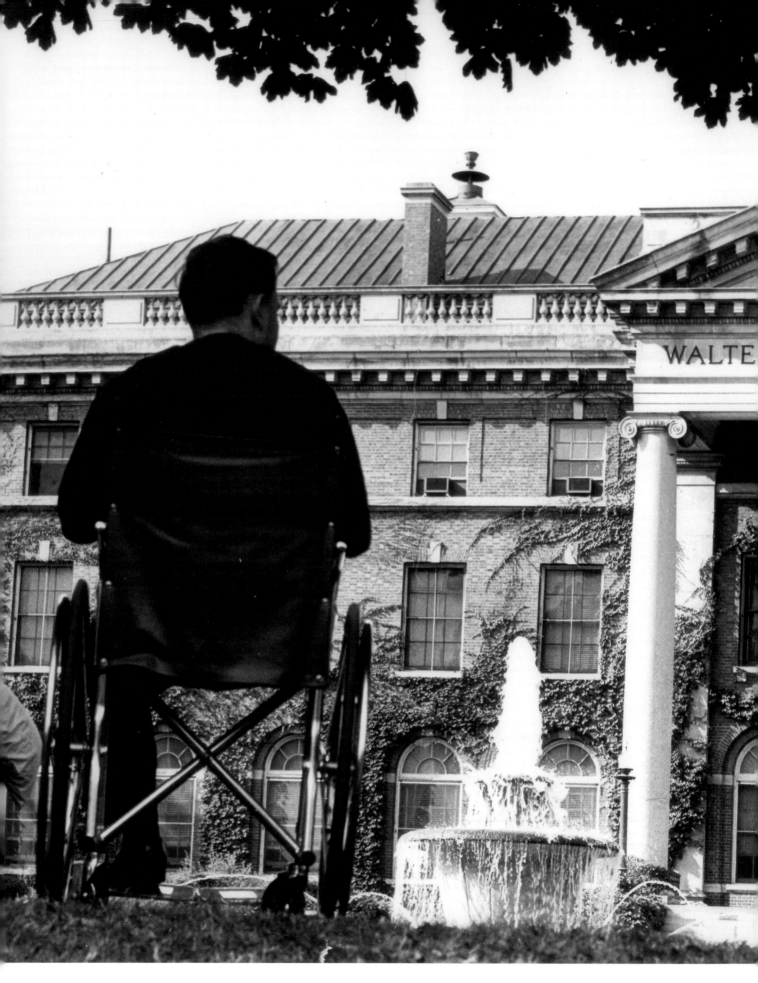

Amputee in wheelchair in front of Walter Reed General Hospital.
Source: National Museum of Health and Medicine, AFIP, NCP 2545

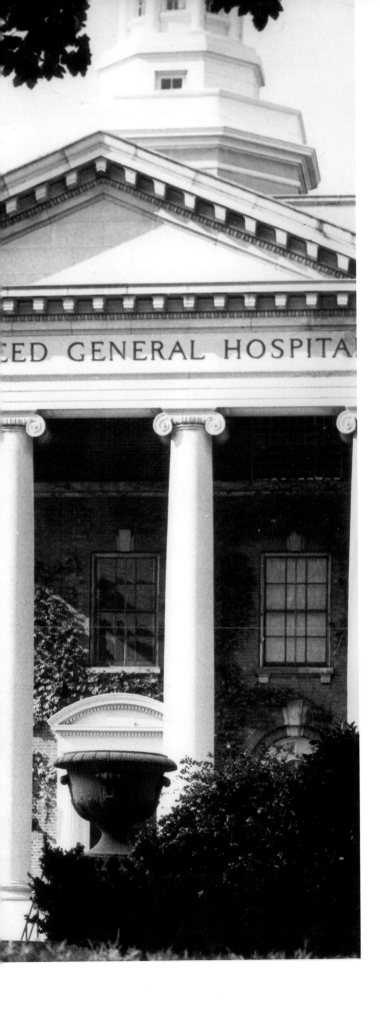

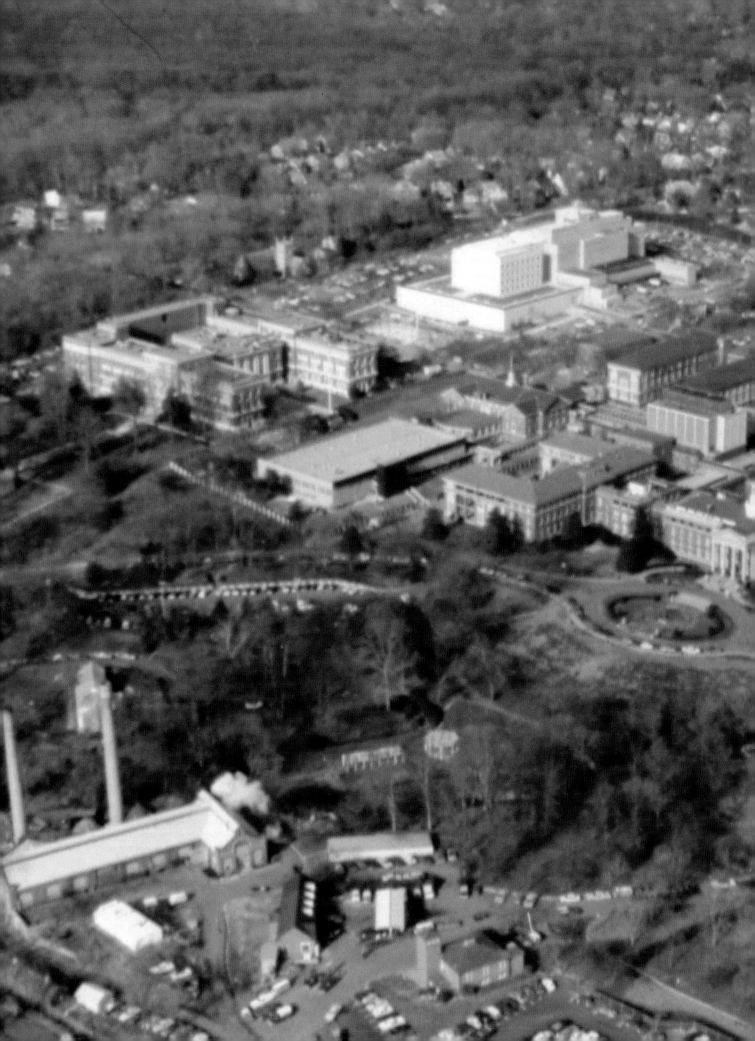

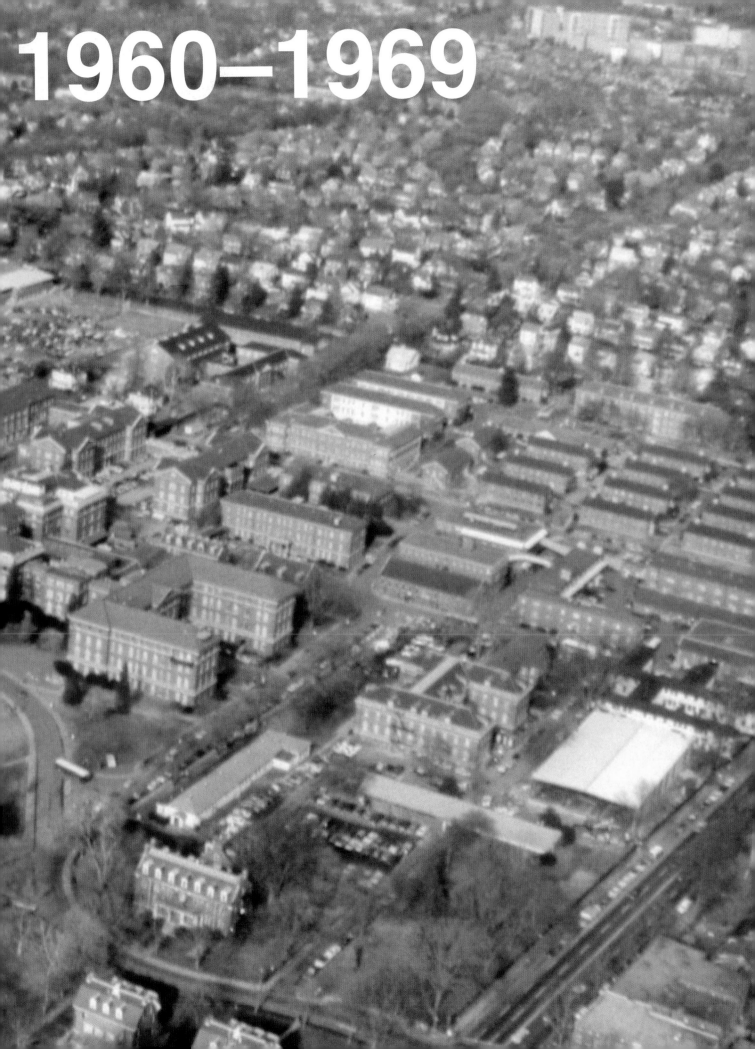

1960–1969

Title page - This aerial photograph, taken in the late 1960s, looks northwest and shows several new structures on the Walter Reed campus. The final permanent addition to the Walter Reed Army Institute of Research (WRAIR — Building 40) can be seen on its west elevation. The Siler wing contained a nuclear reactor for medical research; the reactor was decommissioned in the late 1970s. Just north of the WRAIR building, the new addition to the Armed Forces Institute of Pathology (AFIP) building can be seen under construction. South of Red Cross Hall and east of Building 7 are two new temporary buildings that exist to this day. On the third floor of the far eastern end of Building 1 can be seen what appears to be a dark line. This structure is actually a balcony or small porch that was added to the building during President Eisenhower's 11-month inpatient stay at Walter Reed where he used to get fresh air and sunshine. It was removed about 20 years later.
Source: Walter Reed Army Medical Center, Directorate of Public Works Archives

▶ A new 2,000,000 volt X-ray machine was installed in 1961. The new machine, demonstrated by Col. Albert J. Bauer, the hospital's Chief of Radiation Therapy and an X-ray Technician, weighs in at 6 tons. Its rays are absorbed by 36-inch concrete walls. The patient is alone in the room under treatment as the radiologist views the room from the outside via a specially constructed television camera and monitor. The machine can be elevated and tilted by the operator to any desired position. (Original caption)
Source: Walter Reed Army Medical Center History Office, PAO Historical Collection

After the shocking death of Major Walter Reed at age 51 in 1902, the Walter Reed Memorial Association was formed. The association's goal was to provide support to Reed's widow, Emilie, and daughter, Blossom, and to erect a suitable memorial to Walter Reed. The first meeting was held in August 1903 less than a year after Walter Reed's death. A veritable "Who's Who" of physicians, scientists, and business executives were present at this initial meeting. Among them were Dr. Daniel C. Gilman, President of Johns Hopkins University; Dr. William Welch, noted pathologist from Johns Hopkins; Dr. C.A. Herter, Professor of Pharmacology at Columbia University; Dr. Alexander Abbot, Professor of Hygiene at the University of Pennsylvania; Dr. L. F. Barker, Professor and Head of Anatomy at Rush Medical School at the University of Chicago; Dr. Edward G. Janeway of Bellevue and Dr. Charles P. Putman of Boston. Others in attendance were John Stewart Kennedy, capitalist and philanthropist, Morris J. Jessup, banker and Bishop William Lawrence.

The Walter Reed Memorial Association was not idle while Mrs. Reed and her daughter lived out their lives. The Association sponsored Walter D. McCaw to write a brief history of Reed's life and work. It also commissioned a bust of Walter Reed by Mr. Hans Schuler of Baltimore. The Schuler bust remains on display in the lobby of Building 1. The group also undertook the preservation of Camp Lazear, outside Havana, where the classic yellow fever experiments took place. The Association assisted in the enshrinement of Walter Reed in the Hall of Fame of Great Americans of New York University.

Dedicated on November 21, 1966, The Walter Reed Memorial included the de Weldon bust of Walter Reed and a 25 foot high shaft of white-amoco cream marble with terrace steps of Georgian marble. The dedication was attended by Walter Reed's granddaughter, Mrs. Daisy Reed Royce, and former President and Mrs. Eisenhower.

The end of Walter Reed Hospital's sixth decade would bring the wounded of another war, this time in Southeast Asia, to its historic grounds. Wars always increase the need for qualified medical and nursing personnel and this one was no exception. Because of a lack of qualified nursing personnel, the Walter Reed Army Institute of Nursing (WRAIN) was opened in 1968. A cooperative program with the University of Maryland, the WRAIN produced over 1,200 bachelors prepared nurses for the Army during its years of existence. With the Vietnam War over, WRAIN became "a luxury the Army could no longer afford" and was closed in 1978.

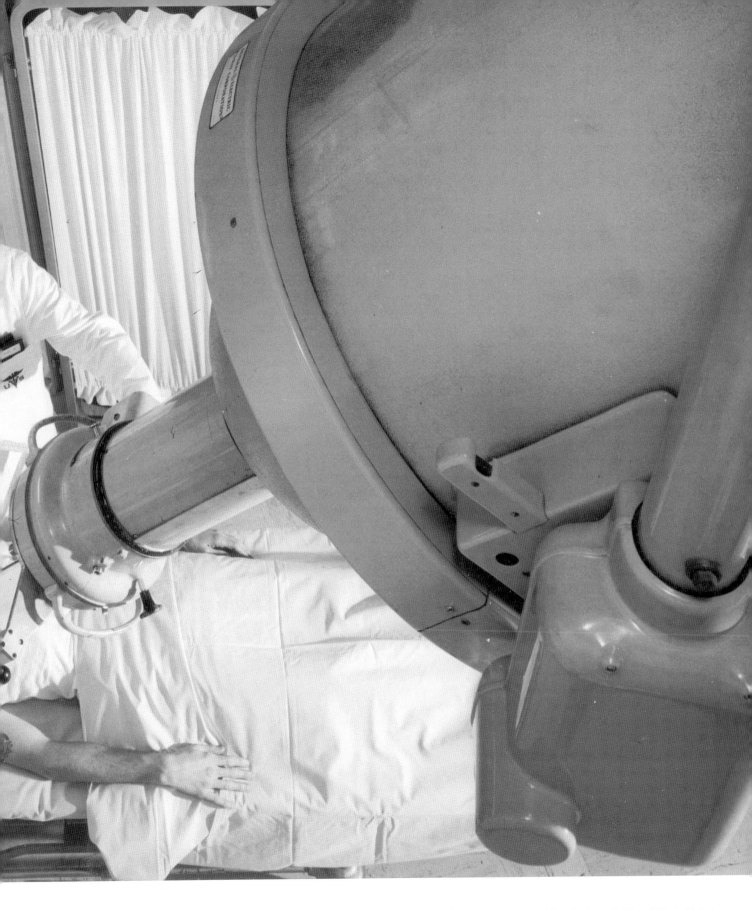

On March 28, 1969, one of Walter Reed's most famous patients died. Dwight D. Eisenhower had been hospitalized on Ward 8 in the Presidential Suite for 11 months (May 1968 - March 1969) because of illness due to coronary artery disease and congestive heart failure. Mrs. Eisenhower resided in an adjacent room. He died following his 14th episode of ventricular fibrillation on March 28, 1969 as there was no intervention, complying with his request. The beloved Ike, West Point Class of 1915, Supreme Commander Allied Expeditionary Force in World War II, General of the Army and twice elected President of the United States was dead at 78 years old.

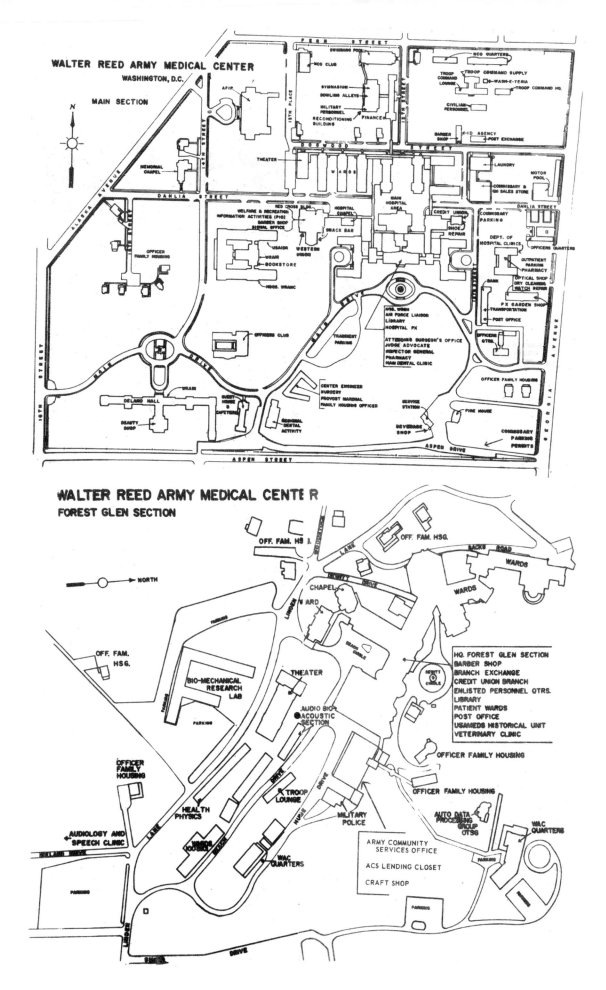

▲ Source: National Museum of Health and Medicine, AFIP, WRAMC History Collection

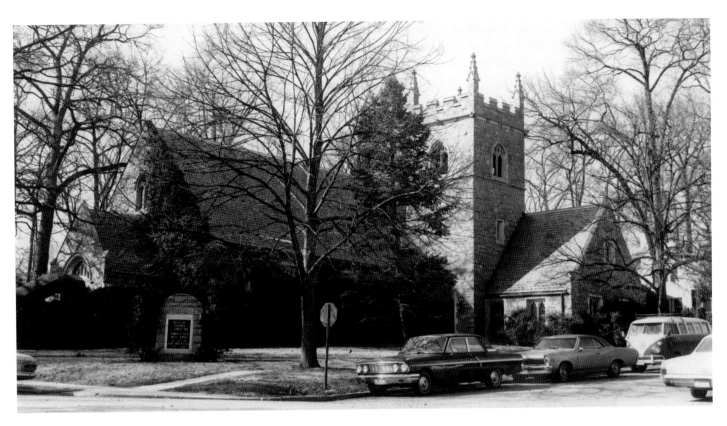

▲ Little changed from the 1930s, the Memorial Chapel, scene of many weddings for patients and staff thirty years after its dedication.
Source: National Museum of Health and Medicine, AFIP, WRAMC History Collection

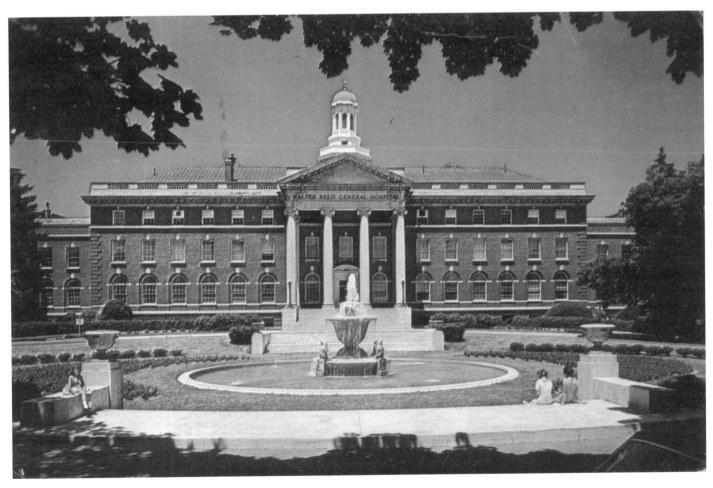

▲ Postcard reads: "A beautiful spring view of the hospital and the Hoff Fountain."
Source: Pierce Collection

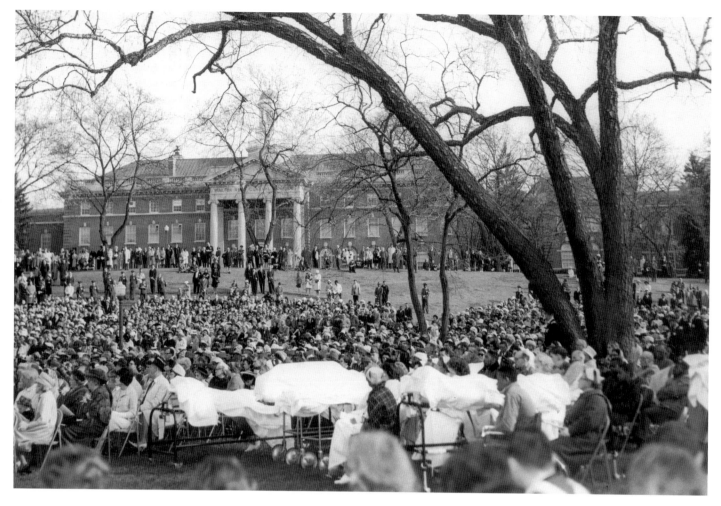

▲ The traditional Easter Sunrise Service was well attended in 1965.
Source: Walter Reed Army Medical Center History Office

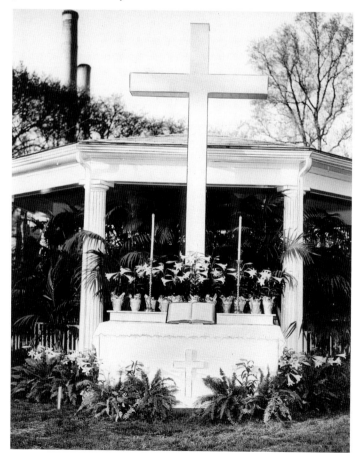

◀ An altar was set in front of the Gazebo for Easter Sunday in 1965.
Source: National Museum of Health and Medicine, AFIP, WRAMC History Collection

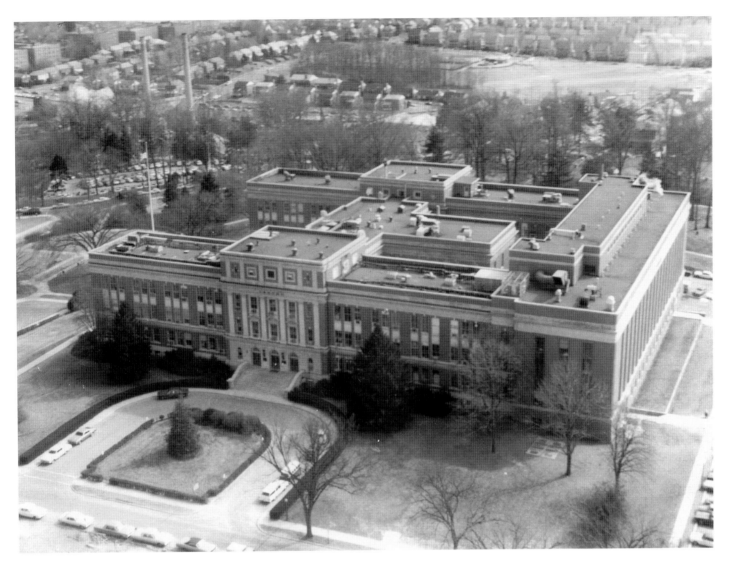

▲ Building 40, now known as Walter Reed Army Institute of Research (WRAIR) with new Siler addition that contained a nuclear reactor for medical research. This new wing, named after Col. Joseph F. Siler, MC, is visible on the right side of the complex.
Source: Walter Reed Army Medical Center History Office, PAO Historical Collection

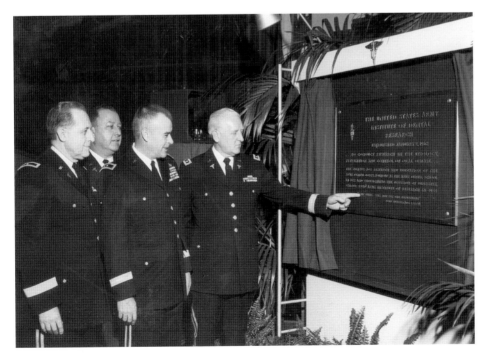

◀ The Dental Research Institute was dedicated March 3, 1962. Viewing the plaque at the dedication of the U.S. Army Institute of Dental Research, Walter Reed Army Medical Center, Washington, D.C., are from left: Brig. General James H. Forsee, Commanding General, U.S. Army Medical Research and Development Command; Col. George H. Timke, Jr., Director of the Institute; Maj. General Dwight E. Beach, Deputy Chief, U.S. Army Research and Development, who dedicated the Institution; and Maj. General Joseph L. Bernier, Chief of the Army Dental Corps. (Original caption)
Source: Walter Reed Army Medical Center History Office

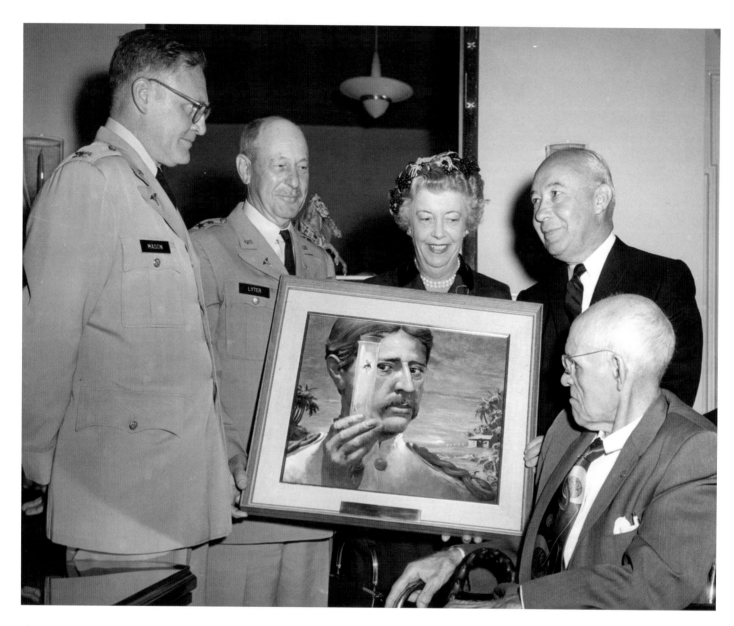

▲ Walter Reed painting presented to Walter Reed Army Medical Center. Just sixty-one years to the day after the Yellow Fever Commission was formed, special tribute was paid to the commission's leader, Maj. Walter Reed. The occasion was the presentation to the Medical Center bearing his name, of an original oil painting of the famed Army doctor. Shown above (left to right) are Col. Richard P. Mason, Director of the Walter Reed Army Institute of Research; Maj. General Clinton S. Lyter, Commanding General of Walter Reed Army Medical Center; Mrs. Charles H. Royce, granddaughter of Major Reed; Dr. Frank A. Warner, Vice-president and Medical Director of the John Hancock Mutual Life Insurance Co., donors of the painting; and Mr. Gustaf E. Lambert, who was an enlisted nurse and cared for the volunteers who developed yellow fever during the experiments in Havana, Cuba. Mr. Lambert praised the likeness of his former leader, but claimed he never "looked that stern." May 24, 1961. (Adapted from original caption)

Source: Walter Reed Army Medical Center, Directorate of Public Works Archives

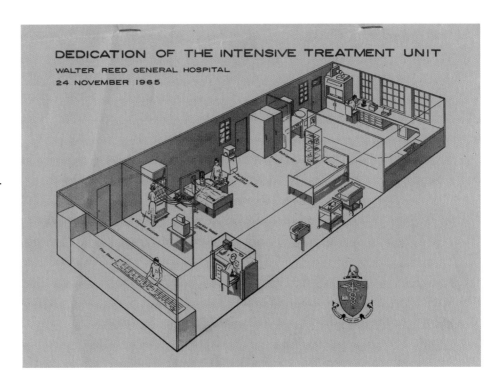

DEDICATION OF THE INTENSIVE TREATMENT UNIT
WALTER REED GENERAL HOSPITAL
24 NOVEMBER 1965

▶ The new Intensive Treatment Unit at Walter Reed General Hospital dedicated November 24, 1965.
Source: National Museum of Health and Medicine, AFIP, WRAMC History Collection

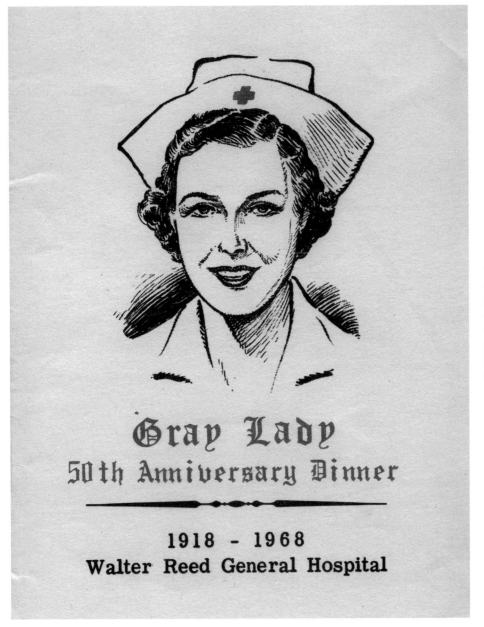

◀ The Gray Ladies, an essential part of the care provided to wounded and sick military personnel since 1918, celebrated its 50th anniversary in 1968. This is the cover for the dinner brochure.
Source: National Museum of Health and Medicine, AFIP, WRAMC History Collection

147

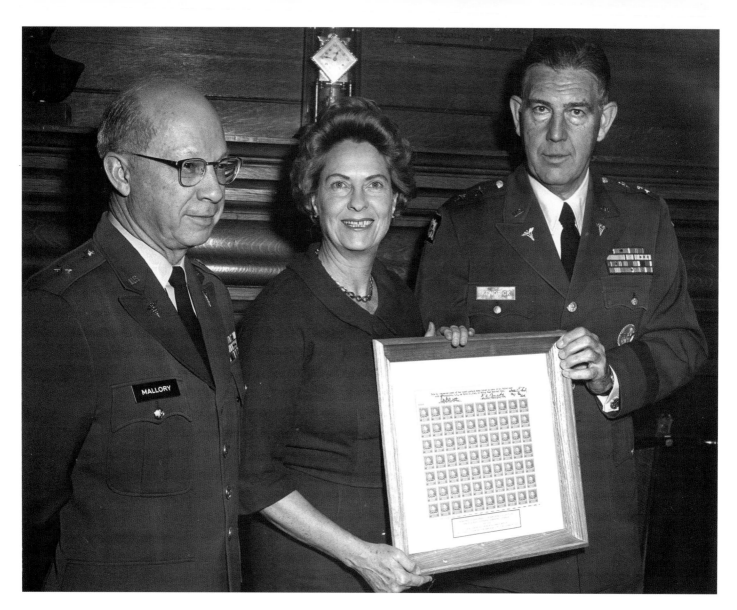

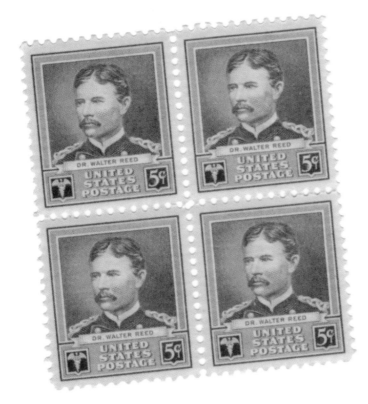

Walter Reed Commemorative Stamps presented to Walter Reed Library. The stamps were originally released April 17, 1940. This sheet of stamps was given by Walter Reed Memorial Association January 13, 1967.
Left to right: Brig. General Philip W. Mallory, Deputy Commanding General; Mrs. Barv, Head Librarian; Maj. General Douglas B. Kendrick, Commanding General WRAMC.
Source: Signal Corps. Pvt. James Reed - photographer

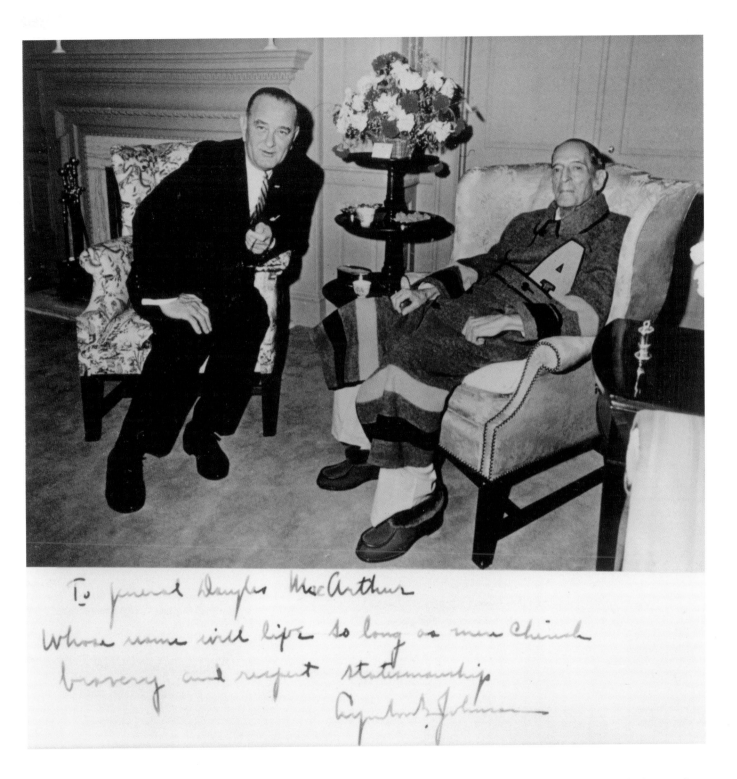

President Lyndon B. Johnson visited General MacArthur on Ward 8 at Walter Reed. The handwritten inscription reads:
"To General Douglas MacArthur
Whose name will live so long as men cherish bravery and respect statesmanship.
                                        Lyndon B. Johnson"

Source: Walter Reed Army Medical Center

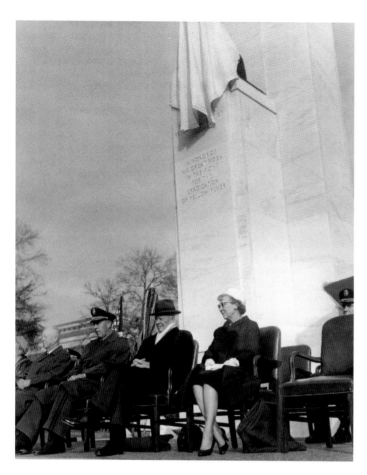

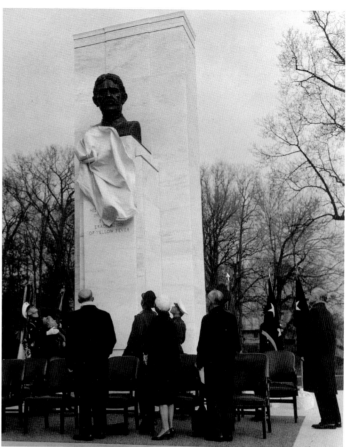

The Walter Reed Memorial in Delano Circle was dedicated on November 21, 1966. The Walter Reed Memorial Association, organized in 1903 to provide support for Mrs. Reed and her daughter, completed its work with the dedication of the Memorial. The Association commissioned Felix de Weldon to sculpt the bust of Walter Reed that sits on top of the column. Special guests at the dedication included Mrs. Daisy Reed Royce, Walter Reed's granddaughter, and former President and Mrs. Dwight Eisenhower.
Source: National Museum of Health and Medicine, AFIP, WRAMC History Collection

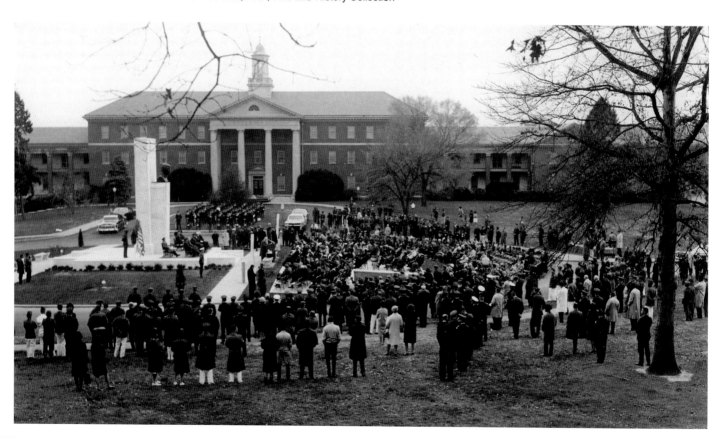

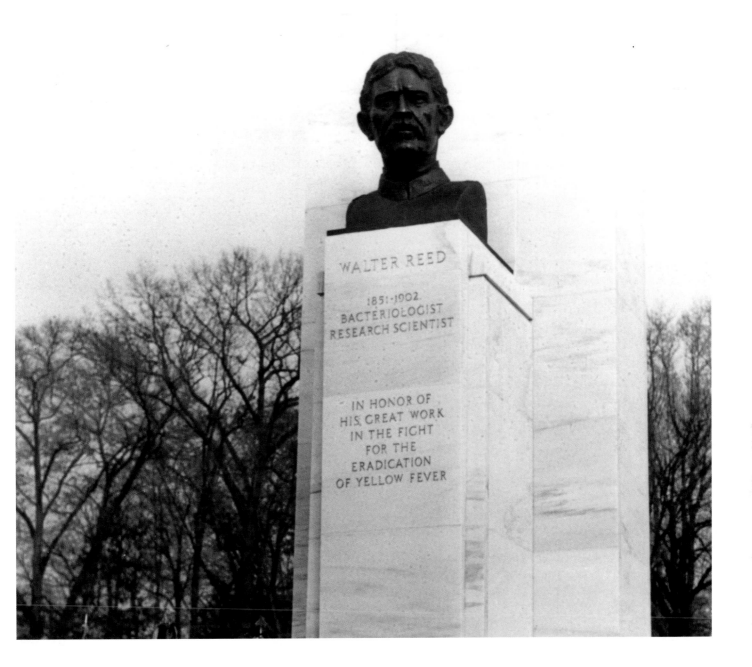

Among the Walter Reed Memorial Association incorporators were industrialist Alexander Graham Bell, former Surgeon General George Miller Sternberg, then current Surgeon General R. M. O'Reilly, and Dr. James Carroll (member of the Army Yellow Fever Board). The goals of the association were to raise $25,000 or more to provide income for Walter Reed's widow and daughter and "to then devote the principal to the erection of a suitable memorial in the City of Washington" to Maj. Walter Reed.

Gifts came in both large and small. John D. Rockefeller and Pierpont Morgan each gave $2,000. Charles W. Eliot, President of Harvard, gave $1,000. Most gifts were, of course, smaller. The goal of $25,000 was reached in 1907. The income from the trust fund was provided to Mrs. Emilie Reed until her death in 1950 at age 96 and to their daughter Blossom until her death in 1964 at age 77.

After Blossom Reed's death, the Association completed its last duty by commissioning Mr. Felix de Weldon to complete the Walter Reed Memorial on the campus of Walter Reed Army Medical Center. Mr. de Weldon, a famous sculptor of Presidents and Kings, had spent nine years completing the enormous Marine Corps (Iwo Jima) War Memorial in Arlington, VA.

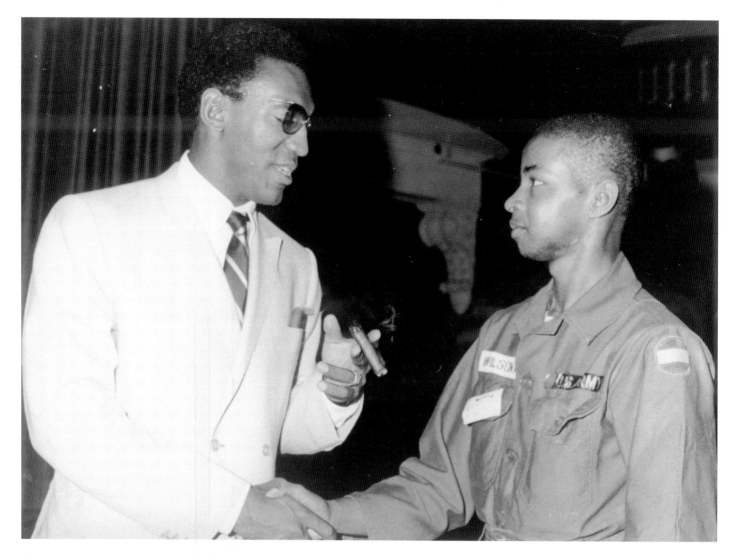

▲ Comedian Bill Cosby visiting with rehabilitation patients at the Forest Glen Annex in 1967. Cosby served four years in the Navy as a physical therapist prior to entering show business.
Source: National Museum of Health and Medicine, AFIP, WRAMC History Collection

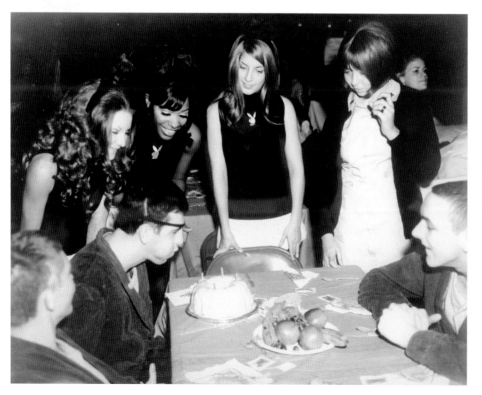

◀ Playboy Bunnies bring cheer and a birthday cake to recovering patients.
Source: National Museum of Health and Medicine, AFIP, WRAMC History Collection

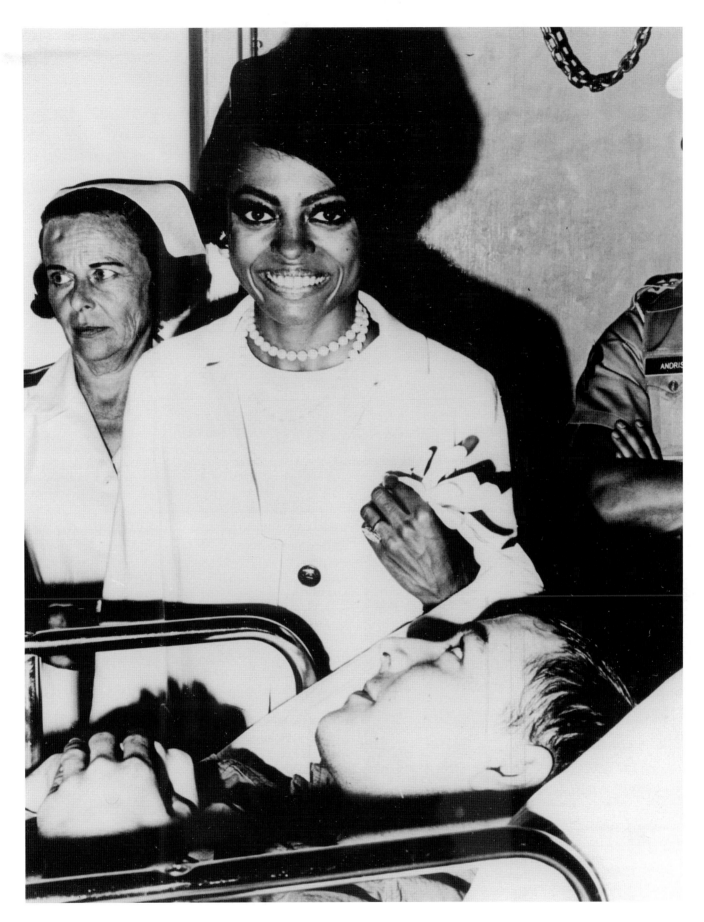

▲ Singer Diana Ross brings a smile to a young soldier.
Source: National Museum of Health and Medicine, AFIP, WRAMC History Collection

153

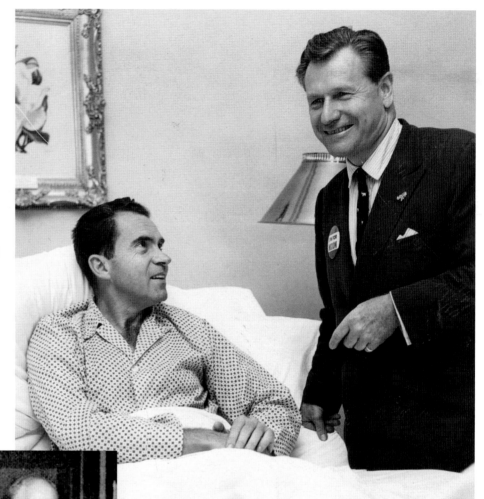

▶ Vice President Richard Nixon, recovering from an infected left knee in the hospital's executive suite, chats with Nelson Rockefeller, then Governor of New York and later Vice President under Gerald Ford.
Source: WRAMC History Office, PAO Historical Collection

At the beginning of its sixth decade, Walter Reed would play a little known role in the historic presidential campaign and election of 1960. Vice-President Richard M. Nixon who was running against Senator John F. Kennedy, injured his left knee in August 1960; the knee ultimately became infected with *Staphylococcus aureus*. Mr. Nixon was admitted to Ward 8 at Walter Reed for treatment with intravenous antibiotics. He left the hospital in early September to begin the campaign in earnest. A few days later, he experienced high fever and chills and was again treated with antibiotics. Nixon had not fully recovered before the first televised debate on September 26, 1960; his general poor physical condition and appearance were apparent to the nation, compared with the apparently robust Kennedy. Nixon did ultimately recover from his infected knee, but never recovered from the poor showing in the debate and lost a close race to John Kennedy.

◀ President John F. Kennedy is shown walking through the hospital with Surgeon General Leonard D. Heaton. In the background to the left is Presidential Press Secretary Pierre Salinger.
Source: Stripe newspaper, April 20, 2006

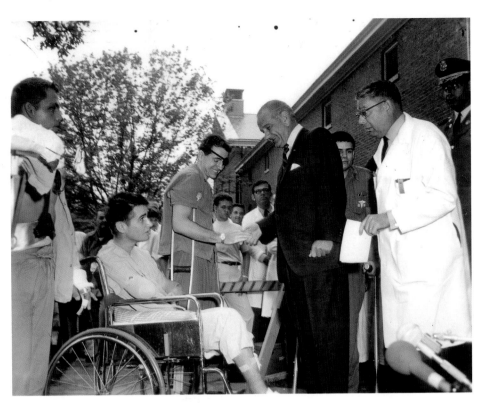

◀ President Lyndon Johnson talks with PFC Allen Lloyd and SP4 Thomas A. Bailey during his visit on June 11, 1968. Looking on is Col. John L. Bradley.
Source: National Archives and Records Administration, SC 646373

▼ President Lyndon Johnson leaving the hospital after a visit with General Douglas MacArthur.
Source: National Museum of Health and Medicine, AFIP, WRAMC History Collection

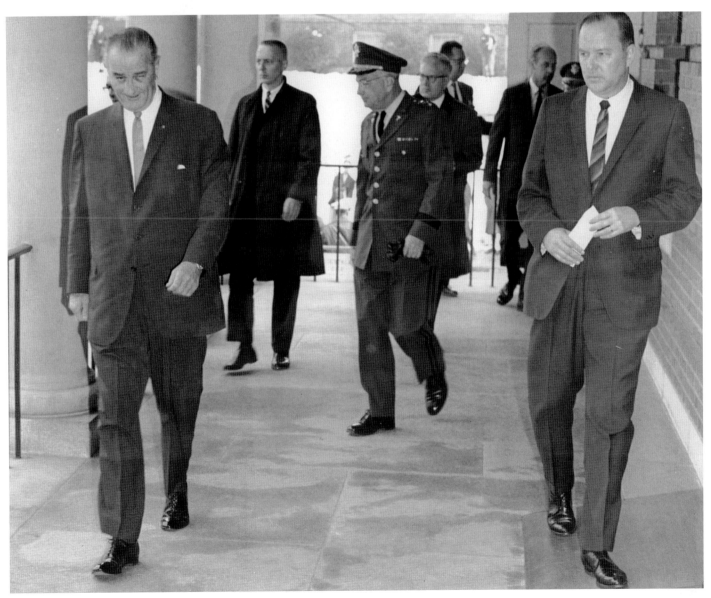

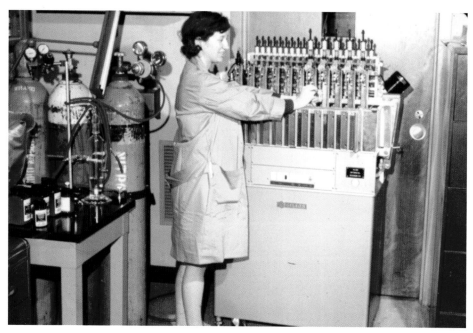

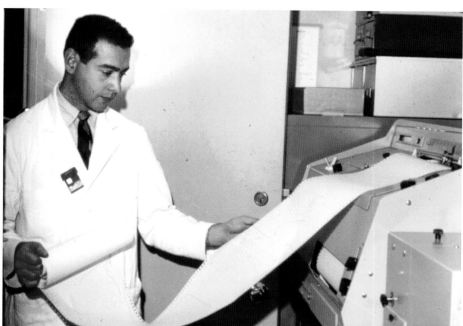

Research and clinical laboratories around the campus of Walter Reed.
Sources: Walter Reed Army Medical Center, Directorate of Public Works Archives

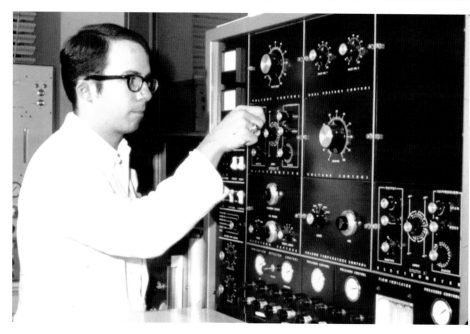

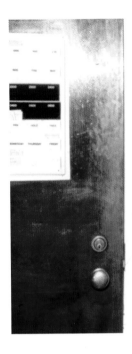
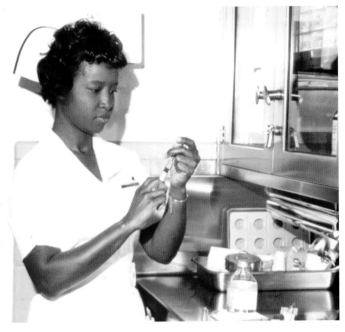
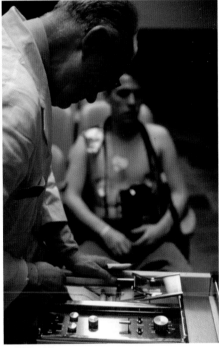

Scenes of patient care at Walter Reed Hospital.
Sources: Walter Reed Army Medical Center, Directorate of Public Works Archives

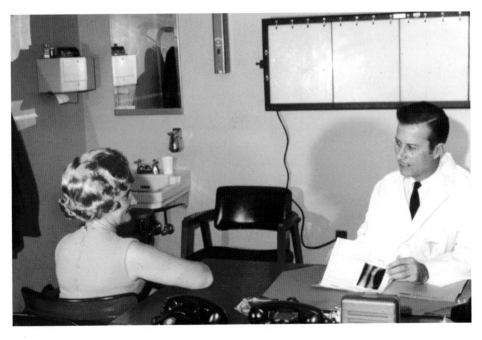

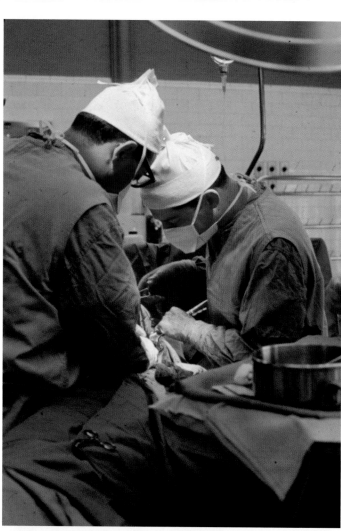

◀ Performing general surgery in the main operating room.
Source: Walter Reed Army Medical Center, Directorate of Public Works Archives

▶ Orthopaedic ward rounds with Col. Walter Metz (left), Chief of Orthopaedics at the time, eventually Chief of Surgery before retiring. Col. George Ivan (G.I.) Baker (center), Assistant Chief. G.I. Baker was promoted to Maj. General in 1977 and served as WRAMC Commander. Monroe Levine (right), then a resident, became the Chief of the Hand Surgery Service in the mid-1970s.
Source: Walter Reed Army Medical Center, Directorate of Public Works Archives.

▼ Filming oral surgery.
Source: Walter Reed Army Medical Center, Directorate of Public Works Archives

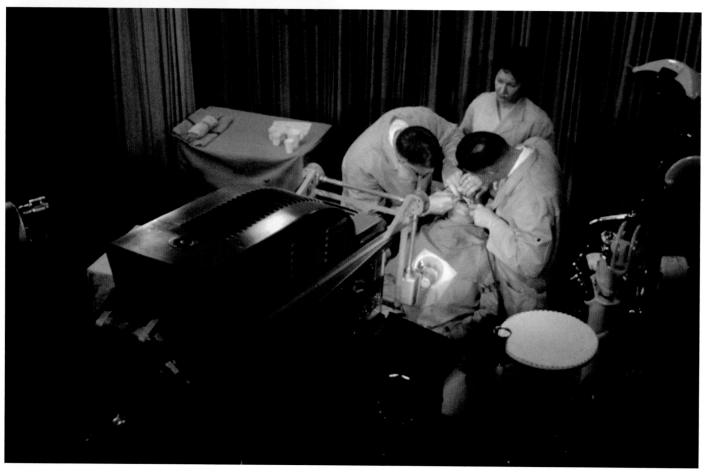

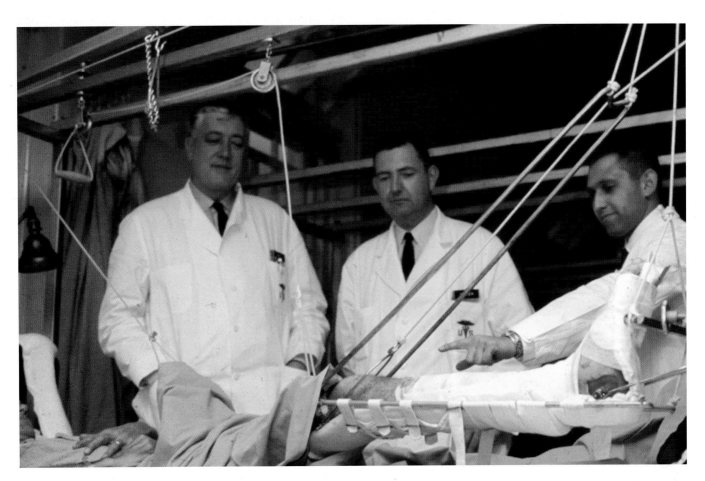

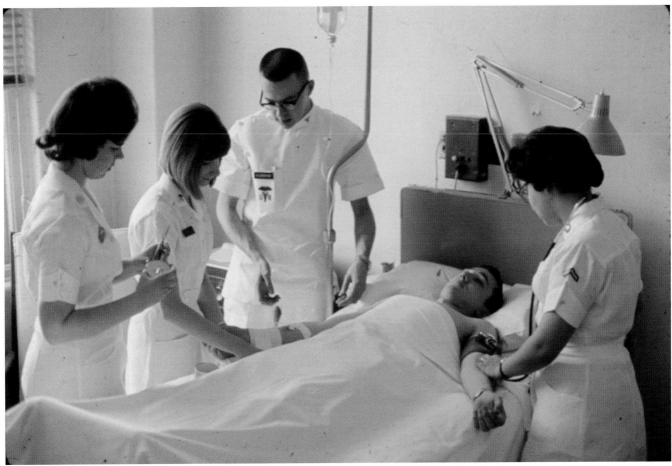

▲ Inspecting an intravenous site and taking vital signs.
Source: Walter Reed Army Medical Center, Directorate of Public Works Archives

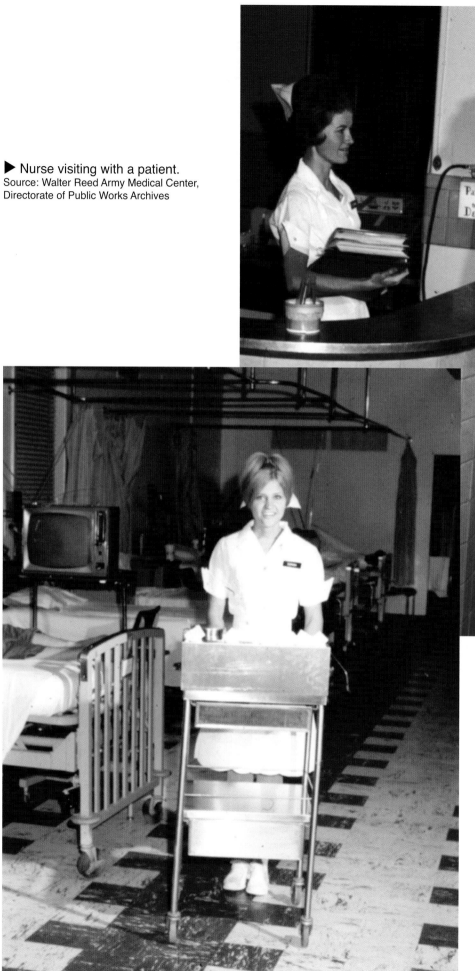

► Nurse visiting with a patient.
Source: Walter Reed Army Medical Center, Directorate of Public Works Archives

◄ Nurse tending to patients on an open bay ward.
Source: Walter Reed Army Medical Center, Directorate of Public Works Archives

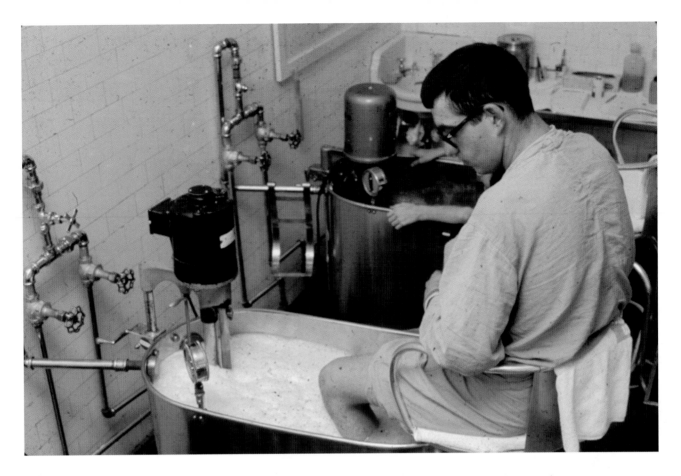

▲ Wound treatment with a whirlpool bath. The circulating water helped debride open wounds.
Source: Walter Reed Army Medical Center, Directorate of Public Works Archives

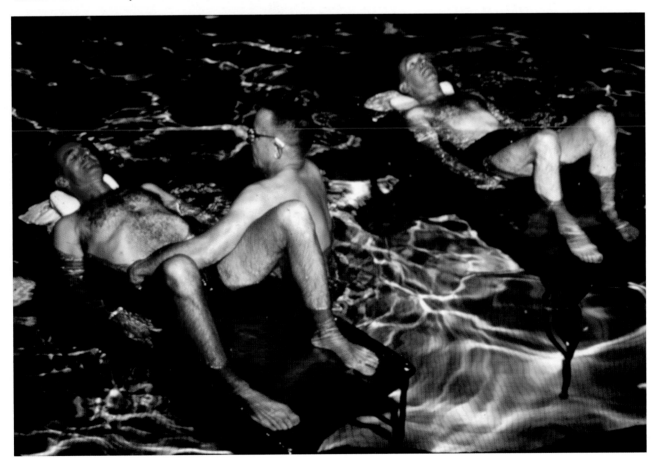

▲ Hydrotherapy for patients with back injuries. The patients are positioned on tables in the pool.
Source: Walter Reed Army Medical Center, Directorate of Public Works Archives

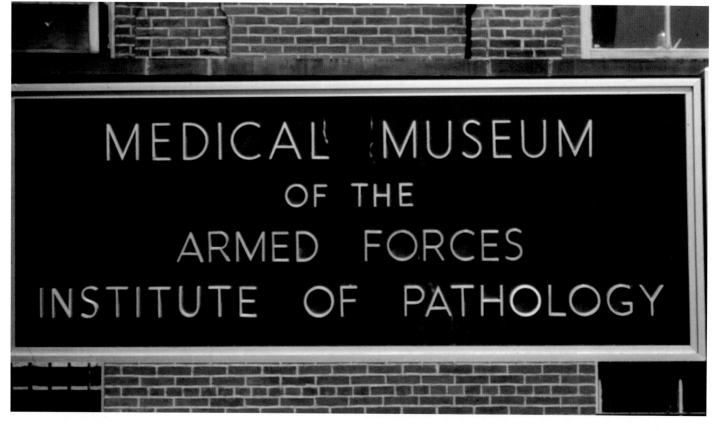

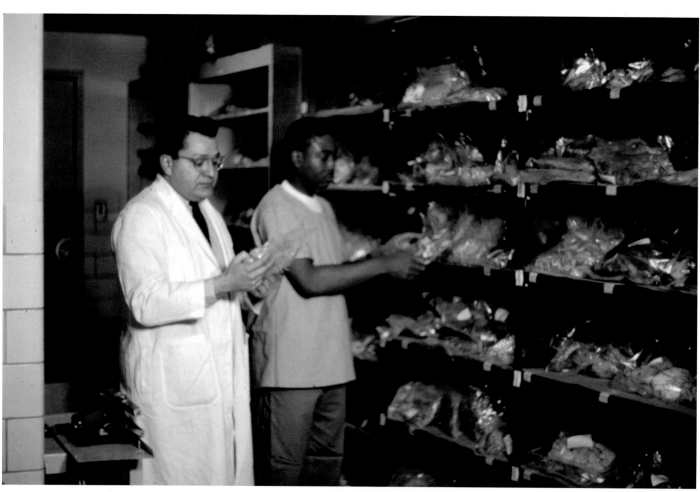

▲ Pathological specimens stored in the Armed Forces Institute of Pathology in the 1970s. As 1975 began, 1,502,688 cases had been accessioned with samples stored for research.
Source: Walter Reed Army Medical Center, Directorate of Public Works Archives

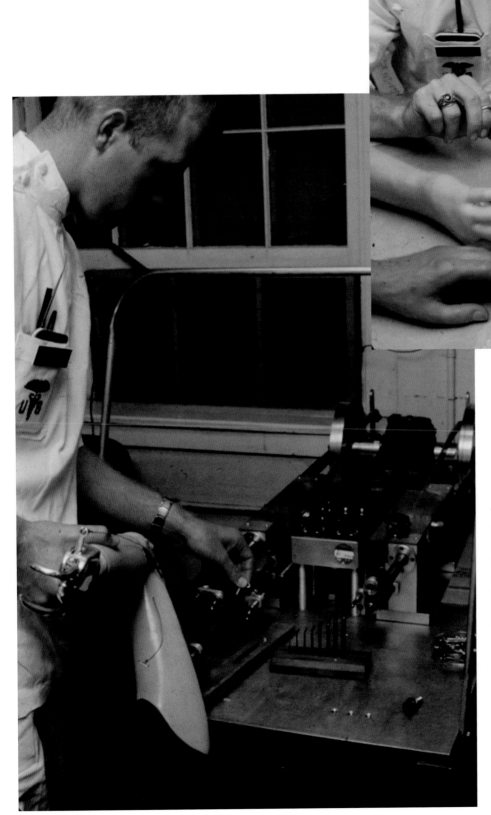

◄ Sign on the museum building at 7th and Independence Avenues, NW. The building was demolished in 1968, and the museum was moved to the WRAMC main campus.
Source: Walter Reed Army Medical Center, Directorate of Public Works Archives

Technician working on prosthetic arms and hands in the Army Prosthetic Research Lab at Forest Glen. Creating cosmetic hand covers (top). Attaching control cables to an upper extremity prosthetic (left).
Source: Walter Reed Army Medical Center, Directorate of Public Works Archives

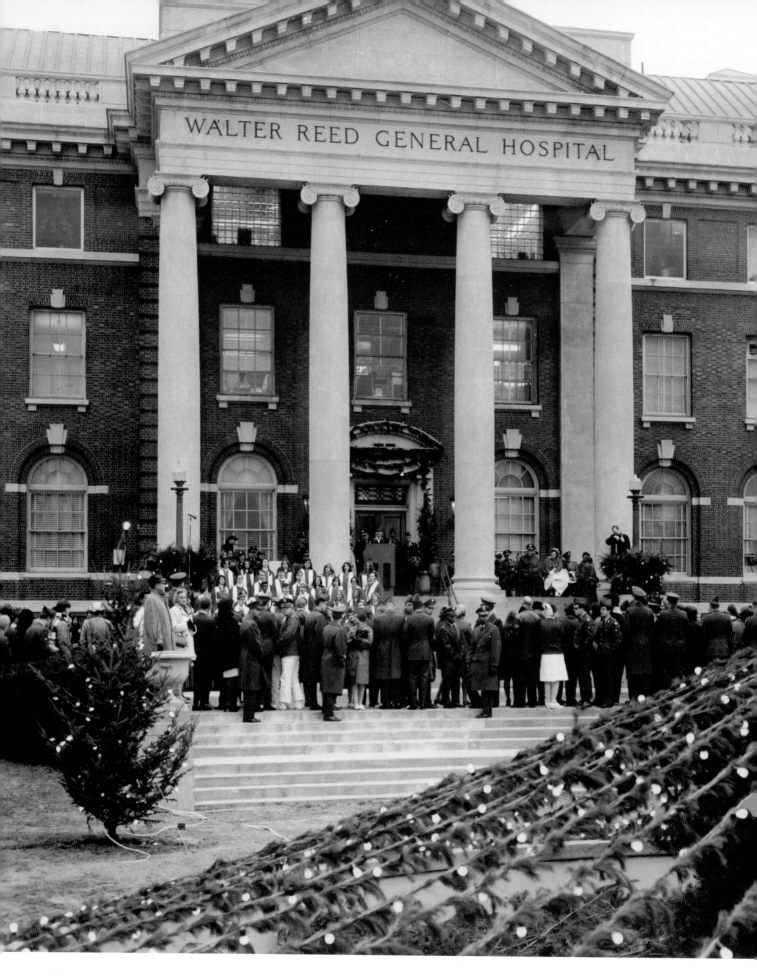

A Christmas choral concert on the front steps of the hospital.
Source: National Museum of Health and Medicine, AFIP, WRAMC History Collection

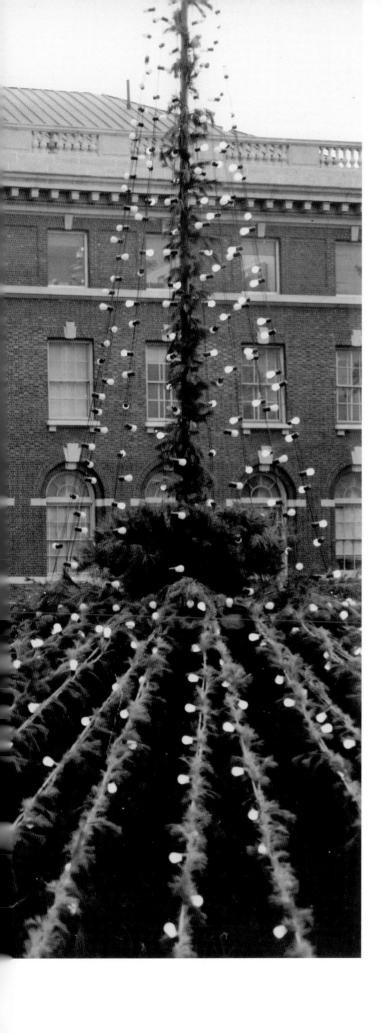

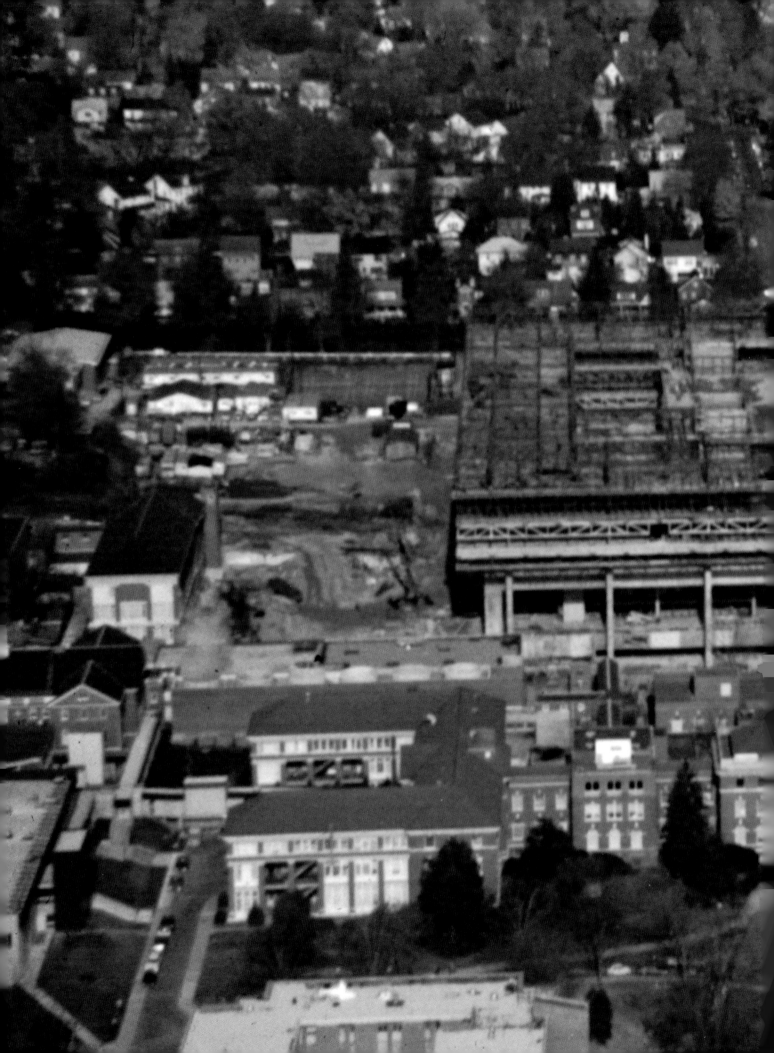

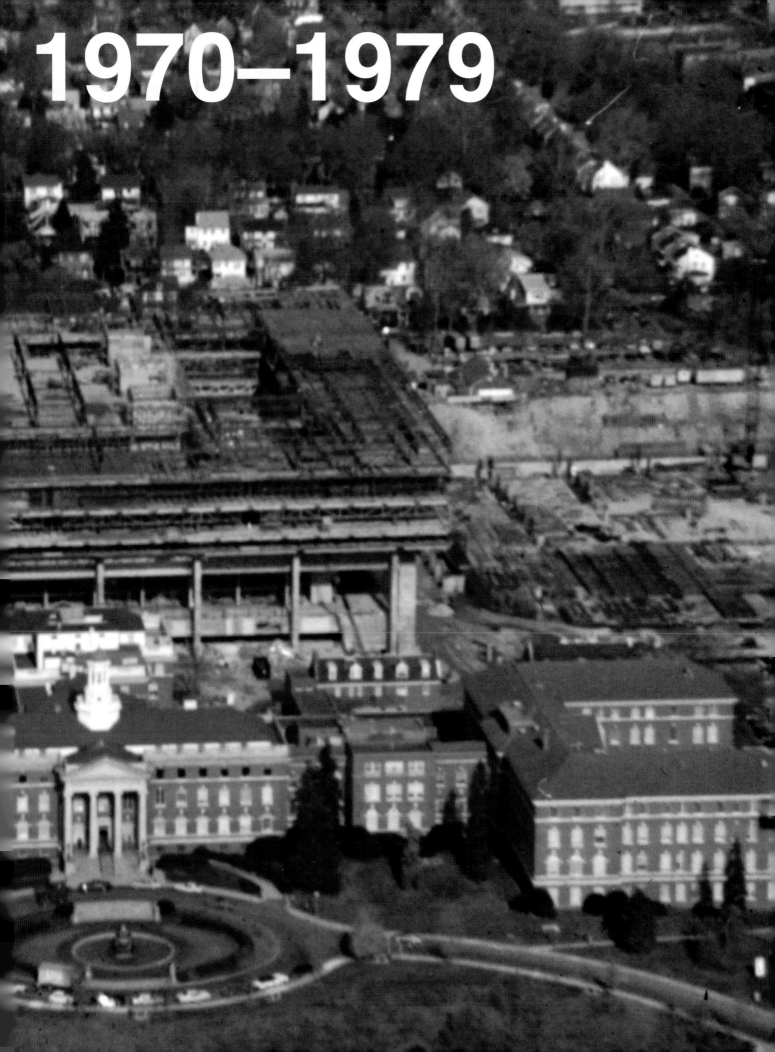

1970–1979

Title page - Looking north, this photograph demonstrates construction of the new clinical building well underway. The underground parking garage can be seen to the right of the main building and appears to be at about the fifth floor level. Construction would take 5 years and 1 month, from groundbreaking on August 26, 1972 until dedication on September 26, 1977.
Source: National Museum of Health and Medicine, AFIP, WRAMC History Collection

▶ Architect's model of the new hospital building, showing its relationship to the rest of the campus. The model resides in the National Museum of Health and Medicine.
Source: Walter Reed Army Medical Center, Directorate of Public Works Archives

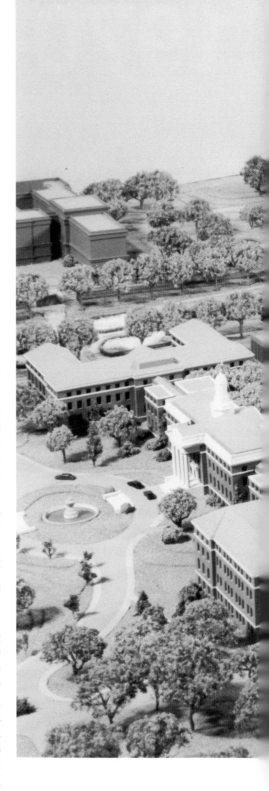

The events of this decade clearly focus on the construction and occupancy of the new clinical building, designated Building 2. In 1967 with the assistance of Senators Dirksen, Russell and Stennis, Army Surgeon General and former Walter Reed Commanding General Leonard D. Heaton procured funds from Congress to start planning for a new hospital facility. The construction of Building 2 changed the face of the entire medical center. In actuality, work had begun several years earlier when a new commissary and post-exchange complex were planned and construction begun at Forest Glen. These services were moved from Walter Reed's main campus to make room for the new hospital building. The motor pool, engineer shops and laundry were also moved to new facilities at Forest Glen. To provide for enlisted housing, Abrams Hall was constructed during the same time period and opened in 1975. Before ground was broken for the new hospital, two temporary buildings (T-2 and T-20) were built to house important facilities that could not be moved to Forest Glen. Thirty-five plus years later both these temporary buildings still remain in use. Under the supervision of the Baltimore District of the U.S. Army Corps of Engineers, the official groundbreaking ceremony took place on August 26, 1972. Those in attendance included Secretary of the Army, Robert Froehlke, the Deputy Chief of Staff for Personnel, Lt. General W. T. Kerwin, the Surgeon General,

Lt. General Hal B. Jennings and WRAMC Commander Maj. General William H. Moncrief.

Complete construction took over five years. During construction the amount of dirt that was moved would have completely filled and buried RKF Stadium. The trucks used to move the earth would have extended from Washington to 40 miles past New York City. The steel used to reinforce the 110,000 cubic yards of concrete used would have stretched from Washington to Denver. The completed building had 5500 rooms, 28 acres of floor space, 1280 patient beds and 16 operating rooms. Construction included an electrical generating plant capable of providing enough power for a city of 50,000 people and an underground garage for more than 1000 cars. There were over 800 workers on site each day and toward the end of construction when finishing work had to be completed on the inside, there were over 1200 workers each day. Unique features included an interstitial floor that included air conditioning, heating, electrical, plumbing and life support systems and was where 80% of the maintenance work would take place. The interstitial space also included a monorail track system that was to handle linen and medical supplies, as well as, a first in the industry patient food cart system. A separate tele-lift system was to carry administrative materials, laboratory samples, x-ray records and patient records. More than 1100 additional

civilian employees were hired to work in the new facility.

Special guest of honor for the dedication ceremony that took place on September 26, 1977 was Daisy Reed Royce, granddaughter of Maj. Walter Reed, the medical center's namesake. Also in attendance was former First Lady Mamie Eisenhower, Senator

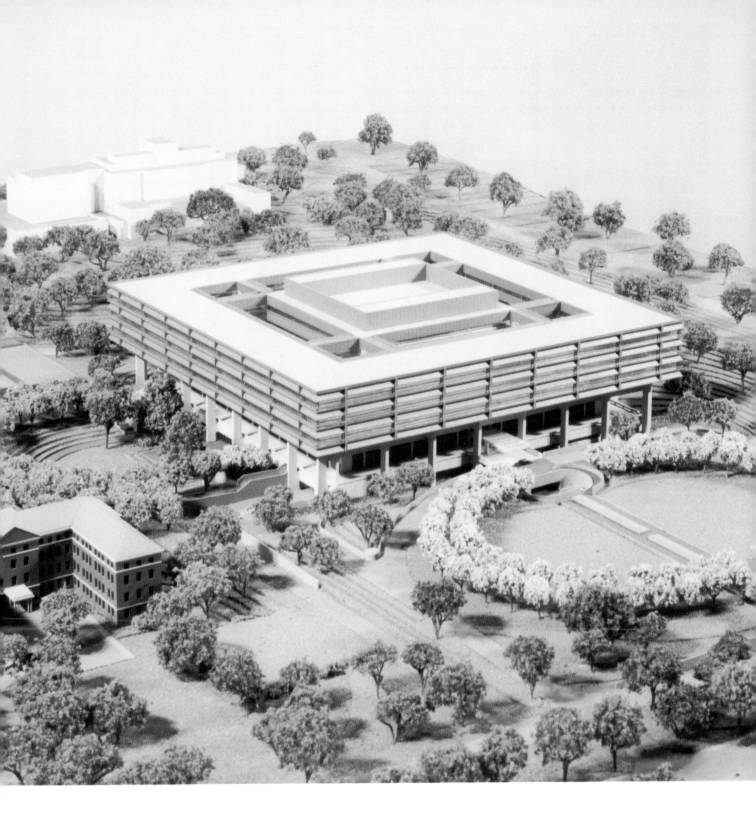

John Stennis, Secretary of the Army, Clifford Alexander, Army Chief of Staff, General Bernard Rogers, chief of the Corps of Engineers, Lt. General John Morris, the Surgeon General, Lt. General Richard Taylor and Walter Reed Commanding General, Maj. General Robert Bernstein. Moving into a building of this size did not happen overnight; the actual move took almost

a year during 1977-1978, mostly on the weekends. The continued functioning of the medical center during these years of construction and moving is truly a remarkable monument to the dedication and service of the soldiers and civilians of WRAMC.

Other construction also took place in the early 1970s with an addition to the

Armed Forces Institute of Pathology (AFIP) building. In contrast to the original AFIP building that was built without windows, this addition to the south elevation had numerous windows. Opened in 1972, in addition to offices and other space for AFIP it housed the National Museum of Health and Medicine, the former Army Medical Museum that dated back to 1862.

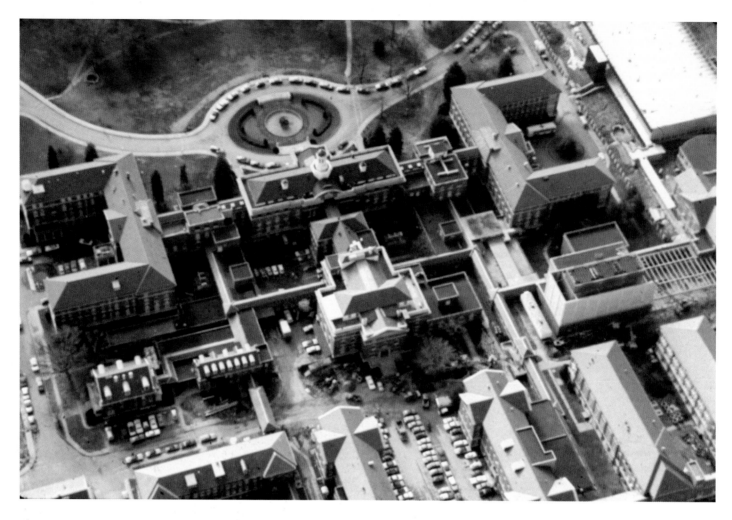

▲ Aerial view of old hospital facing south. The buildings at the bottom of the picture were demolished to make room for the new hospital.
Source: Walter Reed Army Medical Center, Directorate of Public Works Archives

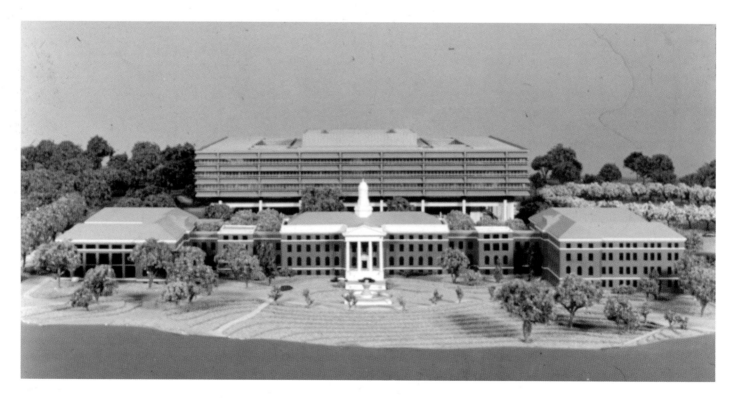

▲ Architect's model of the new hospital rising above the old.
Source: Walter Reed Army Medical Center, Directorate of Public Works Archives

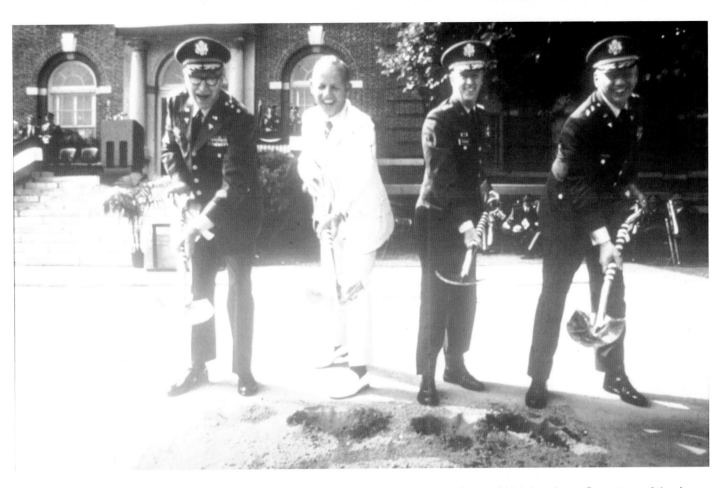

Groundbreaking ceremony for the new hospital. From left to right are: Surgeon General Hal Jennings; Secretary of the Army, Robert Froehlke; Lt. General W. T. Kerwin; and Maj. General William H. Moncrief, WRAMC Commander. August 26, 1972.
Sources: Walter Reed Army Medical Center, Directorate of Public Works Archives

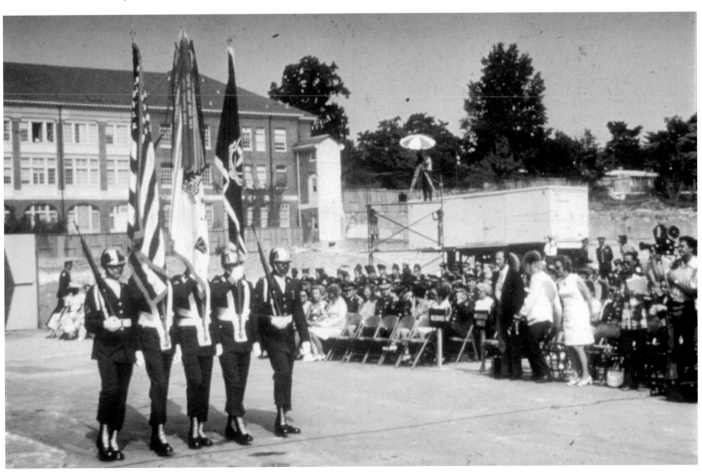

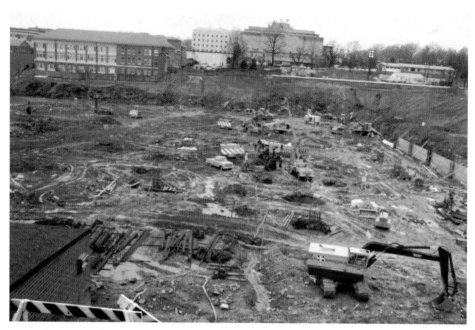

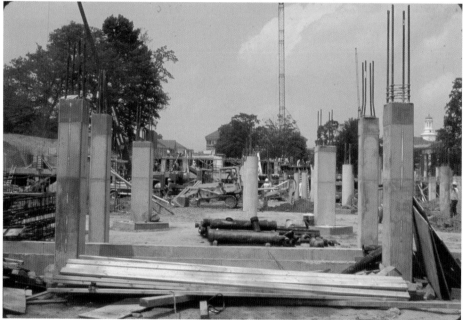

Various stages of construction of the new hospital, 1973–1976.
Sources: National Museum of Health and Medicine, WRAMC History Collection

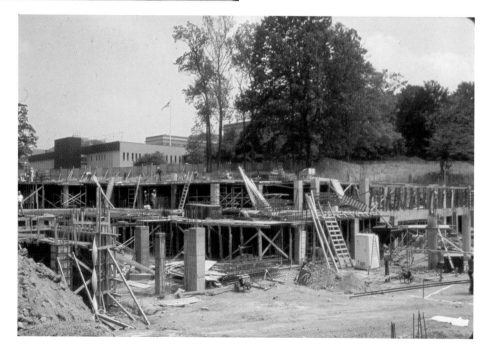

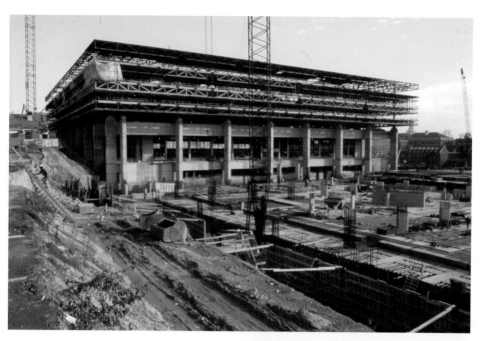

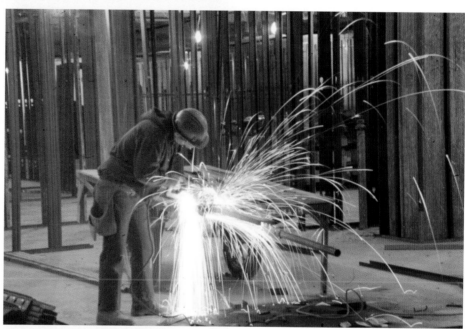

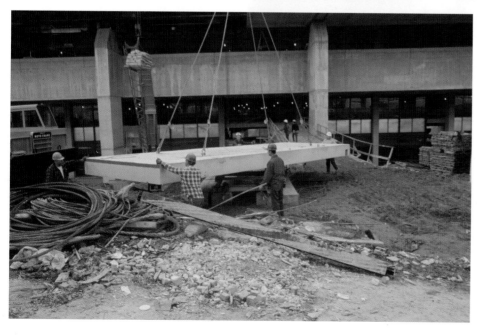

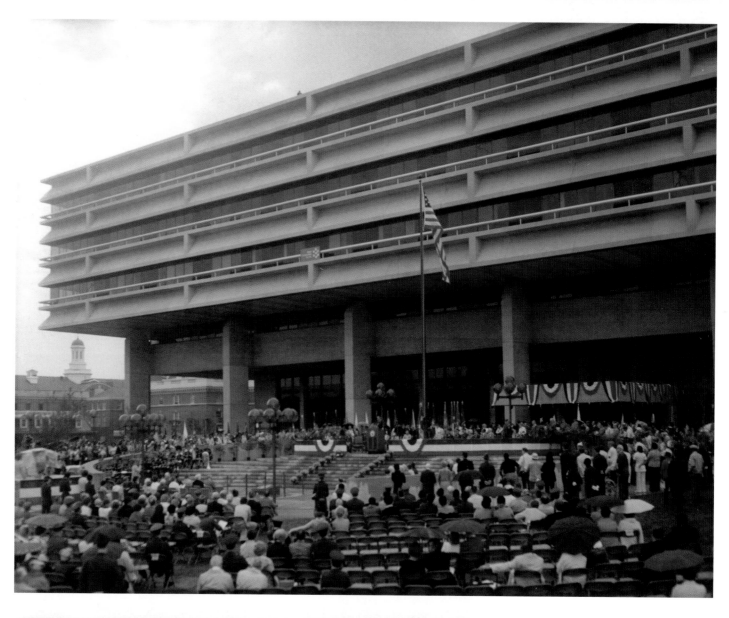

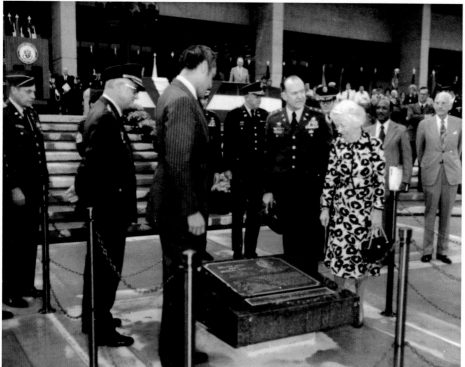

▲ Dedication and opening ceremonies for the new hospital building on September 26, 1977.
Source: National Museum of Health and Medicine, WRAMC History Collection

◄ Setting the dedication plaque of the hospital are Maj. General Robert Bernstein and Daisy Reed Royce, granddaughter of Maj. Walter Reed.
Source: National Museum of Health and Medicine, WRAMC History Collection

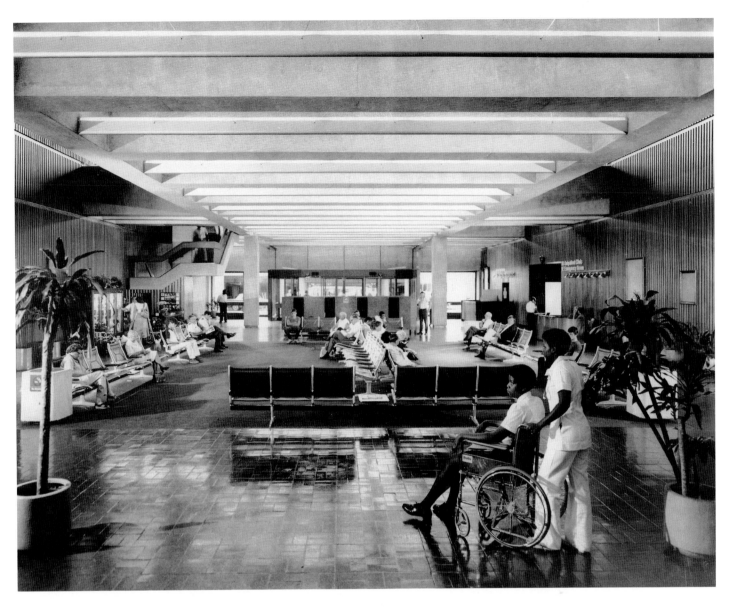

▲ The lower entrance lobby to the new hospital, with plenty of waiting area when it opened in 1978.
Source: National Museum of Health and Medicine, WRAMC History Collection

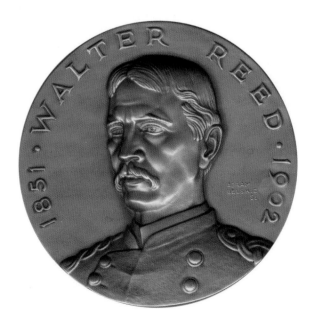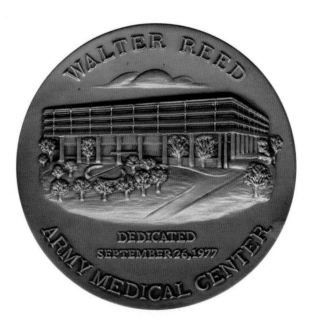

▲ A commemorative coin minted to celebrate the opening of the new hospital. Sept. 26, 1977.
Source: Pierce Collection

ABRAMS HALL

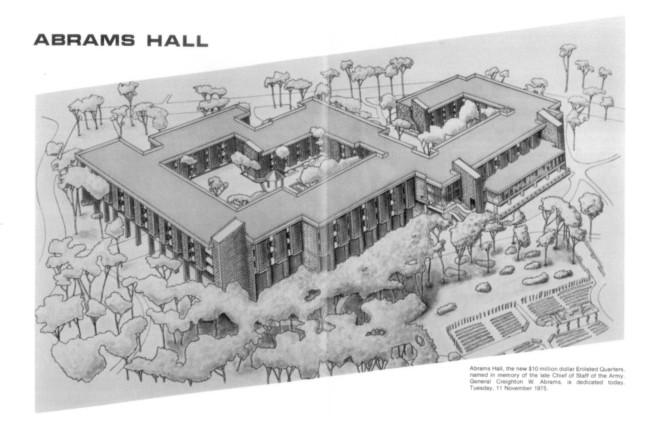

Abrams Hall, the new $10 million dollar Enlisted Quarters, named in memory of the late Chief of Staff of the Army, General Creighton W. Abrams, is dedicated today, Tuesday, 11 November 1975.

Architect's renderings of Abrams Hall.
Sources: Pierce Collection

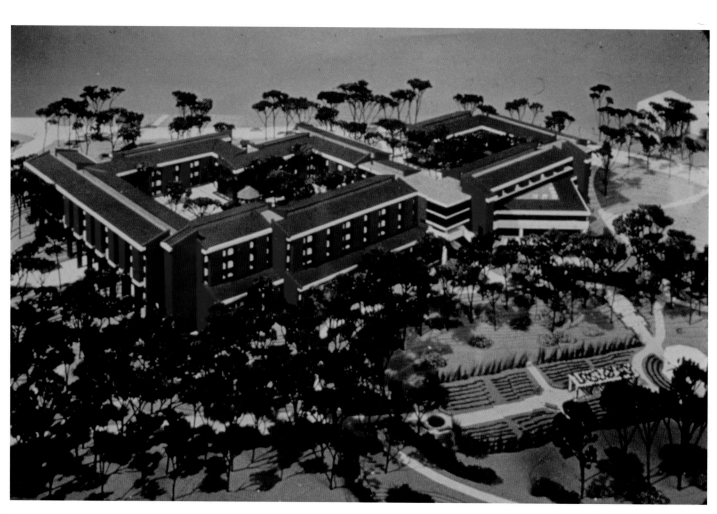

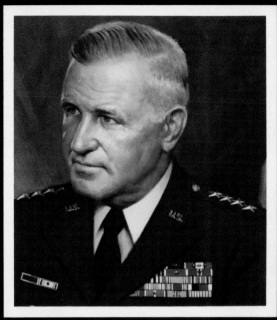

11 NOVEMBER 1975

GENERAL CREIGHTON W. ABRAMS

ABRAMS HALL DEDICATION

WALTER REED ARMY MEDICAL CENTER
WASHINGTON, D.C. 20012

◀ Cover of the program for the Abrams Hall dedication. Abrams Hall was dedicated in 1975 as the primary residence for single enlisted men and women. It was named in honor of General Creighton W. Abrams, Army Chief of Staff from 1972 until his death in 1974 at the hospital. Mrs. Abrams attended the ceremony and unveiled the plaque officially naming and opening the building.
Source: Pierce Collection

▼ Abrams Hall was dedicated in 1975. It was designed to be the primary residence for single enlisted men and women. This photograph is circa 1985, when the building had been in use for a decade.
Source: National Museum of Health and Medicine, AFIP, WRAMC History Collection

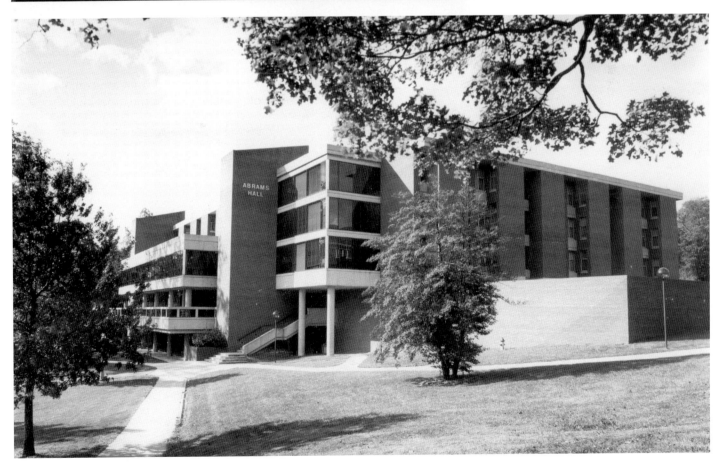

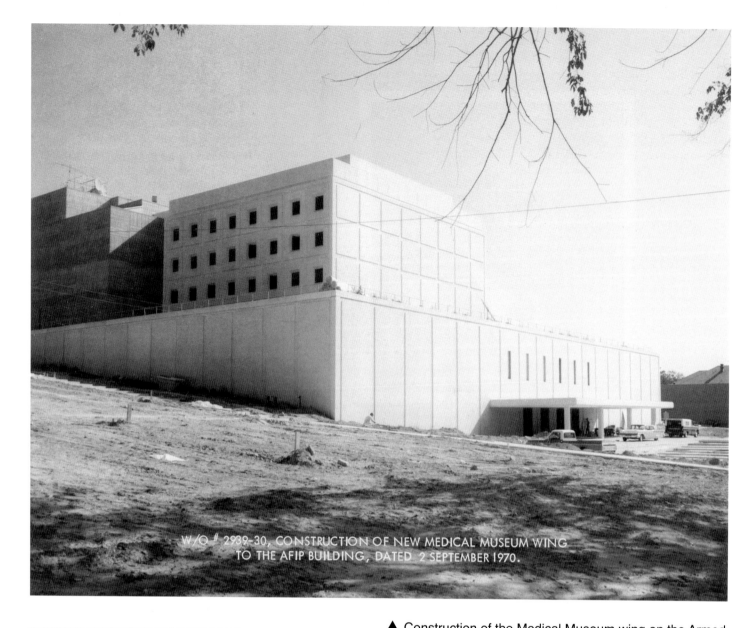

W/O # 2939-30, CONSTRUCTION OF NEW MEDICAL MUSEUM WING TO THE AFIP BUILDING, DATED 2 SEPTEMBER 1970.

▲ Construction of the Medical Museum wing on the Armed Forces Institute of Pathology's A-bomb-proof building.
Source: National Museum of Health and Medicine, AFIP Files, Rededication of Museum Folder 1971

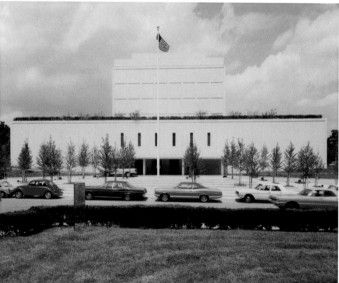

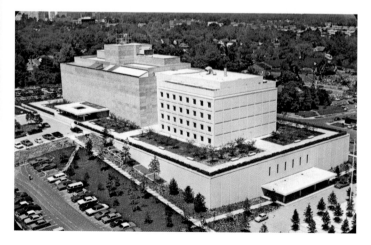

▶ Postcard showing the Armed Forces Institute of Pathology and its new Medical Museum wing.
Source: National Museum of Health and Medicine, AFIP Files, Rededication of Museum Folder 1971

In 1971, the Medical Museum of the Armed Forces Institute of Pathology, founded in 1862 during the Civil War as the Army Medical Museum, opened on the WRAMC campus. The Museum was displaced from the National Mall, its home since 1887, by the Hirschhorn Museum. Once at WRAMC, it stayed open for three years, and then its space was used by the Uniformed Services University of the Health Sciences until 1976.

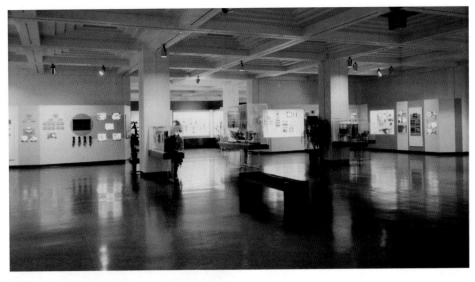

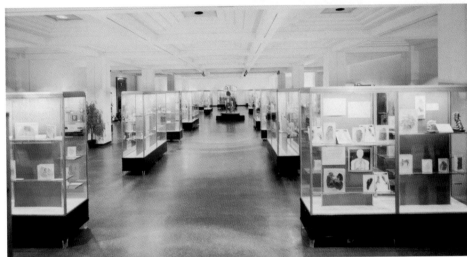

Exhibit space inside the National Museum of Health and Medicine. First, looking right, historical transportation models, a Vietnam War exhibit with an AK-47 and punji sticks, and the history of the microscope. Second, looking left, pathology and anatomy of the human body. Third picture, center of museum showing history of museum exhibit, including one at Walter Reed.
Source: National Museum of Health and Medicine, AFIP, WRAMC History Collection, AFIP Files, Rededication of Museum Folder 1971

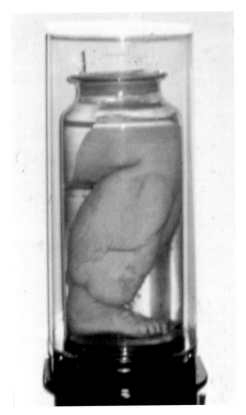

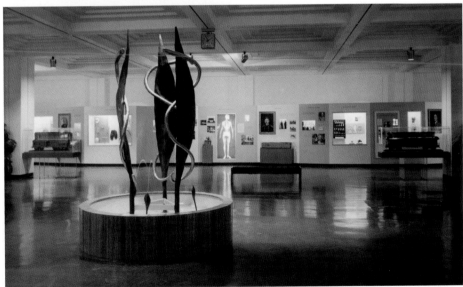

◀ Part of the filariasis exhibit at the museum, 1972.
Source: National Museum of Health and Medicine, AFIP, NCP 2484

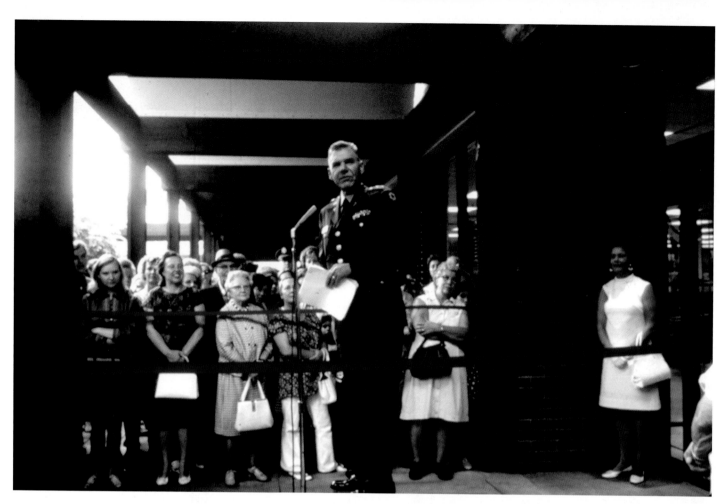

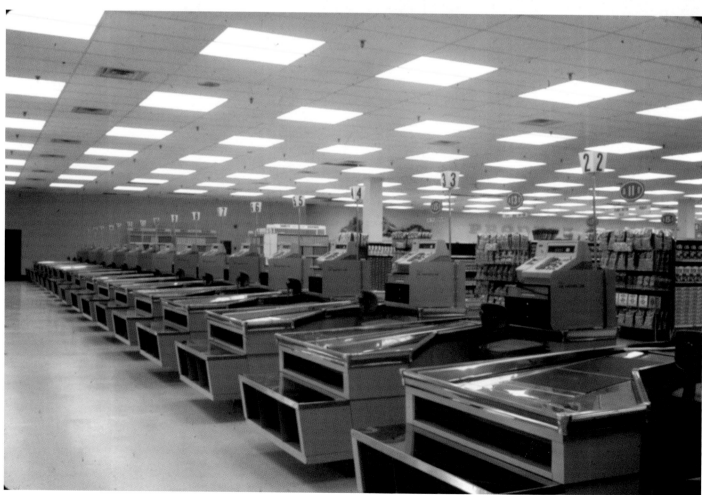

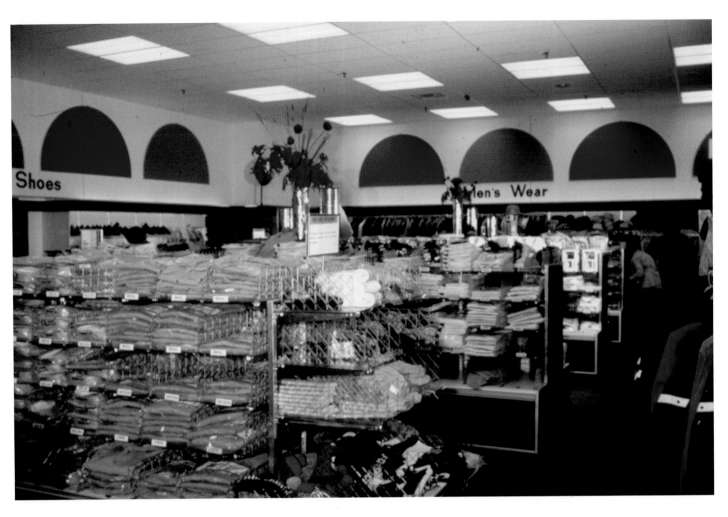

The ceremonial opening of a new shopping center in the Walter Reed Annex at Forest Glen. August 1971.
Source: Walter Reed Army Medical Center, Directorate of Public Works Archives

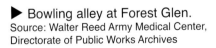 Bowling alley at Forest Glen.
Source: Walter Reed Army Medical Center,
Directorate of Public Works Archives

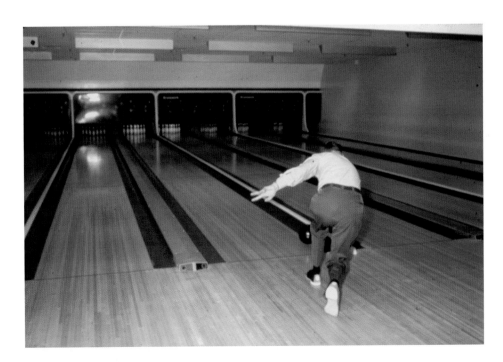

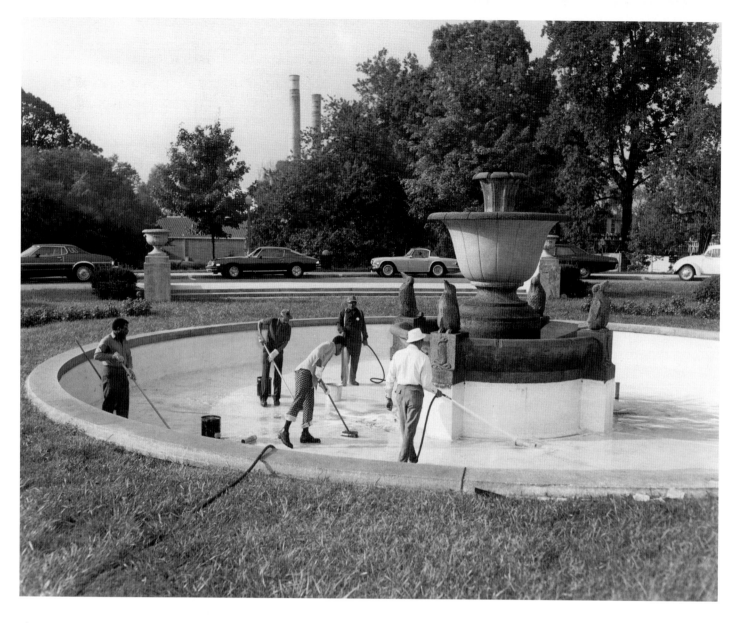

▲ The Hoff Memorial Fountain gets a good cleaning. The penguins were replaced in the 1990s with plastic replicas.
Source: National Museum of Health and Medicine, WRAMC History Collection

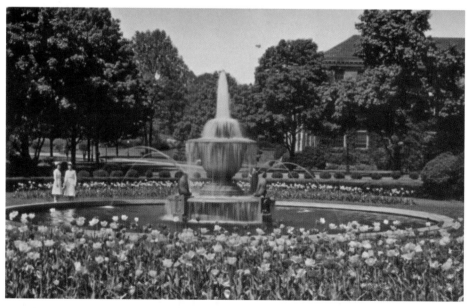

◄ This postcard reads: "Hoff Memorial Fountain, erected in 1935, located at the main entrance to the Administration Building. Walter Reed General Hospital, Army Medical Center, Washington, D.C. Erected in memory of Col. John Van Rensselaer Hoff, MC, U.S.A., famous military surgeon who died in 1920. The fountain is surrounded by tulips of many varieties donated by people of the Netherlands following World War II."
Source: Pierce Collection

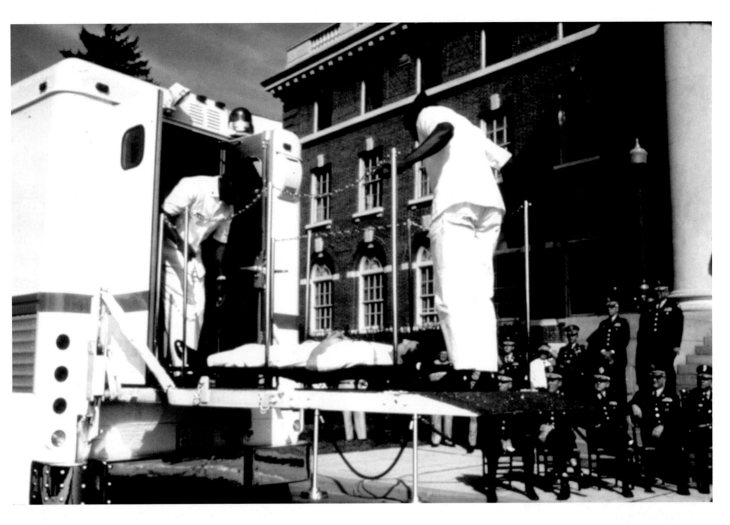

Demonstration of ambulances at the hospital.
Sources: Walter Reed Army Medical Center, Directorate of Public Works Archives

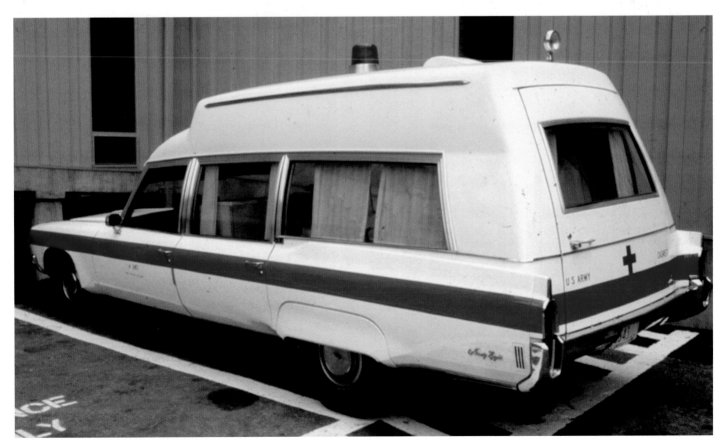

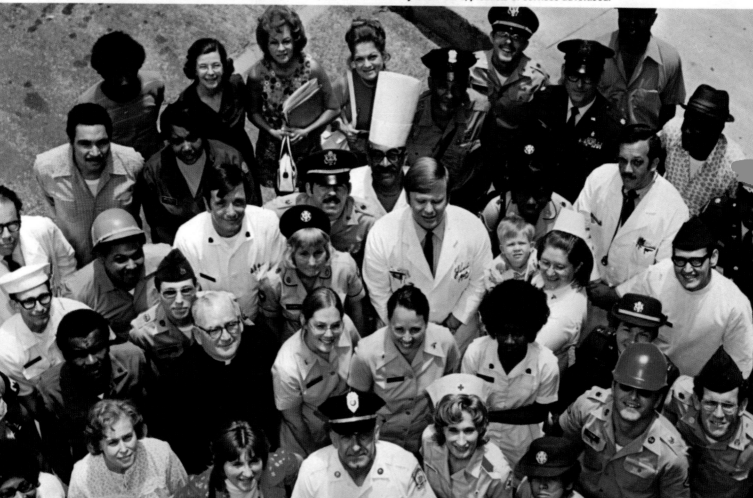

WALTER REED ARMY MEDICAL CENTER

Front cover of the Walter Reed Army Medical Center guidebook, 1979. To the right of the photo, the physician with the stethoscope around his neck is Ronald Blanck. Dr. Blanck would serve as WRAMC Commander from 1992 to 1996 and as Army Surgeon General from 1996 to 2000.
Source: Pierce Collection

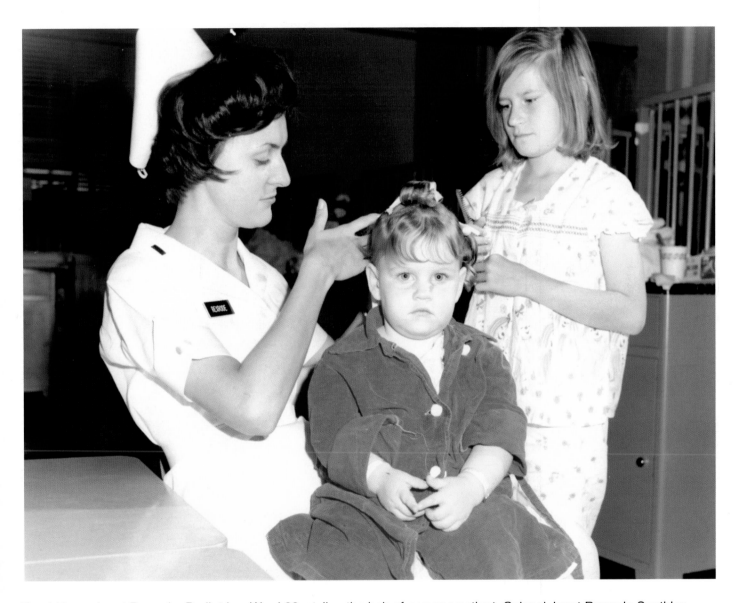

Head Nurse Janet Rexrode, Pediatrics, Ward 22, styling the hair of a young patient. Colonel Janet Rexrode Southby would return to Walter Reed and serve as Chief, Department of Nursing. She has served as President of the Walter Reed Society from 2001 to the present.
Source: Walter Reed Army Medical Center, Directorate of Public Works Archives

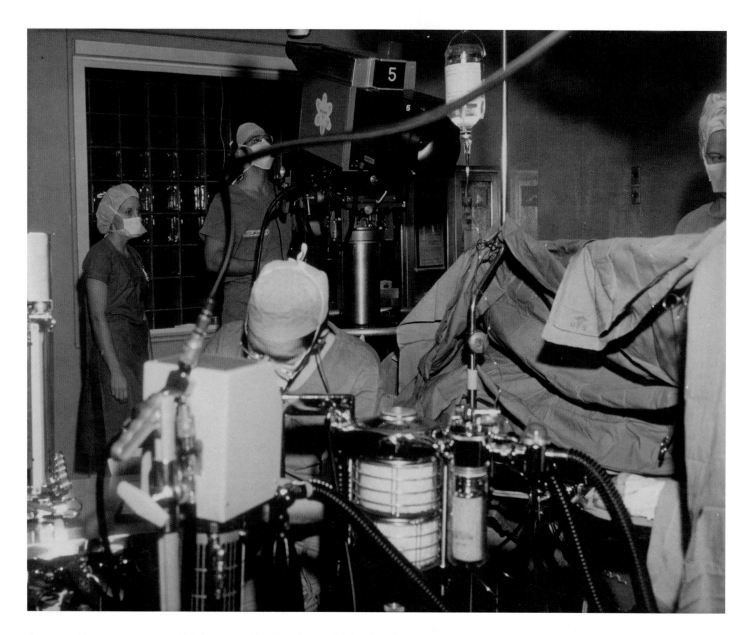

An operating room nurse clinician coordinating the activities involved with the production of an instructional television program, 1973.
Source: National Museum of Health and Medicine, AFIP, NCP 1737

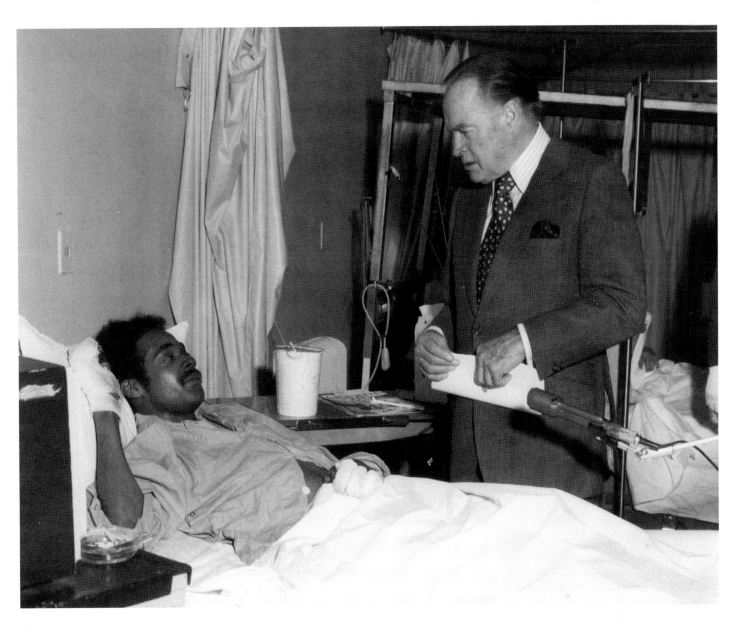

▲ Bob Hope appeared at Walter Reed Army Medical Center on December 30, 1973, with a mini-troop of entertainers to make the holiday season a little more enjoyable for the patients and staff at WRAMC. Hope's troop of entertainers consisted of Betty Joe Grove, Miss Maryland; Priscilla Barnes, Miss San Diego; and Lynda Carter, Miss World—USA 1972. Hope played to a standing-room-only crowd in the Main Post Theatre and then visited Ward 24 before making his trip back to California. (Original caption)
Source: Walter Reed Army Medical Center, Directorate of Public Works Archives

▶ Army Chief of Staff General William Westmoreland visits with a patient at Walter Reed Hospital on Thanksgiving Day, 1970.
Source: WRAMC History Office, PAO Historical Collection

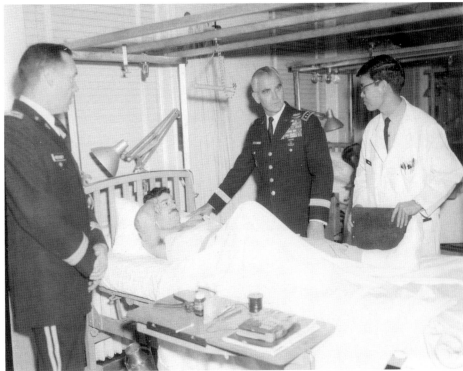

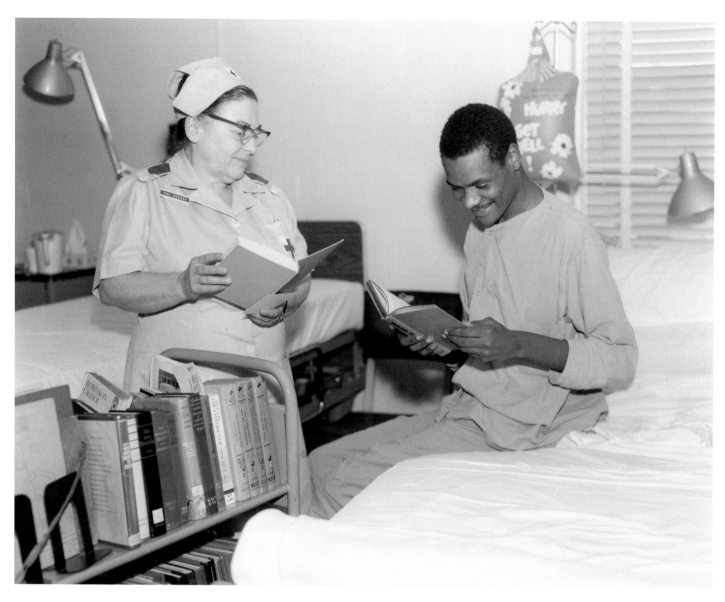

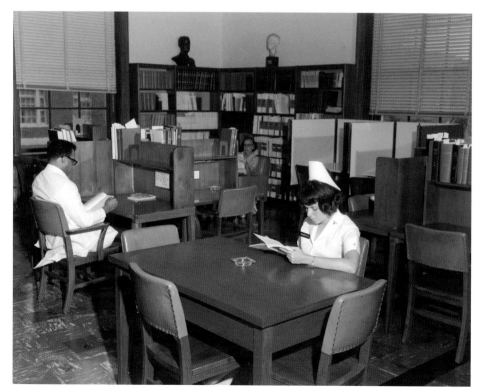

▲ Mrs. Arthur Berger, Red Cross Volunteer at Walter Reed General Hospital, shows a book from the library cart to SSG James L. Broyles (Holly Grove, Ark.) a patient on Ward 28. The cart is taken to the wards by the volunteers for the patients who are unable to utilize the main library facilities. Signal Corp photo by SSG Larry Sullivan. (Original caption)
Source: National Musuem of Health and Medicine, WRAMC History Collection

◄ A section of the Medical Library, Walter Reed General Hospital. The Medical Library is operated as a section of the Main Library of the hospital. Signal Corps photo by SSG Larry Sullivan. (Original caption)
Source: National Museum of Health and Medicine, WRAMC History Collection

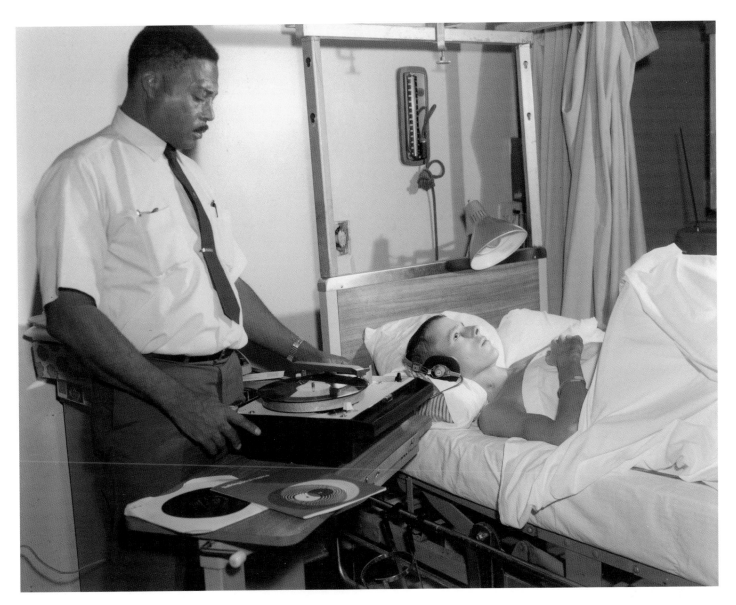

▲ Mr. Charles L. Johnson, Civilian Librarian Aide, at Walter Reed General Hospital plays one of the talking books from the library for SGT Larry J. Whitt (Hunt, WV), a patient on Ward 35. The talking books are provided by the library to be used by patients who are blind or unable to read for other reasons. Signal Corps photo by SSG Larry Sullivan. (Adapted from original caption)
Source: National Museum of Health and Medicine, WRAMC History Collection

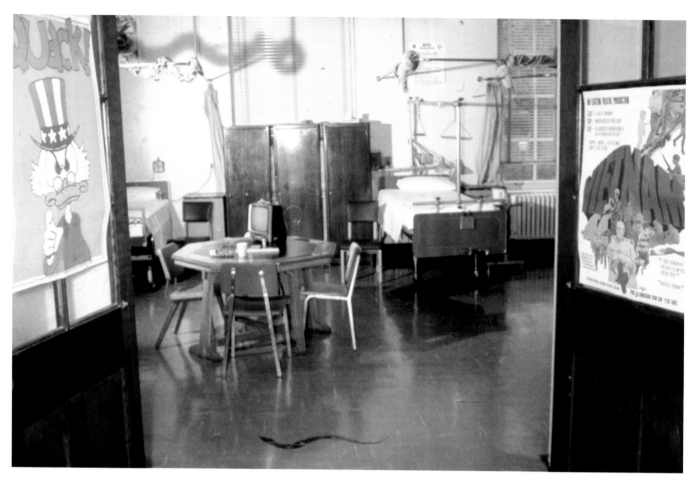

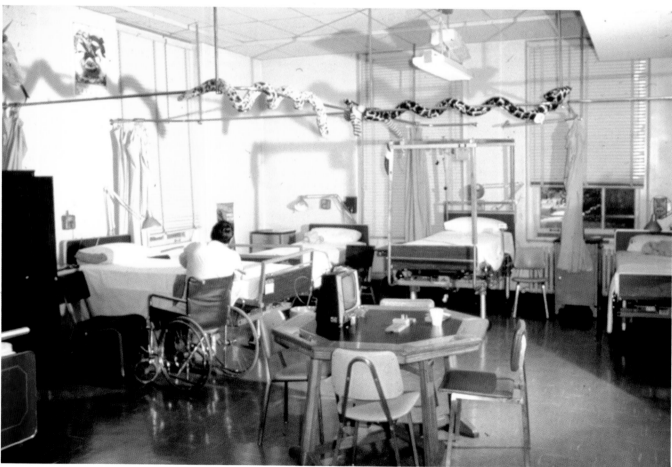

Ward 1, the male officers' Orthopaedic Ward, was known as the "snake pit" during the Vietnam War.
Sources: Walter Reed Army Medical Center, Directorate of Public Works Archives

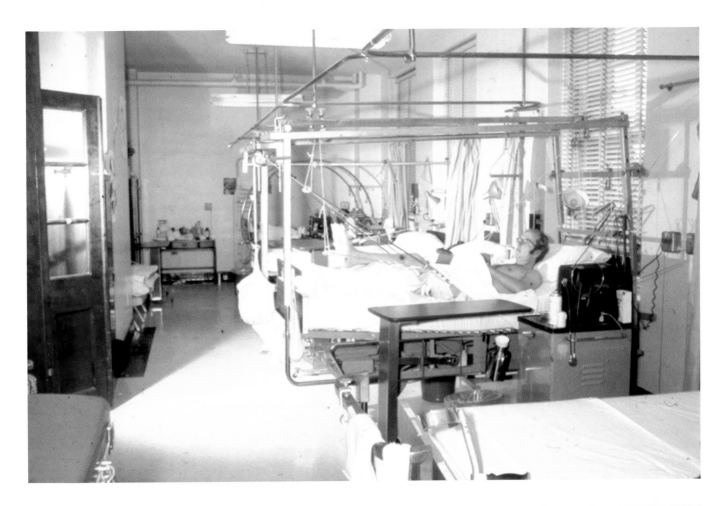

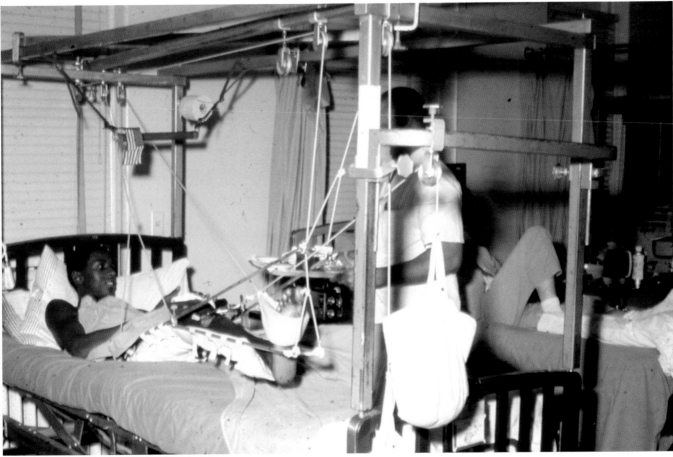

Patients in orthopaedic beds with traction for fracture management.
Sources: Walter Reed Army Medical Center, Directorate of Public Works Archives

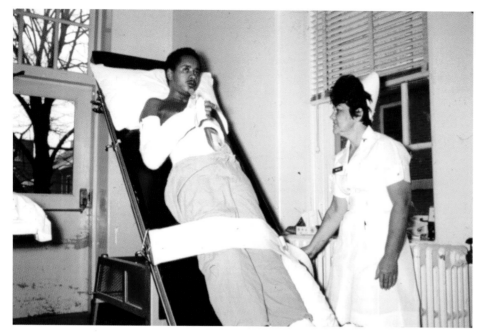

◀ Tilt-table therapy for return to ambulation following bed rest.
Source: Walter Reed Army Medical Center, Directorate of Public Works Archives

▼ Building an upper extremity prosthesis in the hospital prosthetic shop.
Source: Walter Reed Army Medical Center, Directorate of Public Works Archives

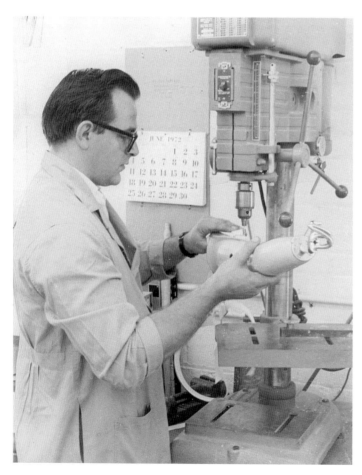

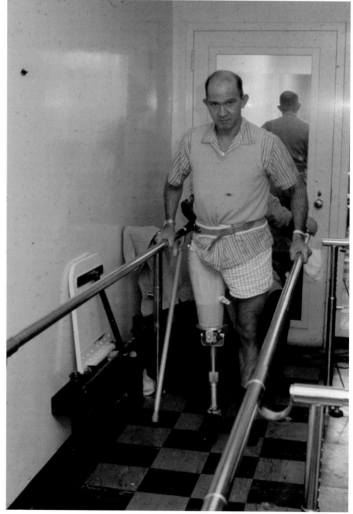

▲ Evaluation of test socket for above-knee amputee.
Source: Walter Reed Army Medical Center, Directorate of Public Works Archives

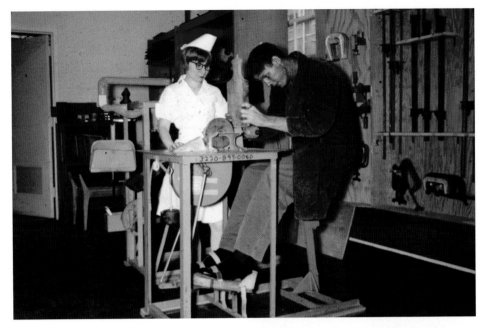

Some forms of occupational therapy are constant. Here, a patient is working on a power wheel just as his predecessors did in earlier decades. Other activities designed to strengthen muscles and improve coordination were performed in the occupational therapy clinic (below).
Sources: Walter Reed Army Medical Center, Directorate of Public Works Archives

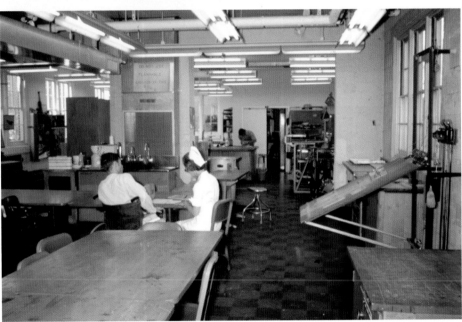

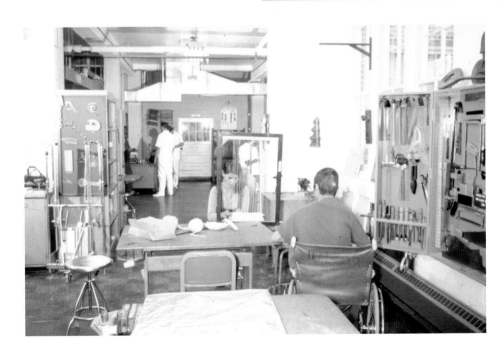

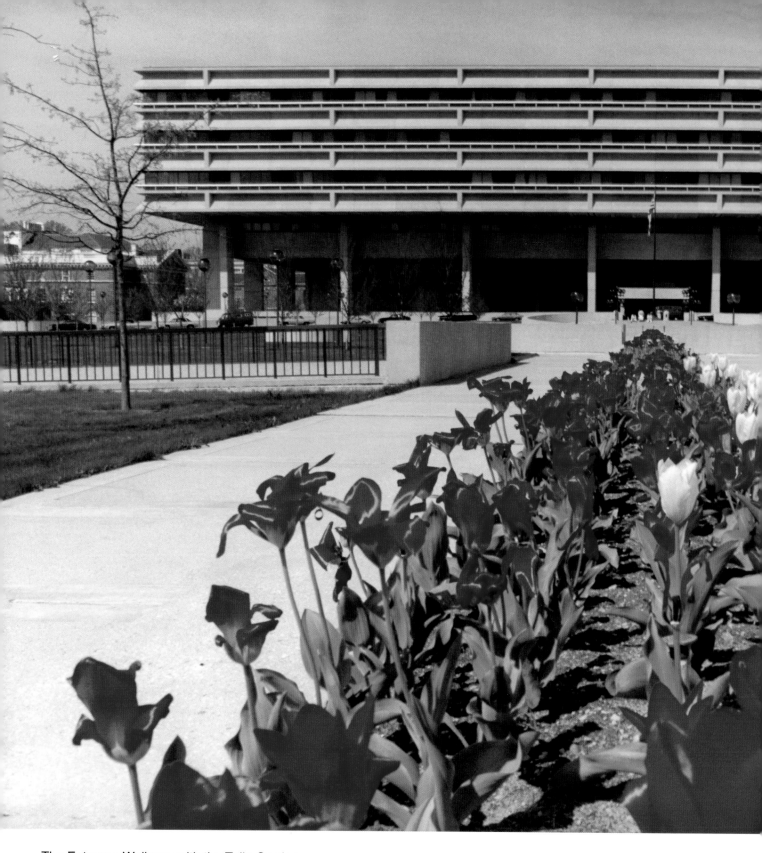

The Entrance Walkway with the Tulip Garden.
Source: WRAMC, History Collection

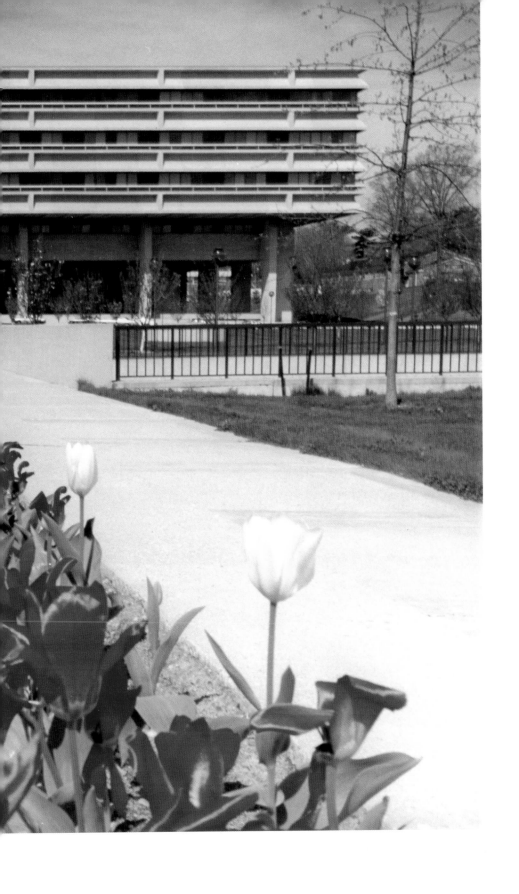

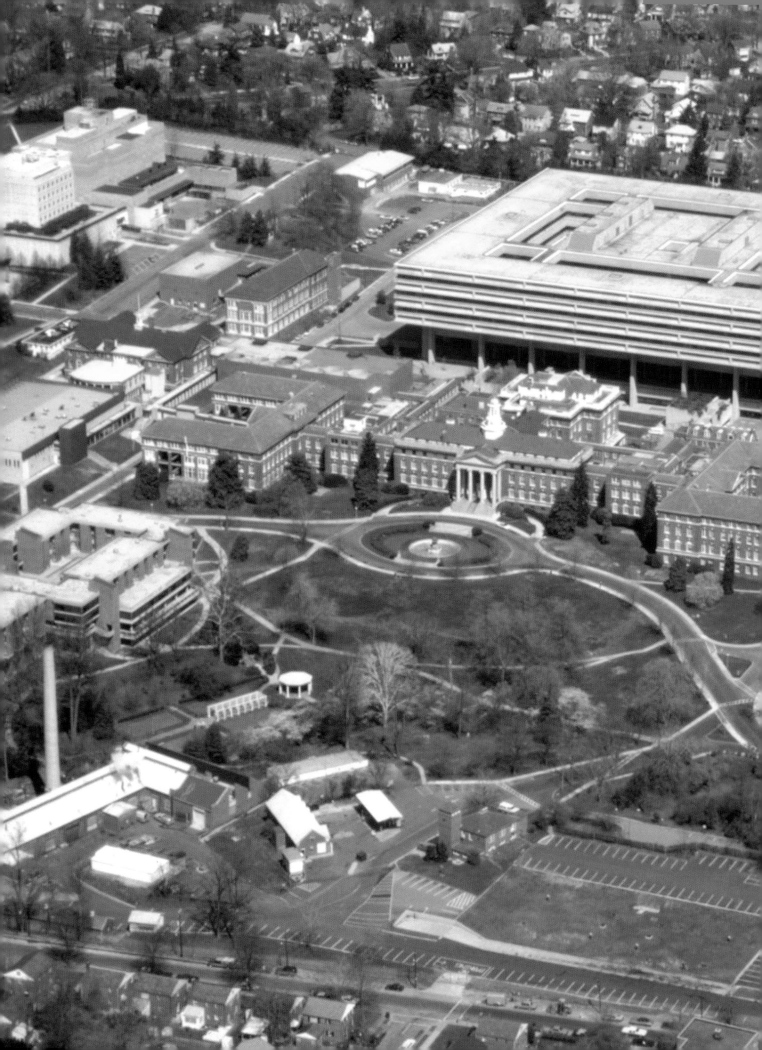

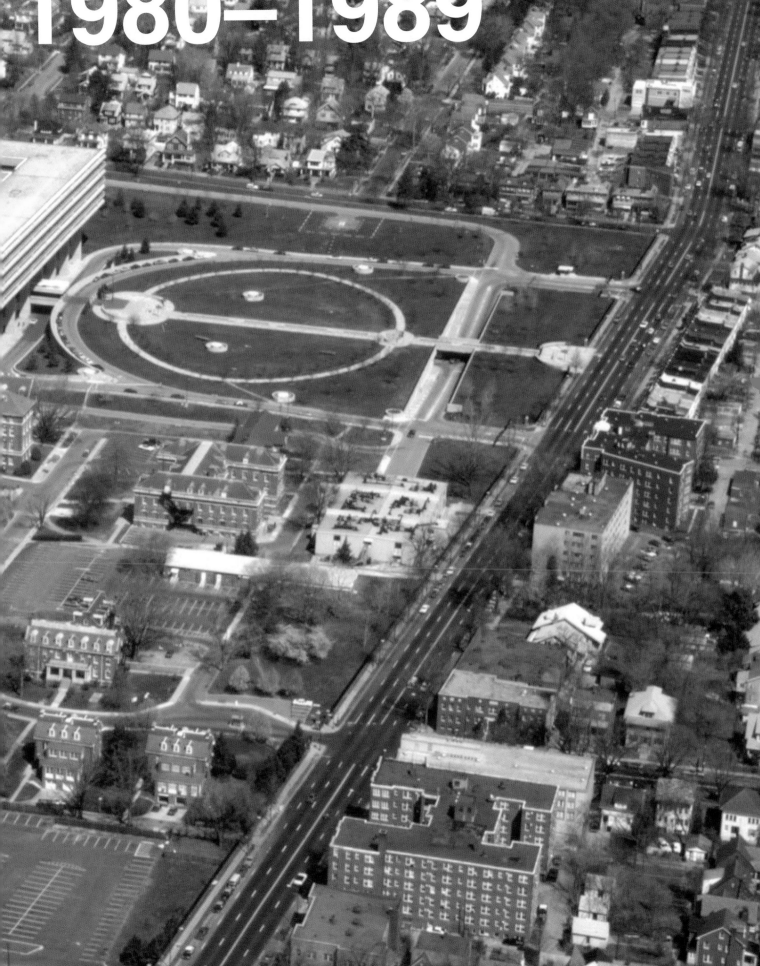

1980–1989

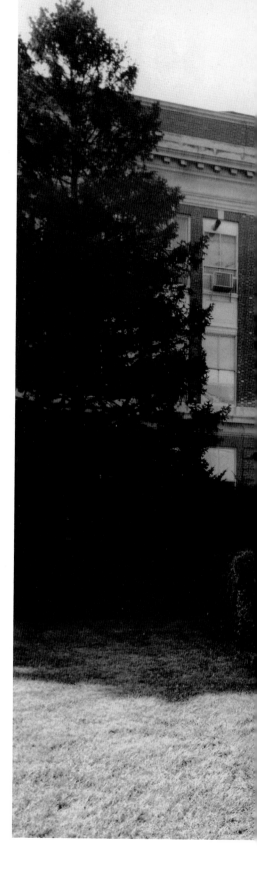

▶ WRAIR Building circa 1985. The North or "Vedder Pavilion" is named for Col. Edward Bright Vedder (1878–1952), one of the Army's leading experts on tropical medicine. He established rice bran extract as a treatment for beriberi.
Source: National Museum of Health and Medicine, AFIP, WRAMC History Collection

With the gleaming new clinical building into which all clinical care was being consolidated, the decade of the 1980s was one of settling into the new structure and providing improved and expanded clinical services. The number of physicians in graduate medical education was growing as more subspecialty clinical services were offered and more fellowships were established in medicine, surgery, pediatrics, obstetrics, gynecology, psychiatry, radiology, pathology, and almost every other field of medical care. Even with the enormous size of the new building, the growing clinical services did cause some space as well as parking issues on campus.

Despite the relative calm of the 1980s, the end of the decade brought very real sadness to the WRAMC family. The deaths of two successive WRAMC commanders within 7 months shocked the soldiers and civilians of the command and of the Army Medical Department. Maj. General Lewis A. Mologne was 56 when he died from complications of liver cancer on August 22, 1988. Dr. Mologne graduated in 1954 from the United States Military Academy at West Point where he had lettered in football and lacrosse as well as won the brigade championship in intramural boxing. He served in the Corps of Engineers before going to medical school. He trained in general surgery at Walter Reed and was renowned for his long

working hours. Prior to coming to Walter Reed he commanded the Army Medical Command in South Korea. He was the first West Pointer to become a General Officer in the Medical Corps. He commanded Walter Reed from June 1983 until just weeks before his death.

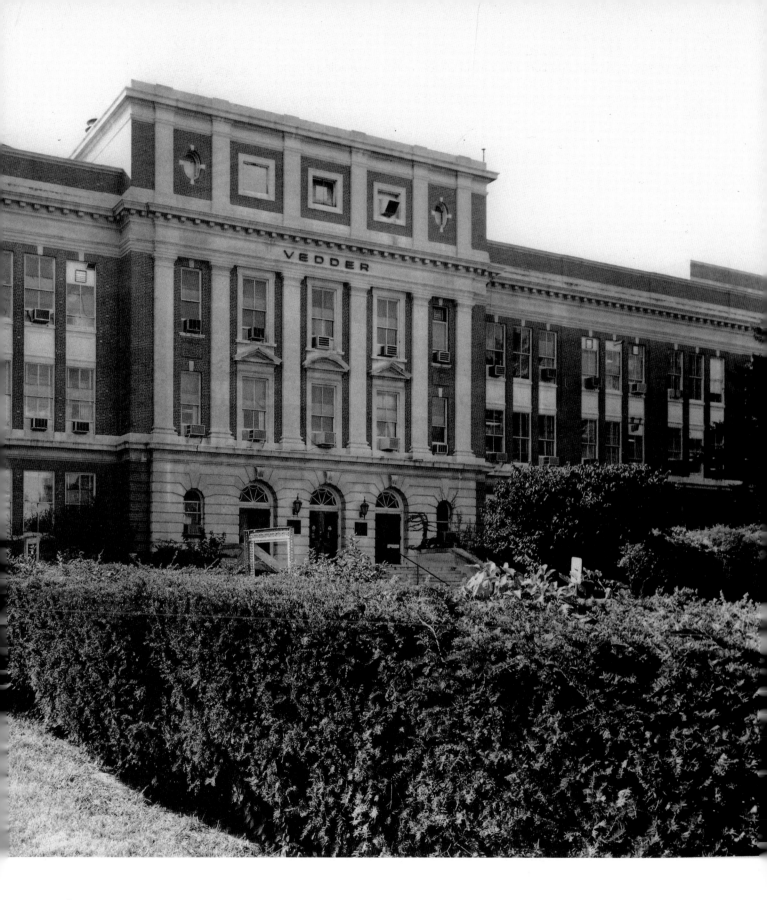

More shocking, as it was completely unexpected, was the death on March 8, 1989, of Maj. General James H. Rumbaugh from injuries sustained in a parachute jump with a surgical team as part of the annual Ahuas Tara 89 exercise in Honduras. Maj.

General Rumbaugh died during air evacuation. He was 49 years old. Dr. Rumbaugh had served his internship and a residency in psychiatry at Walter Reed. He served in Vietnam with the 1st Air Cavalry Division and later had a variety of psychiatry assignments.

He also served as surgeon for the XVIII Airborne Corps at Fort Bragg, NC, home of the 82nd Airborne Division. He had assumed command of Walter Reed in August 1988 following the retirement of General Mologne, and just 7 months before his own death.

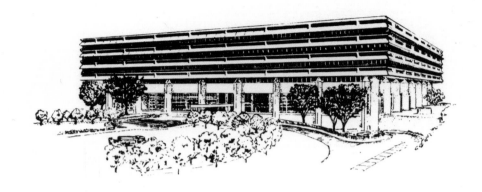

MEMORIALIZATION CEREMONY
DWIGHT D EISENHOWER EXECUTIVE
NURSING SUITE

THURSDAY, 10 JULY, 1980
1030 HOURS

WALTER REED ARMY MEDICAL CENTER
WASHINGTON, DC 20012

Program of the Memorialization Ceremony for the Eisenhower Executive Nursing Suite. The 6-bed suite, also known as Ward 72, serves VIP patients, including heads of state and foreign dignitaries, in a private and secure area of the hospital.
Source: WRAMC History Office, PAO Historical Collection

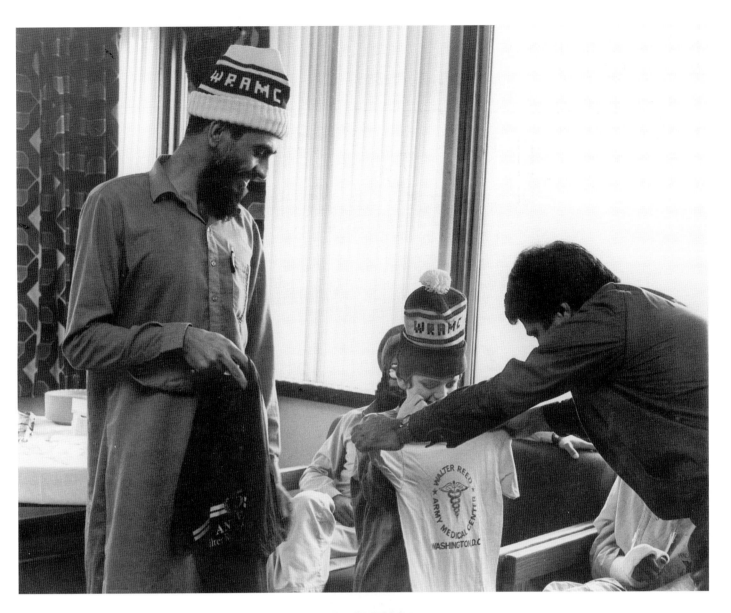

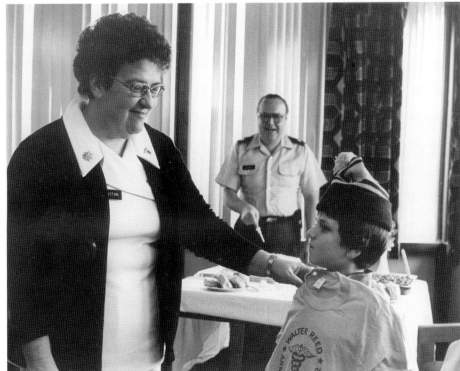

Doctors at WRAMC treated a group of Afghan freedom fighters in 1984, including a 10-year-old boy. They were transported to WRAMC on a mercy flight coordinated by Americares, a charitable organization based in New Canaan, CT.
Source: WRAMC History Office, PAO Historical Collection

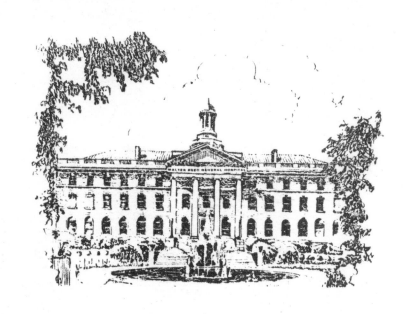

80th
ANNIVERSARY
WALTER REED
ARMY MEDICAL CENTER
1909-1989

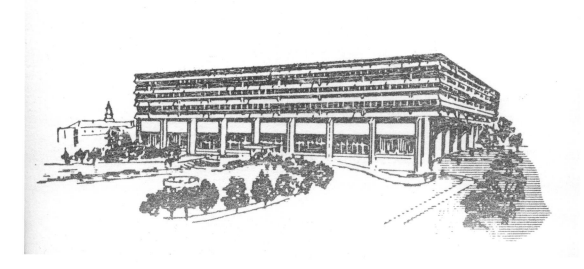

In 1989, Walter Reed Army Medical Center celebrated its 80th anniversary.
Source: National Museum of Health and Medicine, AFIP, WRAMC History Collection

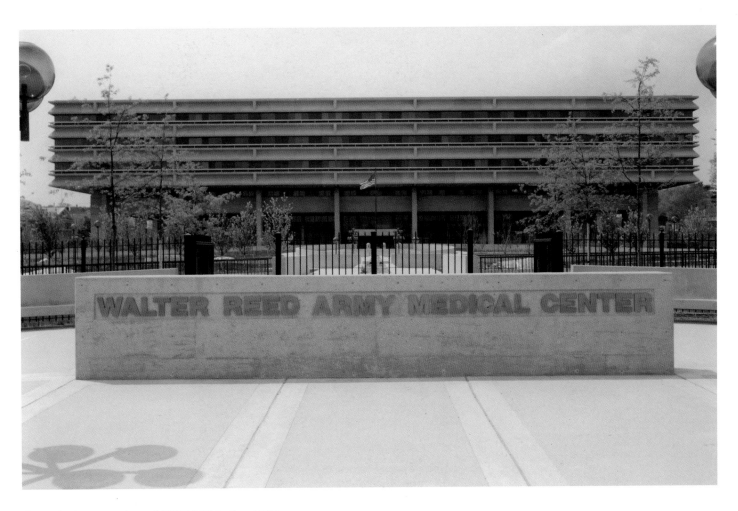

Georgia Avenue view of WRAMC in the 1980s.
Source: WRAMC History Office, PAO Historical Collection

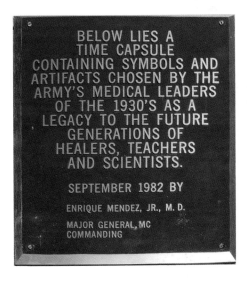

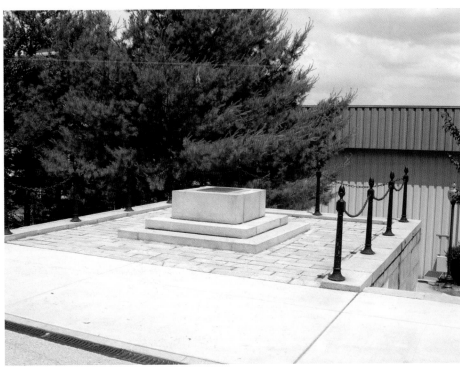

A time capsule replaced the flagpole on the east front of Building 40 when the flagpole was moved to the front of the new hospital (Building 2). The capsule, containing medical items from the 1930s, was dedicated in September 1982 by Maj. General Enrique Mendez. Building T2 stands in the background.
Source: WRAMC History Office, PAO Historical Collection

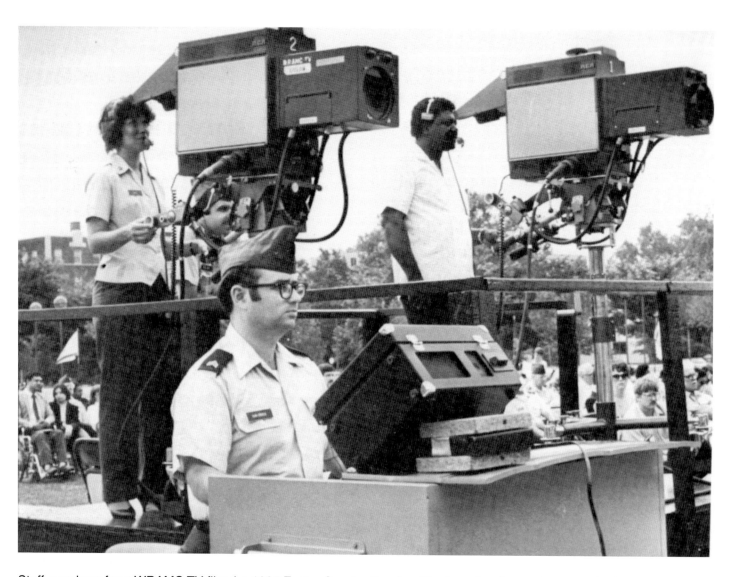

Staff members from WRAMC TV film the 1985 Easter Sunrise Service. The broadcast was shown on the base's closed-circuit TV for patients and servicemen who could not attend in person.
Source: WRAMC History Office, PAO Historical Collection

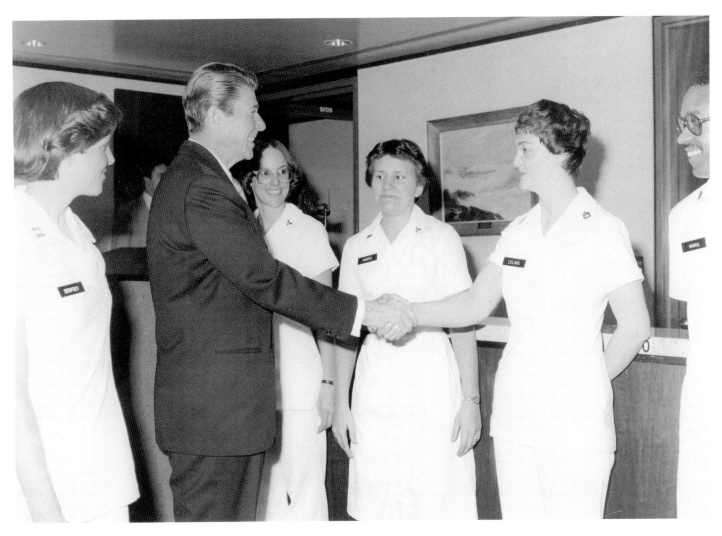

▲ President Ronald W. Reagan greets SFC Billie Leland with the nurses on the VIP Ward (Ward 72) at Walter Reed in the late 1980s. Between the President and SFC Leland are Captain Rebecca Hallberg, and 2nd Lieutenant Barbara Harris.
Source: WRAMC History Office, PAO Historical Collection

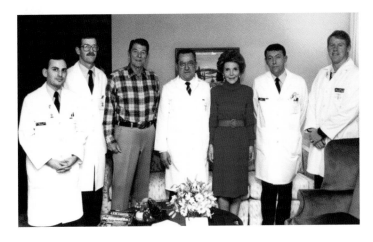

▲ President Ronald Reagan and Nancy Reagan following his surgery at WRAMC in 1989 with Col. George Bogumill (center), Col. Allan Smith, Maj. Paul Perlik, and the anesthesia staff. Dr. Bogumill served as Assistant Chief of the Army Hand Fellowship program at WRAMC and was later Chief of Orthopaedics before going to USUHS as the first Chairman of Anatomy.
Source: Bogumill Collection

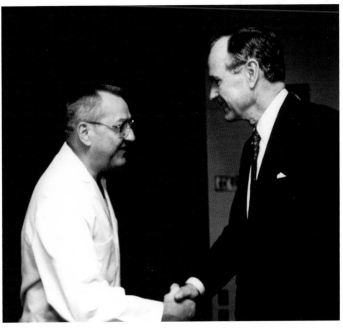

▲ Dr. Bogumill follows up after surgery with President George H. W. Bush at WRAMC.
Source: Bogumill Collection

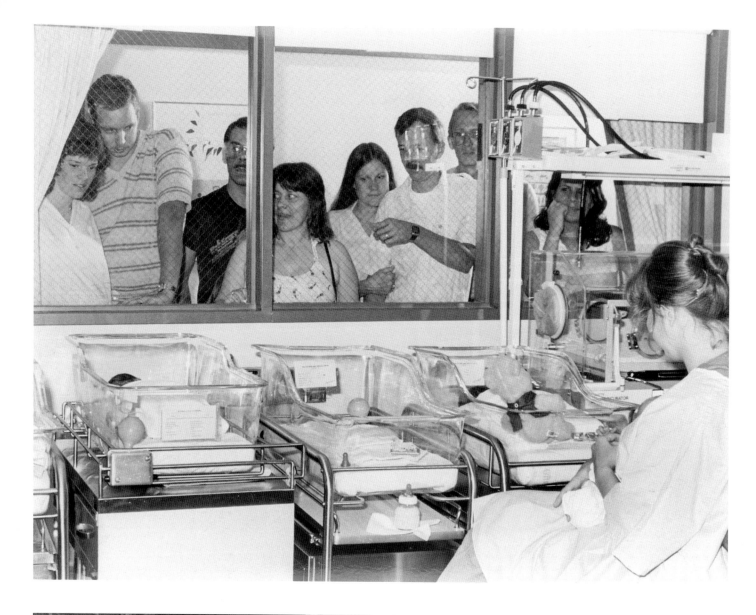

▲ Couples tour the Walter Reed Nursery during a childbirth preparation class at Walter Reed in 1982. The 4-day class covered everything from labor to infant care.
Source: WRAMC History Office, PAO Historical Collection

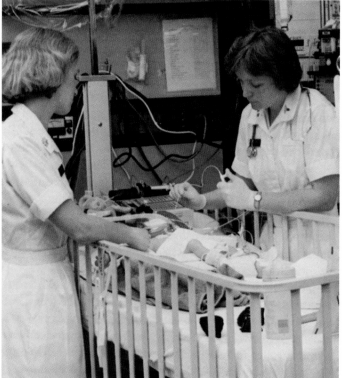

◄ Two Walter Reed nurses care for a tiny patient in the Neonatal ICU at Walter Reed, 1985.
Source: WRAMC History Office, PAO Historical Collection

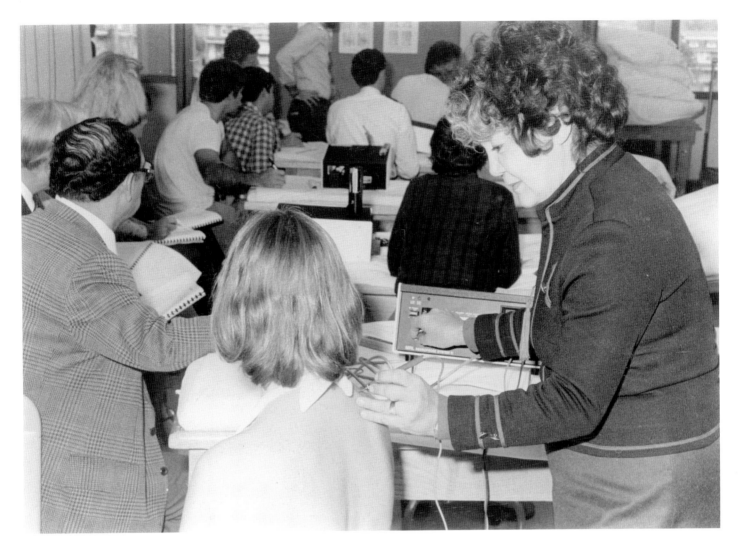

▲ The latest trigger point techniques to relieve chronic pain are demonstrated at a symposium at Walter Reed, 1982.
Source: WRAMC History Office, PAO Historical Collection

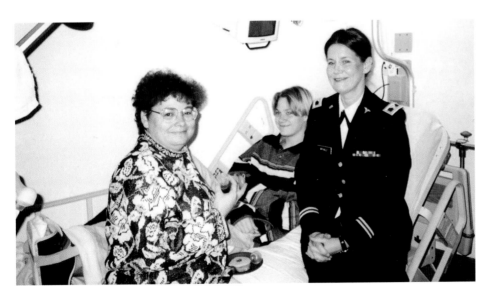

◀ A pediatric patient who underwent Ilizarov fixation is celebrating the holidays with Col. Kathleen McHale, Chief, Pediatric Orthopaedic Surgery.
Source: McIlvaine Collection

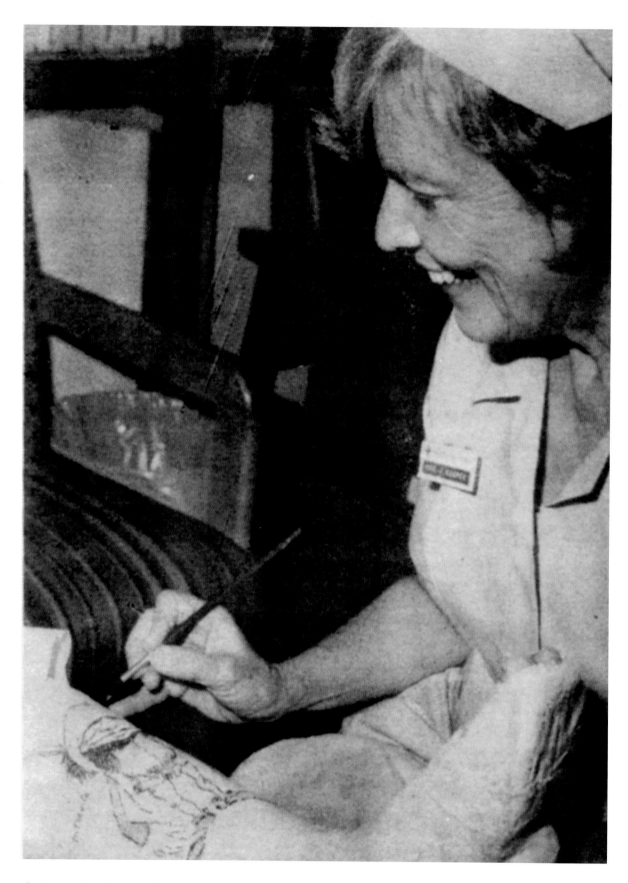

▲ Jacqueline Kasper displays some of her artistic talent on the cast of a patient from Ward 57.
Source: Stripe newspaper, October 10, 1980, Tyrone Milton - photographer

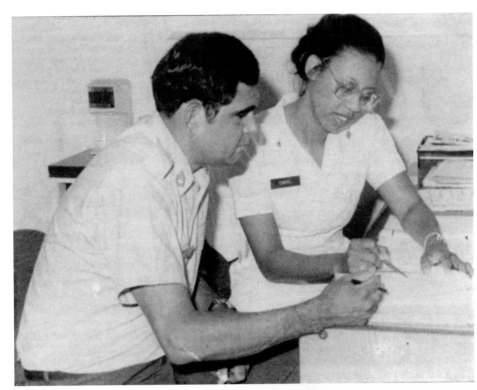

◀ Carolyn Tindal, Director of Nursing Continuing Education, goes over plans for Practical Nurse in-service programs with SFC Francisco Rodriguez.
Source: Stripe newspaper, July 6, 1981, J. D. Fox - photographer

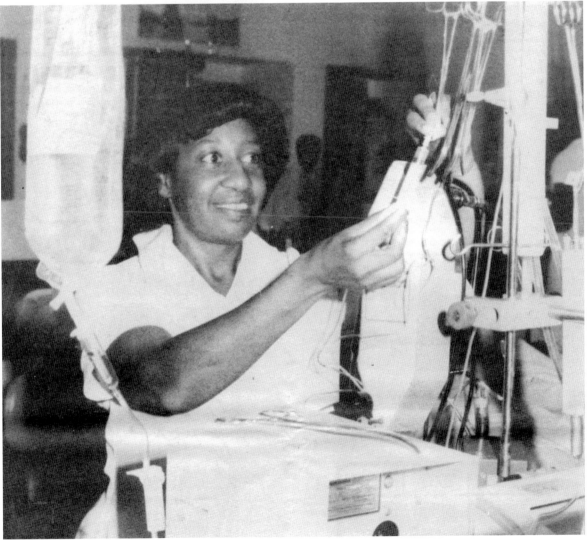

▲ Juanita Wims, Clinical Coordinator for the Dialysis Unit, makes an adjustment to some dialysis equipment to ready it for a patient.
Source: Stripe newspaper, July 6, 1981, J. D. Fox - photographer

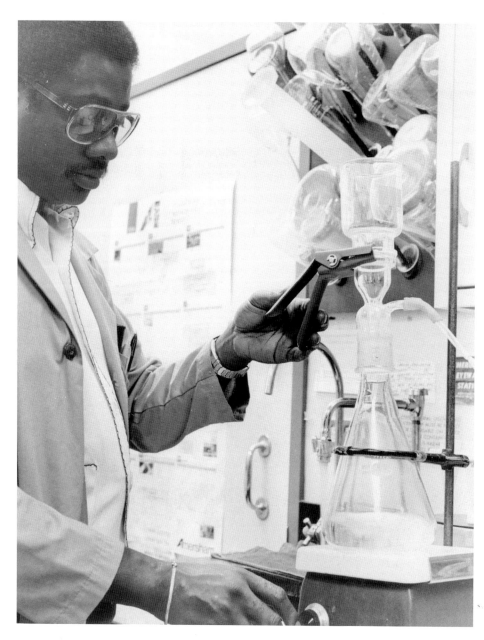

Laboratory personnel at Walter Reed in the 1980s.
Source: WRAMC History Office, PAO Historical Collection

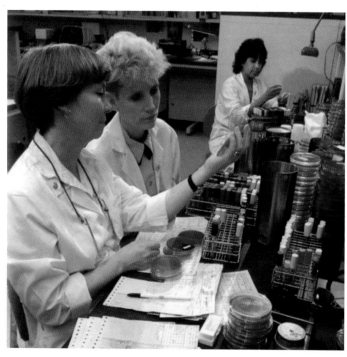

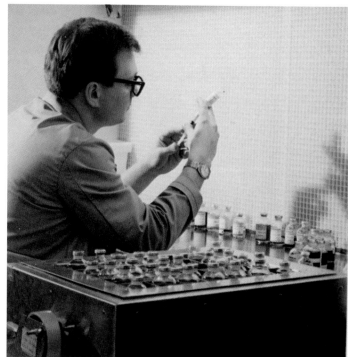

▶ Surgeons perform an open abdominal surgery in the main operating room at Walter Reed in 1985. Separate from the main OR was an Ambulatory Surgery Program that offered certain procedures on an outpatient basis, including tubal ligation and biopsies, beginning in 1980.
Source: WRAMC History Office, PAO Historical Collection

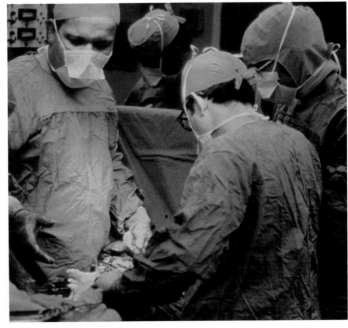

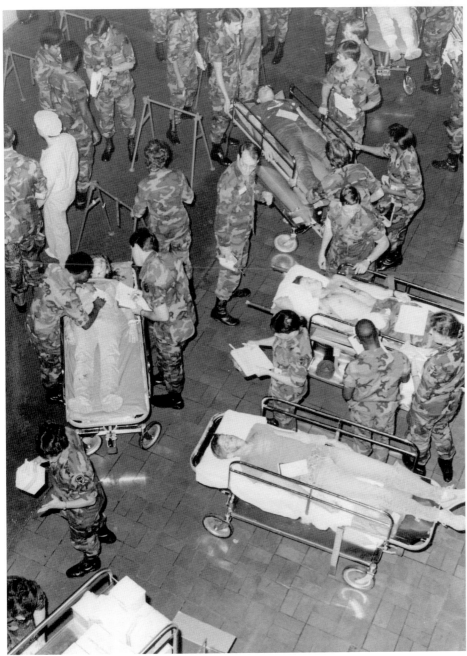

◀ The Walter Reed staff participates in a mass casualty exercise in the hospital lobby in 1986. The scenario for the exercise was an explosion on Post.
Source: WRAMC History Office, PAO Historical Collection

STRIPE

VOL. XXXVI, NO. 45

November 14, 1980

Published in the interest of the patients and staff of The Walter Reed Army Medical Center

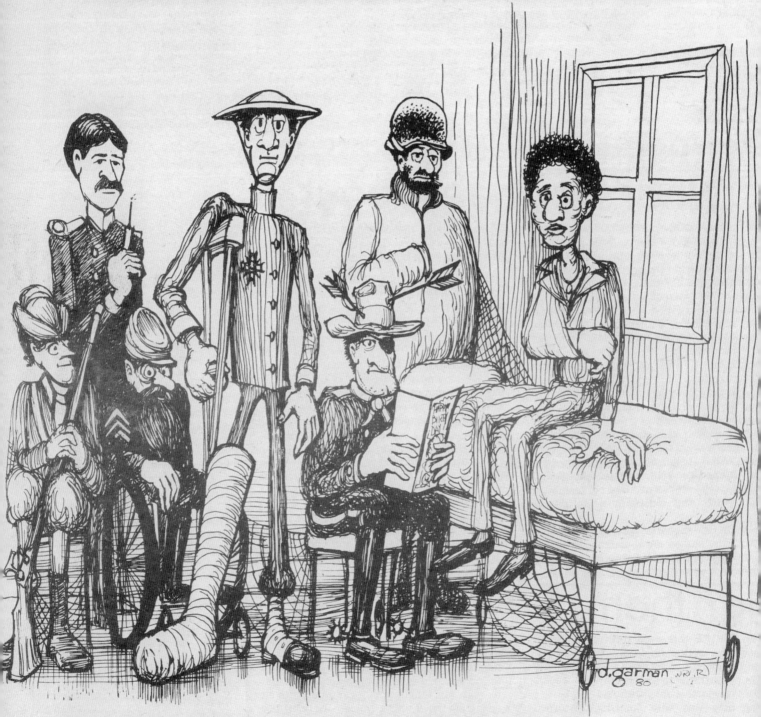

The wait can be long for Medical Hold patients

. . . page 8

Cover of the Walter Reed newspaper *Stripe* illustrates the realities of the Medical Hold process at Walter Reed in 1980.
Source: WRAMC History Office, PAO Historical Collection

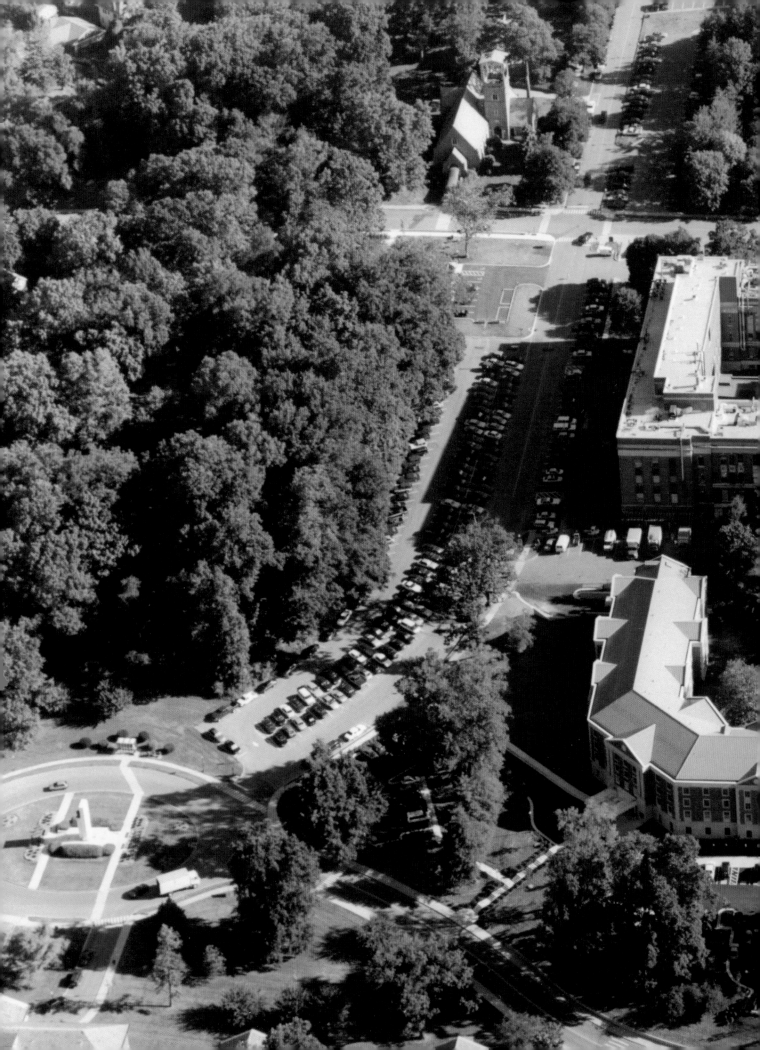

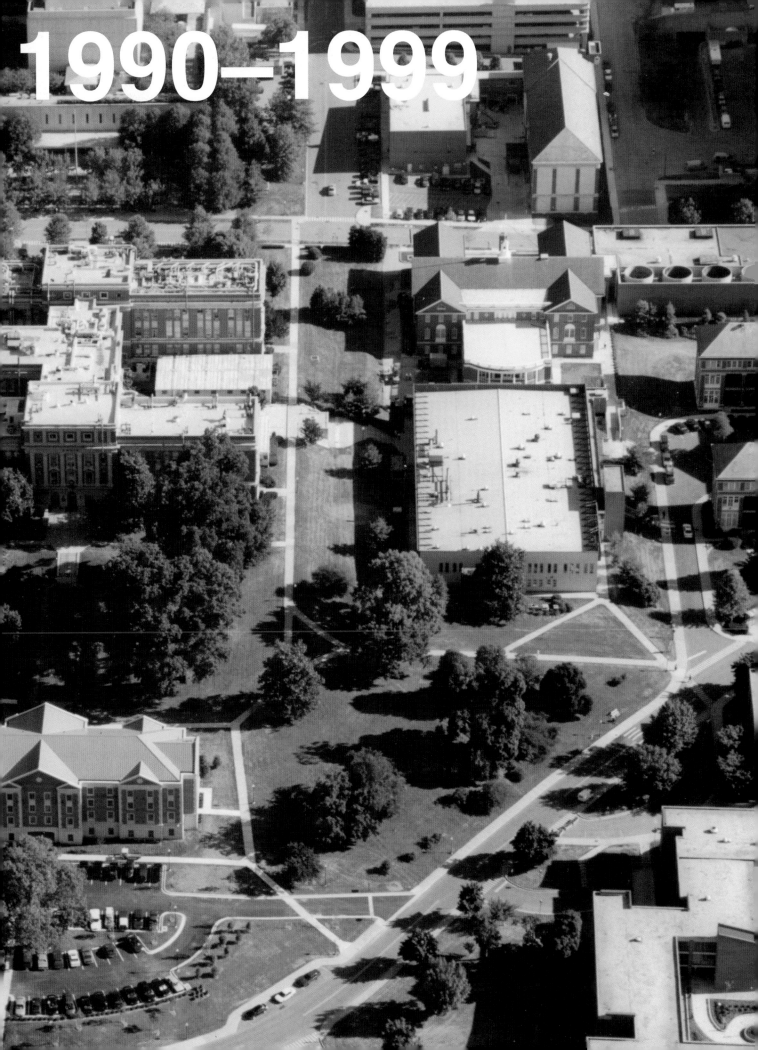

1990–1999

▶ DPW staff members plant begonias in front of the hospital named in honor of former commanding Lt. General Heaton.
Source: WRAMC History Office, PAO Historical Collection

The early 1990's again brought war to the United States Army with the Iraqi invasion of Kuwait and the resultant Persian Gulf War. Despite initial estimates of higher casualties, the war between August 2, 1990 and February 28, 1991, accounted for 151 deaths and 462 wounded among the American forces. Walter Reed was prepared for many more wounded but fortunately for all they did not materialize.

The campus continued to evolve with the addition of several new buildings. A much needed partial solution to the parking issues was answered by the addition of the Rumbaugh Parking Garage in 1993, named in honor of former WRAMC commander, Maj. General James Rumbaugh who helped procure its funding. The Borden Pavilion, built to house behavioral health providers and support personnel as well as clinical investigation activities, was opened in 1995 and named in honor of Lt. Colonel William Cline Borden, Medical Corps, U.S. Army. Dr. Borden was the main mover behind the establishment and naming of Walter Reed General Hospital.

The Mologne House, with 200 rooms and suites, was opened in 1997 and named in honor of former Walter Reed commander, Maj. General Lewis A. Mologne who had a dream of a comfortable, safe, low cost place for soldiers and their families to stay while receiving out patient care or visiting loved ones at Walter Reed.

A long needed new home for the Walter Reed Army Institute of Research (WRAIR) was built at the Forest Glen Annex and opened in 1999. In 2001, it was named in honor of Hawaii Senator Daniel K. Inouye, who in World War II was a member of the famed 442nd Regimental Combat Team one of the most highly decorated units in the history of the Army. For his service in World War II, he was awarded the Bronze Star Medal, the Distinguished Service Cross later upgraded to the Congressional Medal of Honor, and the Purple Heart.

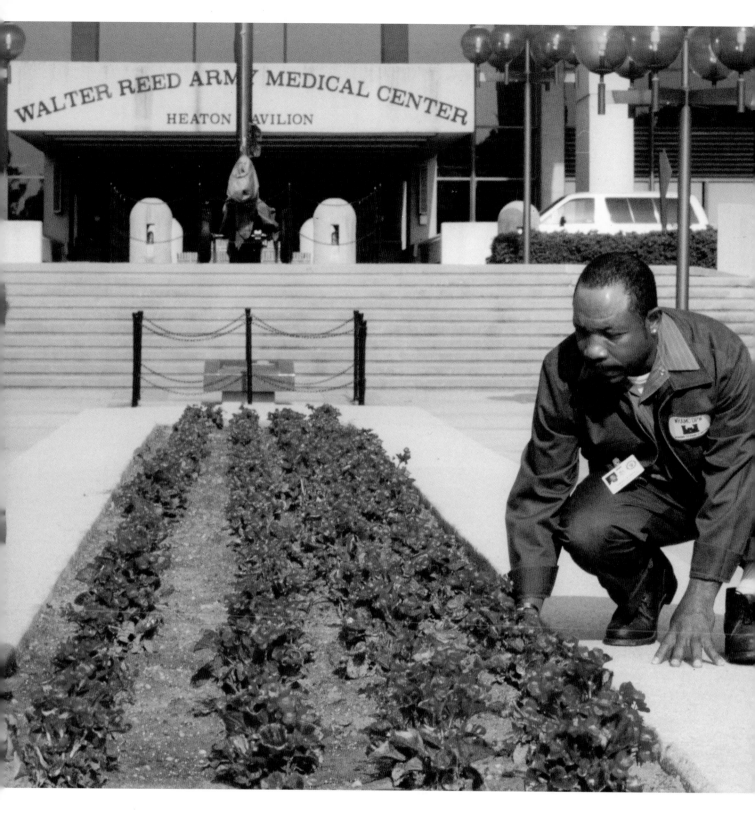

In 1990, Pauline Trost, wife of Chief of Naval Operations Admiral Carlisle Trost, presented to Zachary and Elizabeth Fisher the need for temporary lodging facilities for families at major military medical centers. The Fishers readily accepted the challenge and donated monies to start building two Fisher Houses, one at Bethesda and the other at Walter Reed. In June 1991, President George H. W. Bush dedicated the Fisher House at the National Naval Medical Center, Bethesda, MD. A second house, at the Forest Glen Annex to Walter Reed Army Medical Center, opened a month later. Since that time two additional Fisher Houses have been opened on the main campus at Walter Reed, the second in 1996 and the third in 2004. Altogether the Fisher Foundation has built almost 40 Fisher Houses on military bases and Veteran's Administration hospital grounds. The Foundation plans for more than 60 houses by 2011.

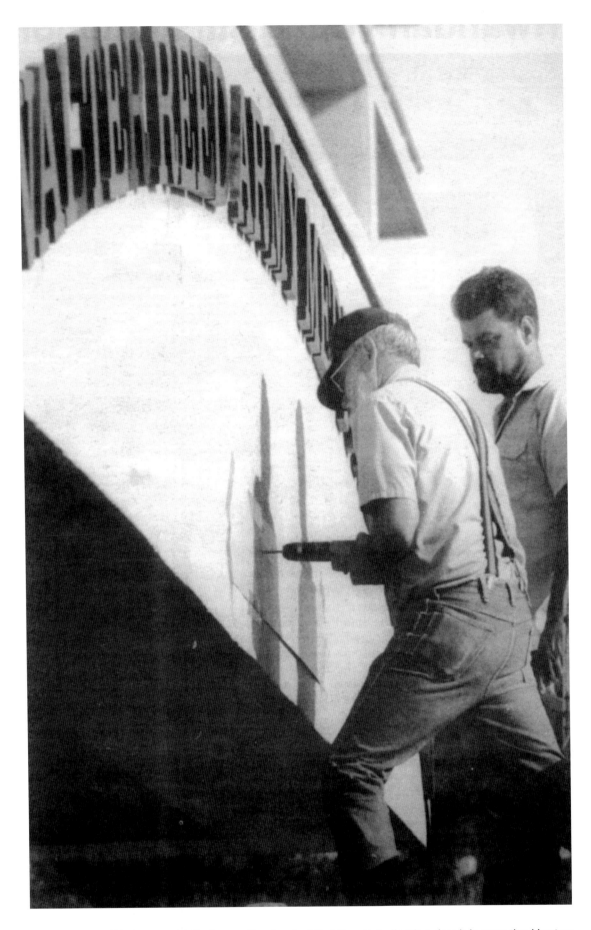

A new name. Workers put lettering on the front of Building 2, indicating that it is now the Heaton Pavilion. The name change honors the late Lt. General Leonard D. Heaton, who was commander at WRAMC from 1953 to 1959, and was Army Surgeon General from 1959 to 1969. A ceremony was held September 14, 1994 for the name change.
Source: Stripe newspaper, September 16, 1994, Jerry Merideth - photographer

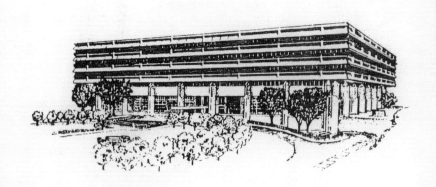

HEATON PAVILION

DEDICATION

WALTER REED ARMY MEDICAL CENTER

14 SEPTEMBER 1994

◄ Building 2, the "new" hospital, was rededicated on September 14, 1994 to honor Lt. General Leonard D. Heaton. Heaton was Walter Reed Commander from 1953 to 1959. He served as Surgeon General of the Army from 1959 to 1969. As a young doctor, he cared for the injured at Pearl Harbor. In 1946, he started the Surgery Program at Walter Reed and became WRAMC Commander in 1952. Lt. General Heaton died in 1983.
Source: National Museum of Health and Medicine, AFIP, WRAMC History Collection

▼ This photo from the 1950s shows Heaton and his most famous patient, President Eisenhower. Heaton operated on the President in 1956 and became his physician until his death in 1969. They were both avid golfers and became fast friends.
Source: Stripe newspaper, September 9, 1994

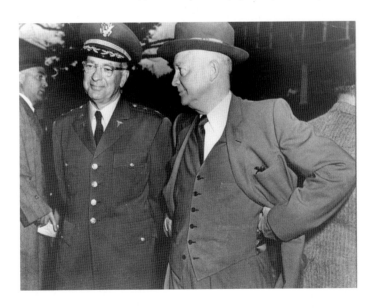

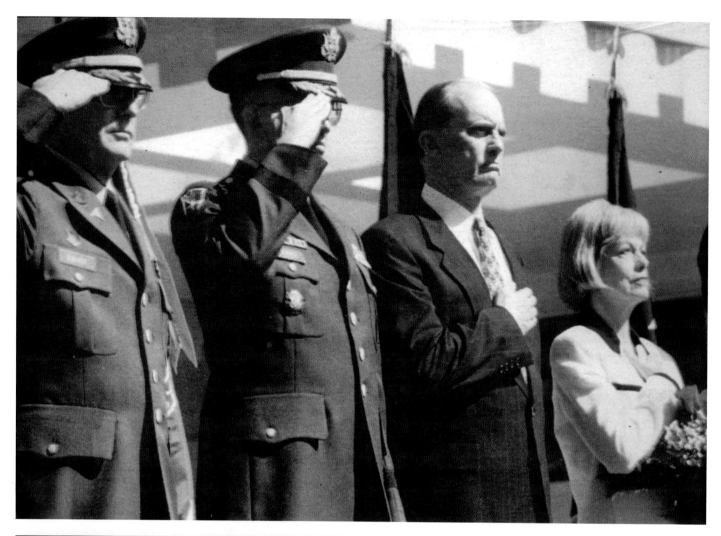

Maj. General Leslie Burger (CG WRAMC), Lt. General Ronald Blanck (Surgeon General of the Army), Lt. General Bernhard Mittemeyer (Ret.) and Mrs. Rose Mologne at the dedication of the Mologne House. Mologne House was dedicated to "a soldier's general."
Source: Stripe newspaper.

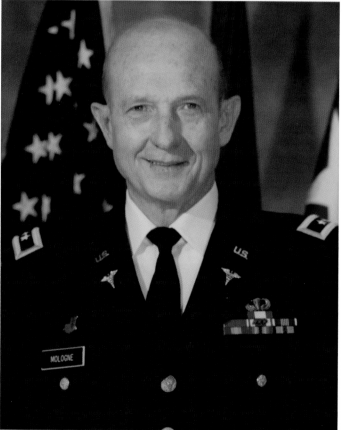

The Mologne House, a 200-room hotel for patients and their families, was dedicated on May 12, 1997. It was named for Maj. General Lewis A. Mologne, Commander of Walter Reed from June 22, 1983 to August 1, 1988. He took command at a time when Walter Reed was experiencing budgetary, personnel, and morale problems. He reenergized a sense of purpose and value, with an increased sense of teamwork and goal sharing.

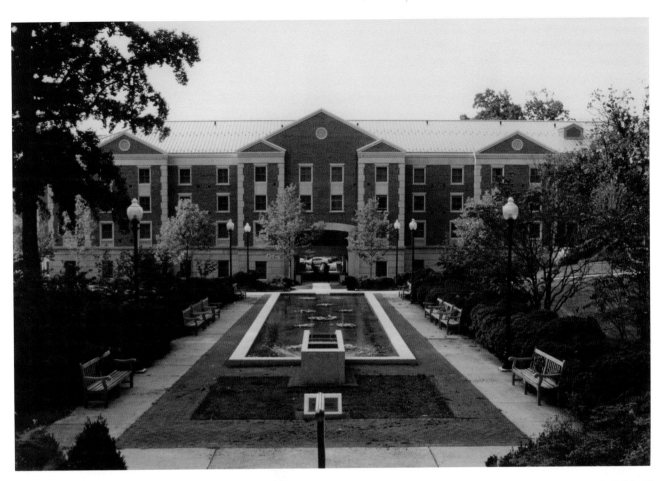

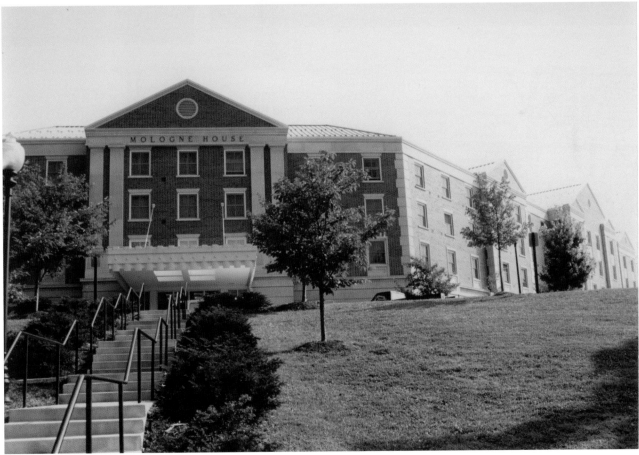

The fountain and courtyard (top) are surrounded by the Mologne House and the old WRAIR building. This staircase leads up to the front entrance of the hotel (bottom).
Source: Walter Reed Army Medical Center, Directorate of Public Works Archives

221

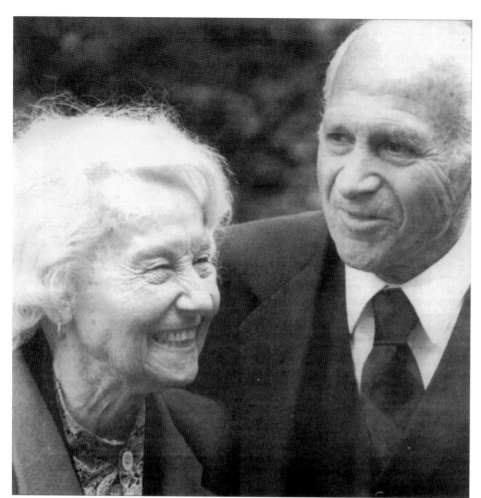

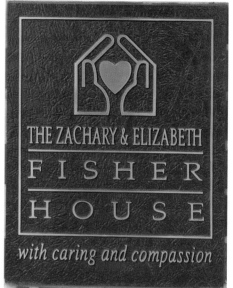

Elizabeth and Zachary Fisher funded Fisher Houses at Walter Reed Army Medical Center. The first house is at the Forest Glen Annex. The Fishers donated funds for houses built for families of patients hospitalized for long-term care at military posts around the country. The second house can accommodate up to 24 family members of very seriously ill patients.
Source: Stripe newspaper, October 6, 1995

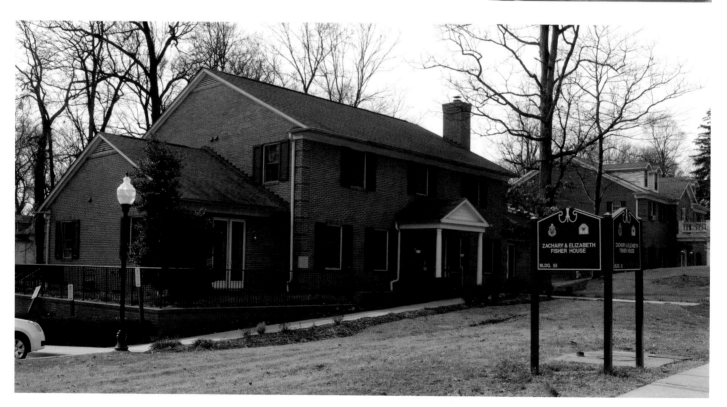

▲ The Zachary and Elizabeth Fisher Houses as they appear today. The groundbreaking for this first house on the Walter Reed campus was October 11, 1995. A second house, shown in the background, was built on campus in 2004.
Source: Borden Institute, Douglas Wise - photographer

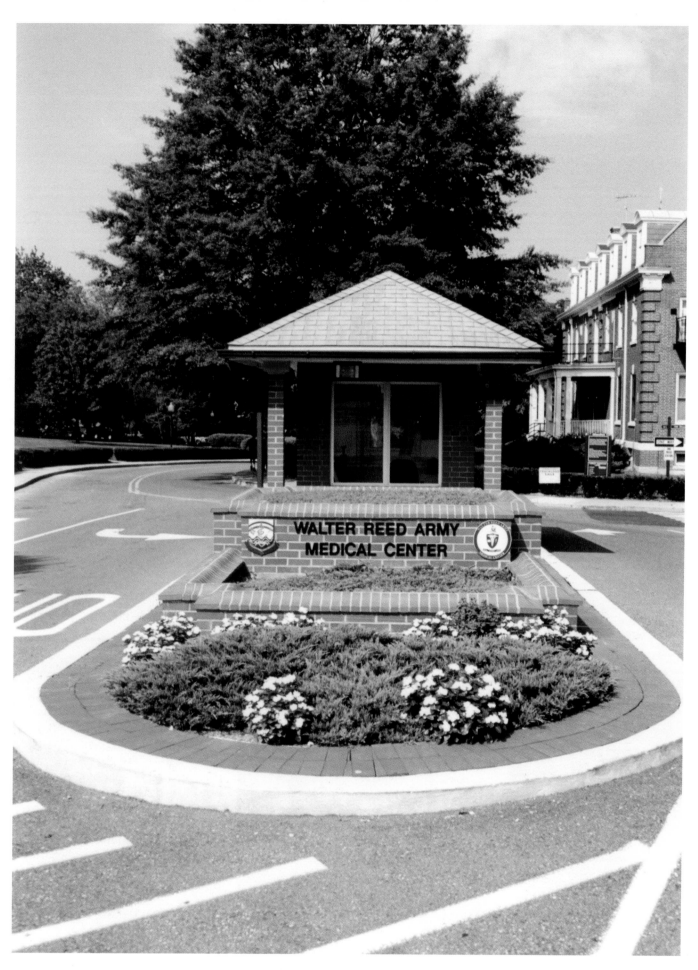

A new guardhouse at one of the Georgia Avenue gates.
Source: Walter Reed Army Medical Center, Directorate of Public Works Archives

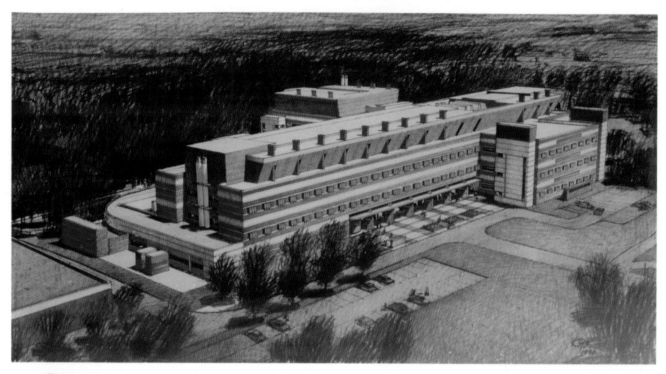

THE WALTER REED ARMY INSTITUTE OF RESEARCH
THE NAVAL MEDICAL RESEARCH INSTITUTE
WALTER REED ARMY MEDICAL CENTER, FOREST GLEN, MD

In 1999, the new Walter Reed Army Institute of Research (WRAIR) building opened at Forest Glen. The building appears much larger than it actually is, as does the hospital (Building 2) on the WRAMC campus. Both were built with interstitial floors to provide access to physical plant and electrical systems.

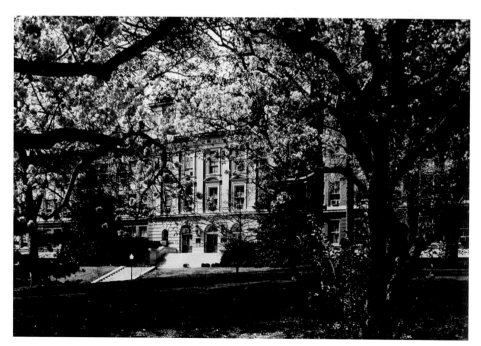

WRAIR and the Naval Medical Research Institute (NMRI) conduct research and development of products, procedures, and practices aimed at management of infectious diseases, combat injuries, operational medical problems, and chemical and biological threats. WRAIR and NMRI will continue the tradition of research at home and abroad, as well as collaborative work with academia and industry. The new research laboratory center serves as the focal point for combined Army-Navy medical research. In 2008, responsibility for WRAIR was transferred to Medical Research and Materiel Command.
Source: National Museum of Health and Medicine, AFIP, WRAMC History Collection

◀ The old WRAIR building (Building 40) on the WRAMC campus viewed through cherry blossoms.

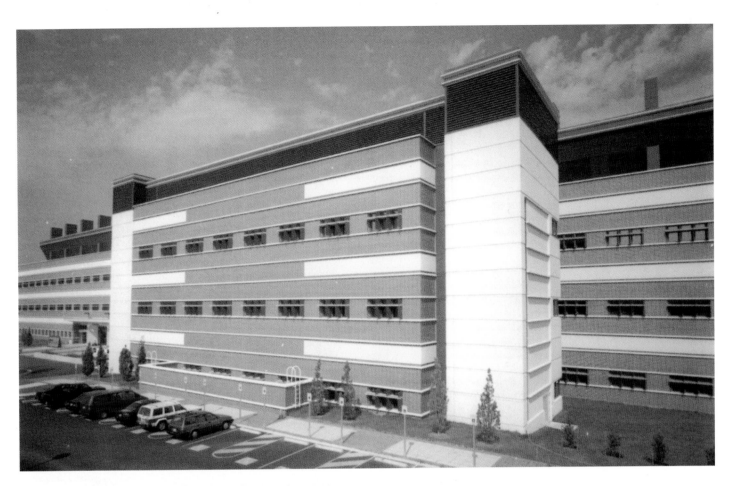

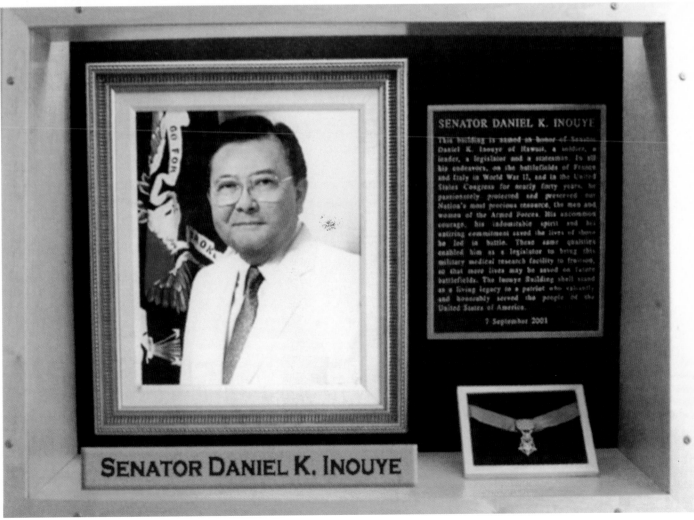

SENATOR DANIEL K. INOUYE

This building is named in honor of Senator Daniel K. Inouye of Hawaii, a soldier, a leader, a legislator and a statesman. In all his endeavors, on the battlefields of France and Italy in World War II, and in the United States Congress for nearly forty years, he passionately protected and preserved our Nation's most precious resource, the men and women of the Armed Forces. His uncommon courage, his indomitable spirit and his untiring commitment saved the lives of those he led in battle. These same qualities enabled him as a legislator to bring this military medical research facility to fruition, so that more lives may be saved on future battlefields. The Inouye Building shall stand as a living legacy to a patriot who valiantly and honorably served the people of the United States of America.

7 September 2001

SENATOR DANIEL K. INOUYE

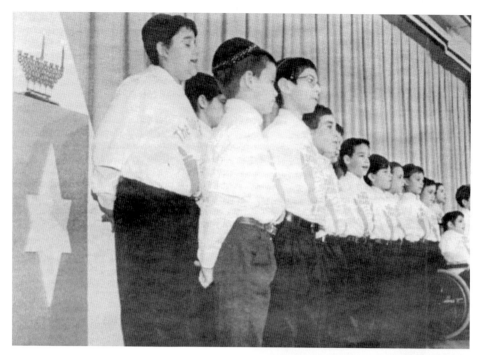

◄ Feast of Dedication. Students from the Torah School of Greater Washington commemorate Chanukah, the "Feast of Dedication," during a cantata in the Walter Reed Hospital's Joel Auditorium.
Source: Stripe newspaper, December 18, 1998, Beau Whittington - photographer

► Dr. Clarence G. Newsome, Associate Dean, Howard University School of Divinity, addresses the congregation at the annual memorial tribute to Dr. Martin Luther King, Jr., January 12 at the Memorial Chapel.
Source: Stripe newspaper, January 19, 1990, Patrick Swan - photographer

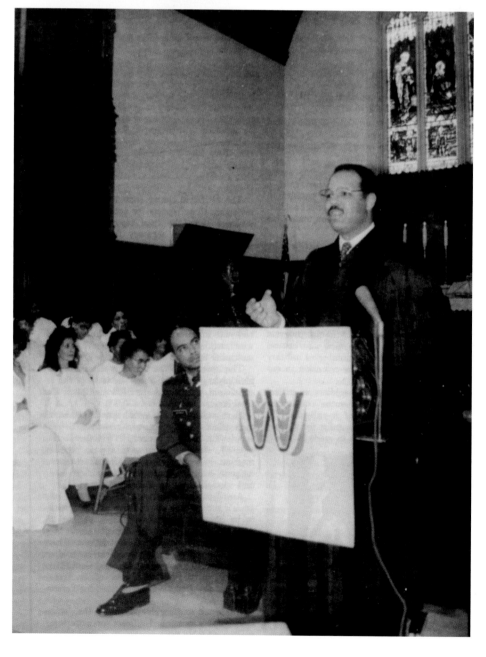

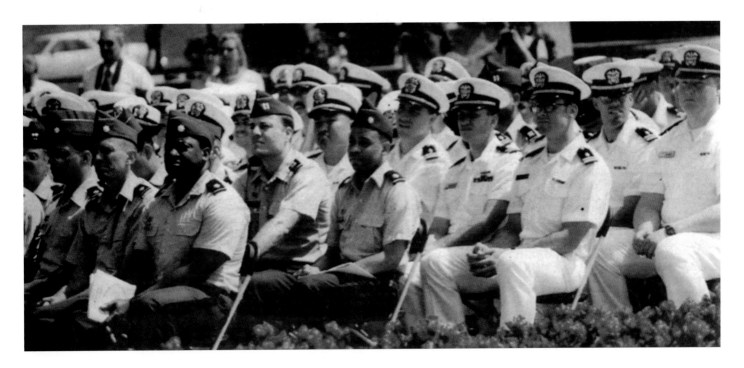

▲ It was a sea of green and white at Walter Reed as the Army's premier medical center hosted the first combined gradu-ate medical education graduation ceremony between itself and the Navy's flagship healthcare facility, the National Naval Medical Center in Bethesda, MD.
Source: Stripe newspaper, June 27, 1997

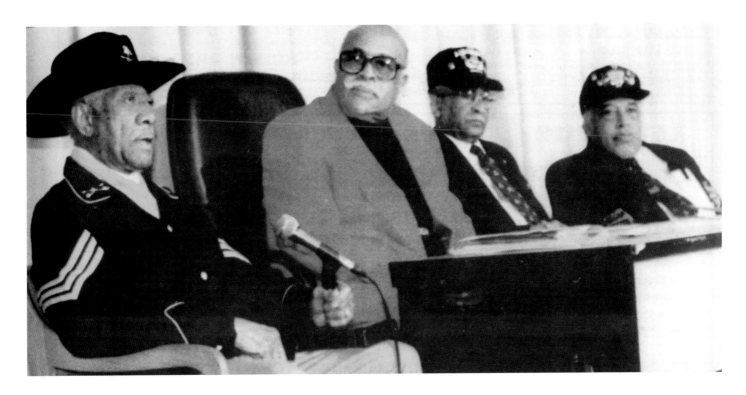

▲ "Buffalo Soldier" SFC John E. Wright of the 9th Cavalry, Tuskegee Airman Leroy A. Battle of the 99th Pursuit Fighter Squadron, and "Buffalo Rangers" George Jackson and Paul Lyles of the 2nd Ranger Infantry Company (Airborne) discuss contributions made by blacks to the armed forces during an African-American Heritage Month program February 4 in the hospital's Joel Auditorium.
Source: Stripe newspaper, February 13, 1998, Bernard S. Little - photographer

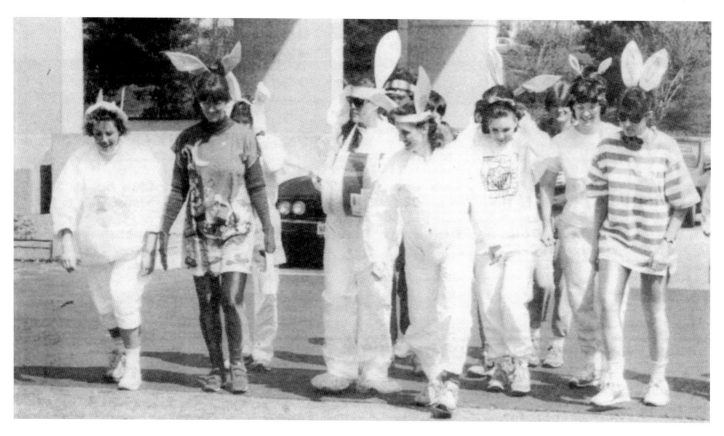

▲ Bunnies begin the first leg of the "Fun Bunny Run" held April 12 at WRAMC (above). The run was sponsored by the Department of Nursing Socialization Association. Students of the Intensive Care Professional Nursing Course and other Department of Nursing personnel participated in the run held for the holiday and for Physical Fitness Readiness Test preparation.
Source: Stripe newspaper, April 20, 1990

▶ Advertisement for the sixty-fourth Easter Sunrise Service.
Source: Stripe newspaper

Walter Reed Army Medical Center

Cordially Invites You to Attend

THE SIXTY FOURTH

Easter Sunrise Service

SUNDAY MORNING, 15 APRIL, 1990
6900 GEORGIA AVENUE N.W.

LOCATION: IN THE ROSE GARDEN

TIME: 7:00 a.m.

SPEAKER:

CH(LTC) DICK DENSON, (RET.)
DIR OF DEPT OF MINISTRY AND
PASTORAL CARE

BAPTIST HEALTH SYSTEM OF
EAST TENNESSE

COME AND ENJOY!

MUSIC BY THE VIERS MILL BAPTIST CHOIR AND THE UNITED STATES ARMY BAND
INCLEMENT WEATHER: HOSPITAL SECOND FLOOR VERANDA (SOUTHEAST CORNER)

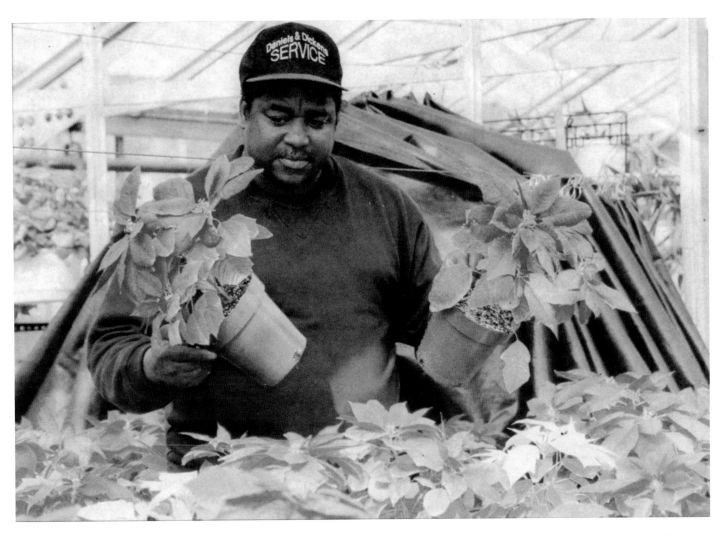

Joe Dickens, head gardener at the Department of Psychiatry's Horticulture Therapy Greenhouse, prepares a few of the facility's 500 poinsettia plants for delivery to Walter Reed wards during the holidays. Dickens, along with co-workers T. C. Williams, George Blevins, and Robert Coram, used many of the plants to create the center's annual poinsettia tree in the hospital's main lobby. The greenhouse was demolished by the end of the decade.
Source: Stripe newspaper, December 17, 1993, Jerry Merideth - photographer

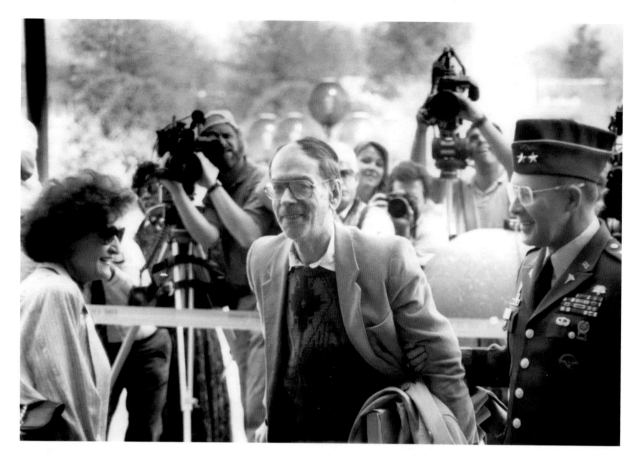

▲ Robert Polhill, accompanied by Maj. General Cameron (WRAMC Commander), entering Walter Reed Hospital following his release from Lebanon, where he had been held hostage for 39 months (from January 24, 1987 to April 1990).
Source: NCP 1262

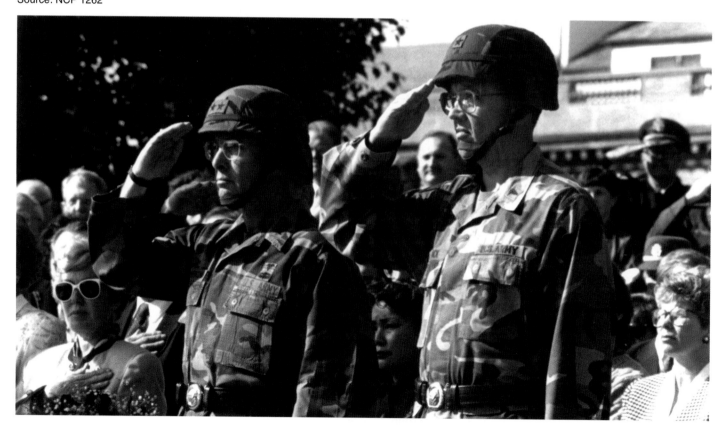

▲ 1992 change of command ceremony in front of the Heaton Pavilion with Maj. General Cameron, outgoing WRAMC Commander and Brig. General Ronald Blanck as incoming Commander.
Source: Blanck Collection

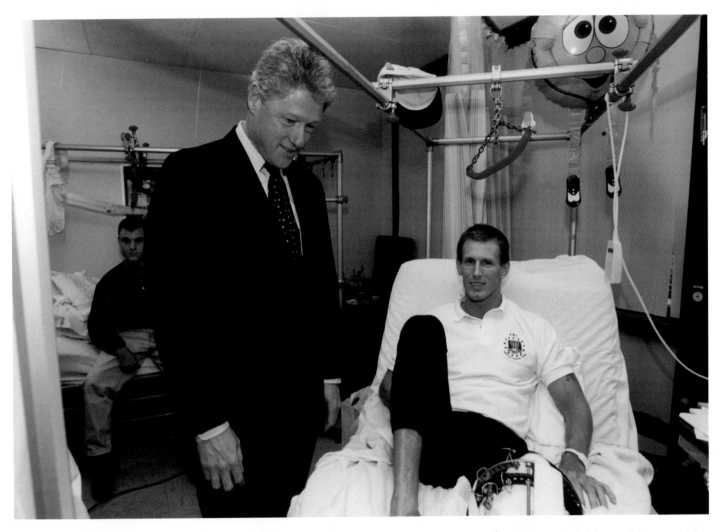

▲ President Bill Clinton visiting a soldier wounded in Somalia.
Source: WRAMC History Office, PAO Historical Collection

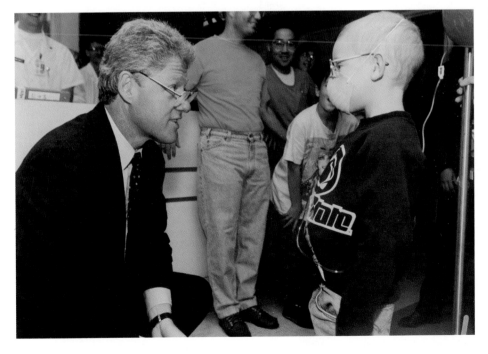

▲ President William J. Clinton is enjoying his conversation with a young patient on Ward 51 during an October 1993 visit to the hospital.
Source: Stripe newspaper, April 28, 2006

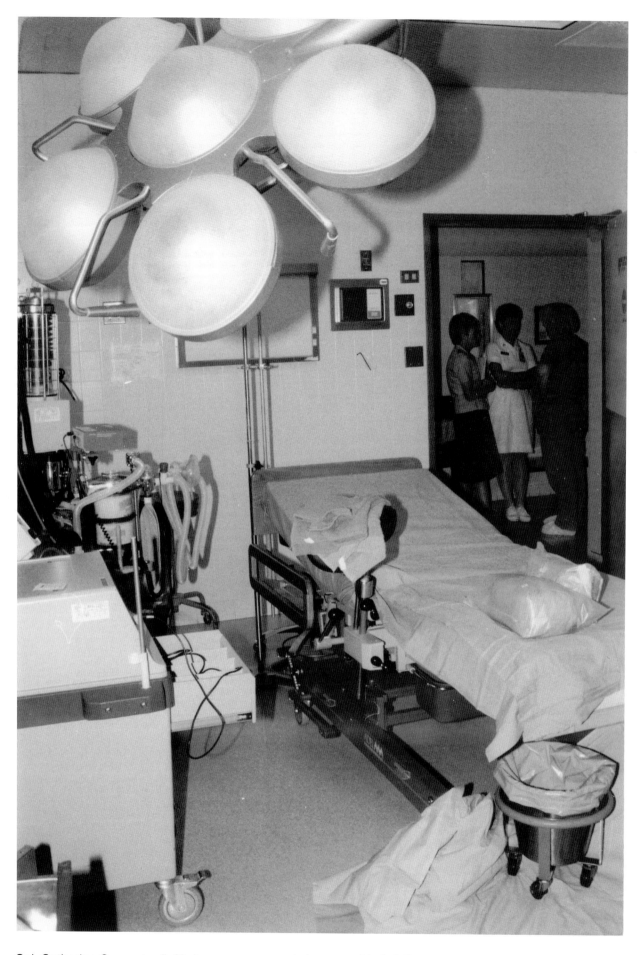

Col. Catharine Carpenter (left) discusses proposal changes with Col. Baird and Maj. Sullivan (in scrubs) that will transform this delivery room into a birthing room.
Source: Stripe newspaper, June 28, 1991, Bonnie S. Heater - photographer

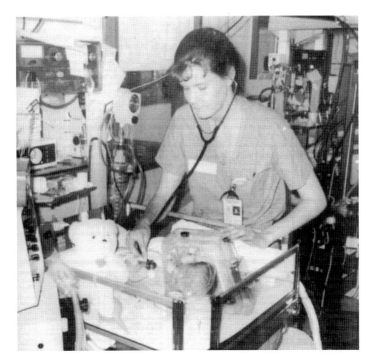

◀ Lt. Lynn Jinishian provides tender loving care to a premature baby.
Source: Stripe newspaper, February 2, 1990

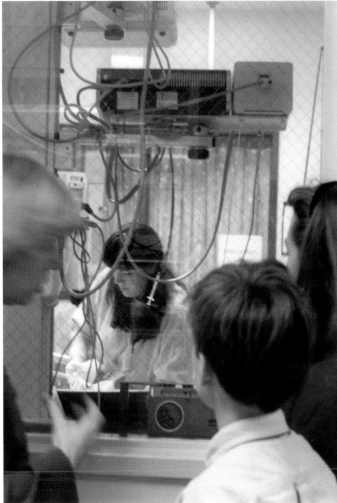

▶ Maj. Lenhart tends to her son in the Newborn Intensive Care Unit.
Source: Cox Collection, 1992

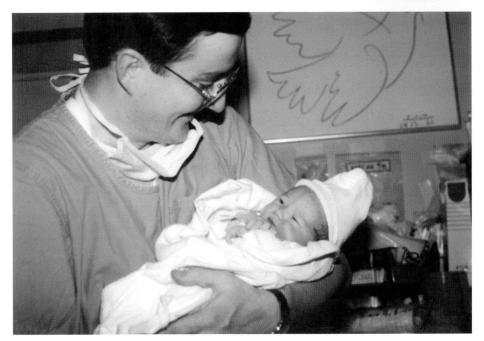

◀ Maj. Dave Mahoney holds newborn in delivery room. 1993.
Source: Murry Collection

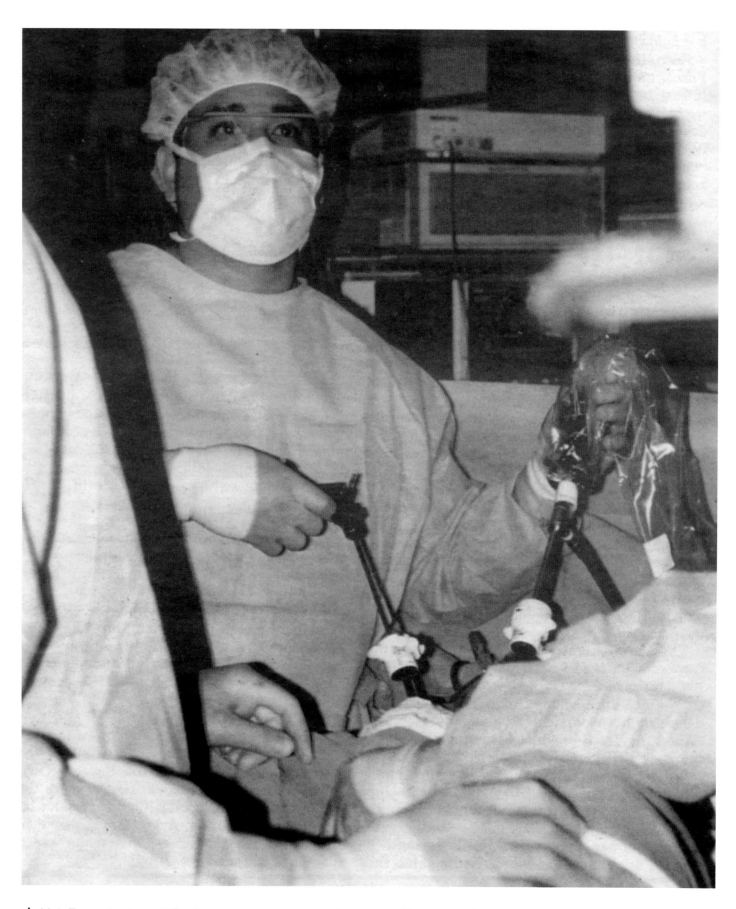

▲ Maj. Ernest Lockrow, DO, views a monitor as he performs a total laparoscopic hysterectomy.
Source: Stripe newspaper, Ramona E. Joyce - photographer

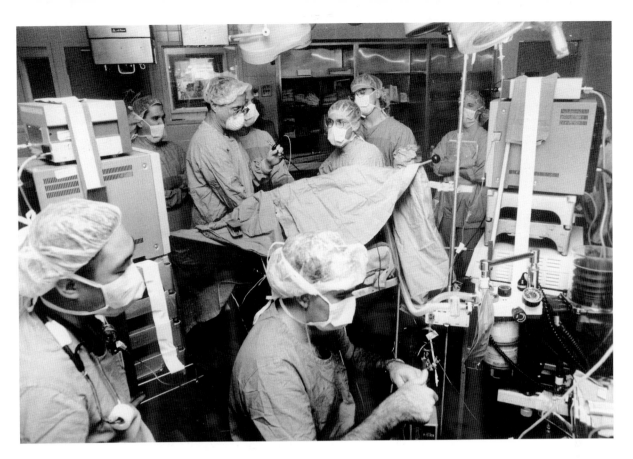

▲ Surgeon, Col. Harold Fenster, performs Walter Reed Army Medical Center's second laparoscopic cholecystectomy for gallbladder removal, October 16, 1990.
Source: Stripe newspaper, October 1990

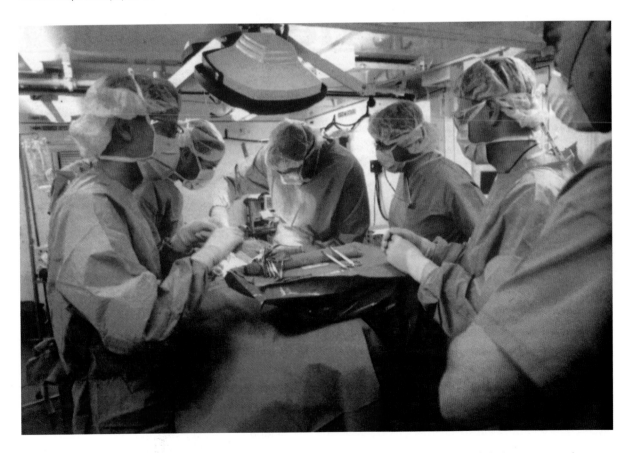

▲ The public was invited to observe how the Army cares for its soldiers in the field during an open house that showcased a Deployable Medical System at Walter Reed.
Source: Stripe newspaper, March 28, 1997

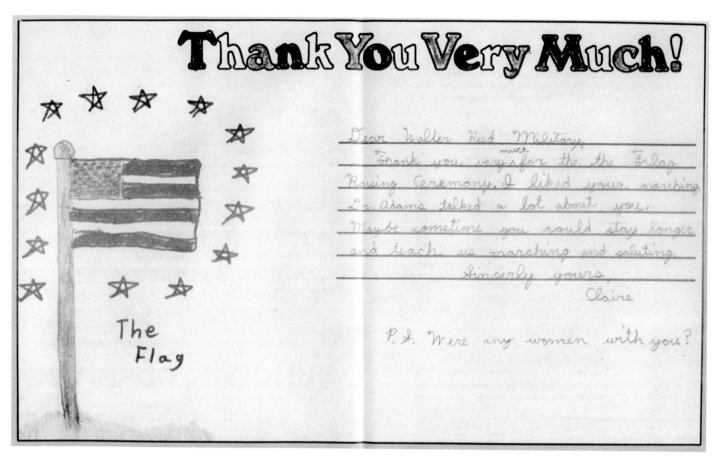

Thank You Very Much!

The Flag

Dear Walter Reed Military,
Thank you very much for the the Flag Raising Ceremony, I liked your marching. Dr. Adams talked a lot about you. Maybe sometime you could stay longer and teach us marching and saluting.
Sincerly yours,
Claire

P.S. Were any women with you?

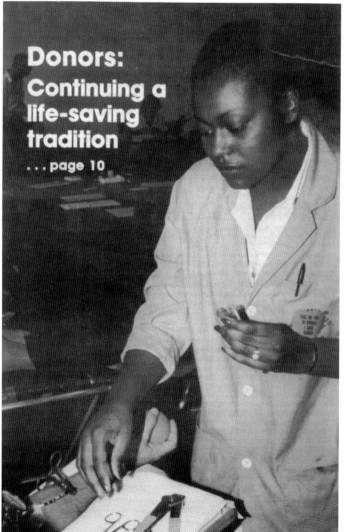

Donors:
Continuing a
life-saving
tradition
...page 10

▲ A letter written by a Glen Haven Elementary School student to the Walter Reed Precision Drill Team. As part of WRAMC's Adopt-A-School program the Medical Center Brigade soldiers had recently performed for the students.
Source: Stripe newspaper, April 20, 1990

◄ The Walter Reed Army Medical Center Blood Donor Center sends out the call for donors.
Source: Stripe newspaper, July 17, 1992

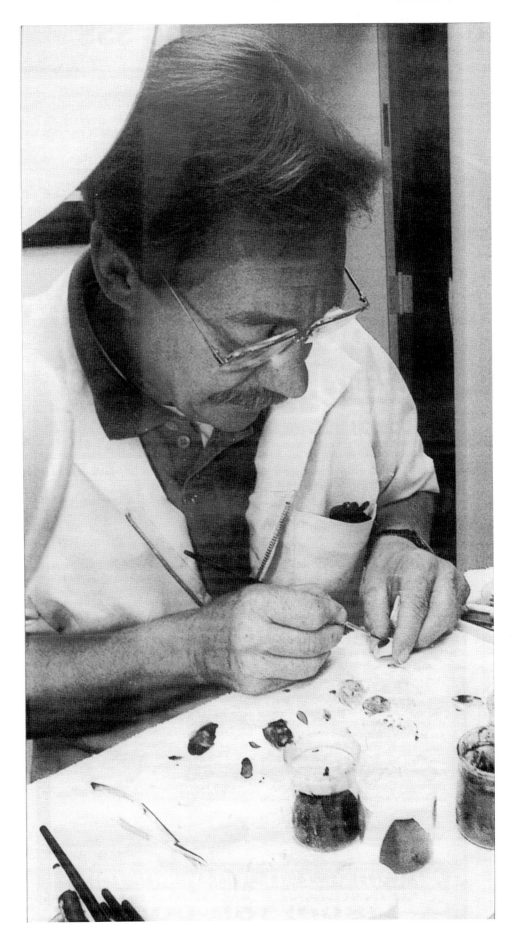

Ocularist Vince Przybyla paints the iris of a plastic eye. Painting the iris requires a very subtle mixing of paints to get a perfect color match with the patient's other eye.
Source: Stripe newspaper, September 10, 1993, Barry Reichenbaugh - photographer

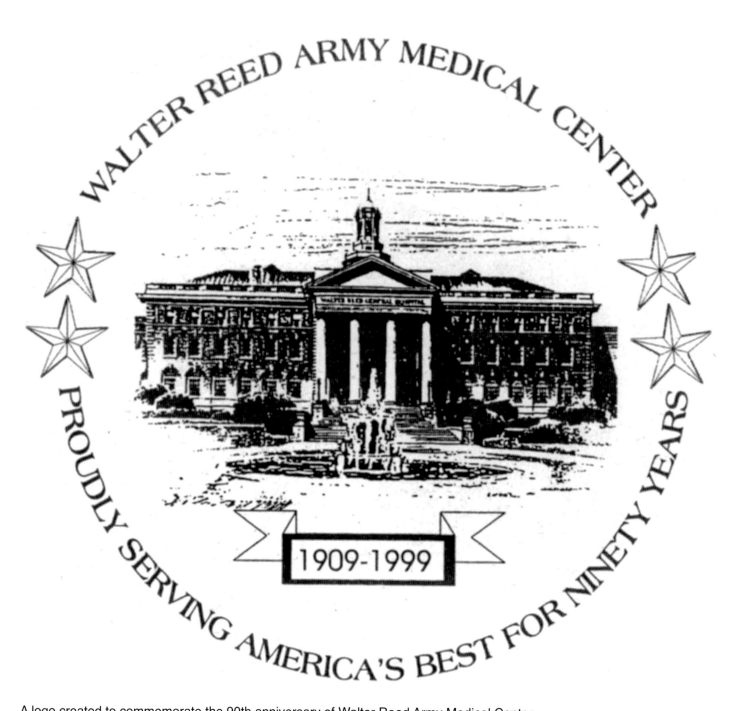

WALTER REED ARMY MEDICAL CENTER

PROUDLY SERVING AMERICA'S BEST FOR NINETY YEARS

1909-1999

A logo created to commemorate the 90th anniversary of Walter Reed Army Medical Center.
Source: Stripe newspaper, April 23, 1999

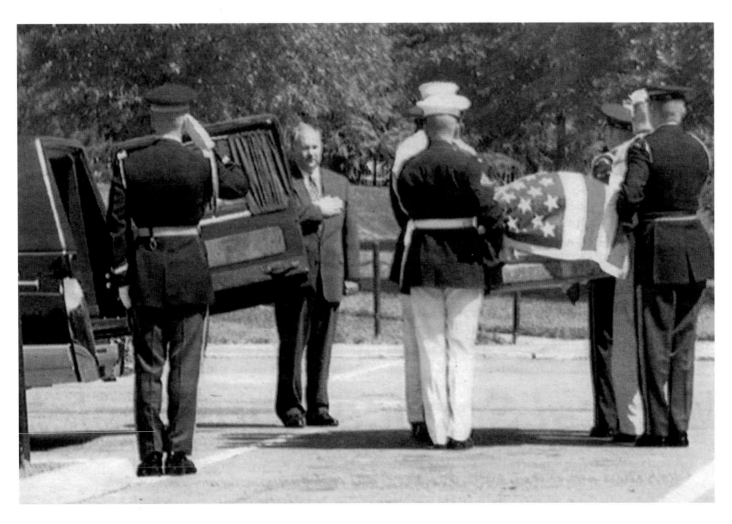

The Tomb of the Unknown in Arlington National Cemetery honors the unknown dead of several wars. Modern science and DNA testing made it possible to identify the bodies of nearly all the military who died during the Vietnam War. On May 14, 1998, the body of the Vietnam War Unknown was disinterred and brought by military escort to the Armed Forces Institute of Pathology, at Walter Reed for testing and identification. Members of the Department of Defense Honor Guard remove the casket of the Vietnam Unknown from a hearse in front of the AFIP Building.
Source: Stripe newspaper, May 15, 1998, Veronica Ferris - photographer

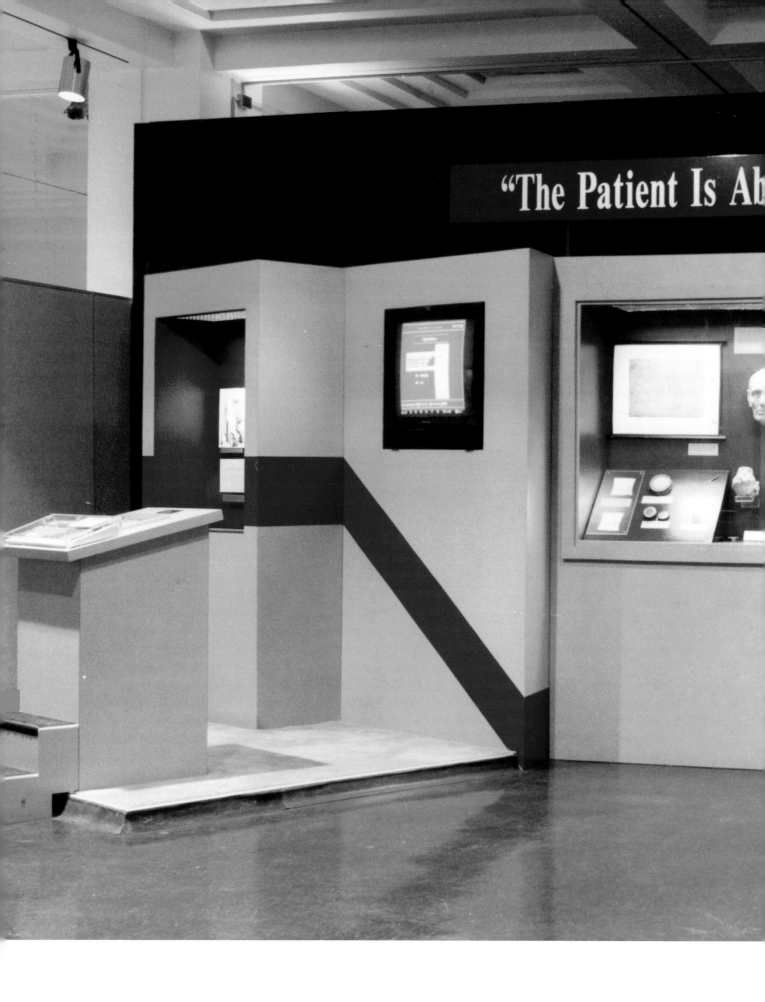

"The Patient Is Ab

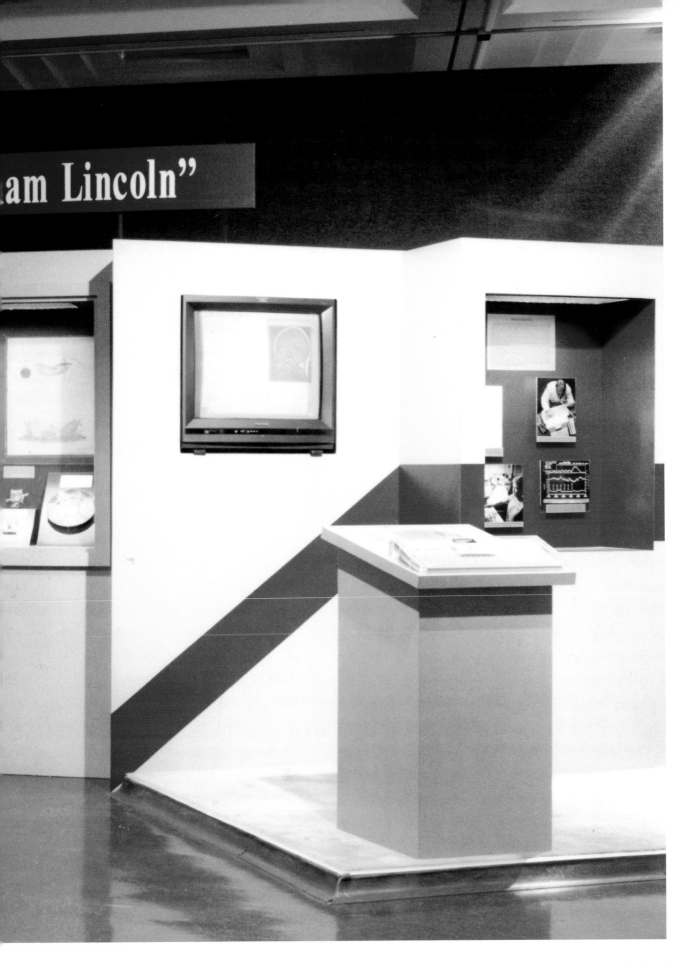

This collection of artifacts from the treatment of President Abraham Lincoln remains on display today at the National Museum of Health and Medicine.

Source: National Museum of Health and Medicine, AFIP, NCP 3395, Mike Rhode - photographer

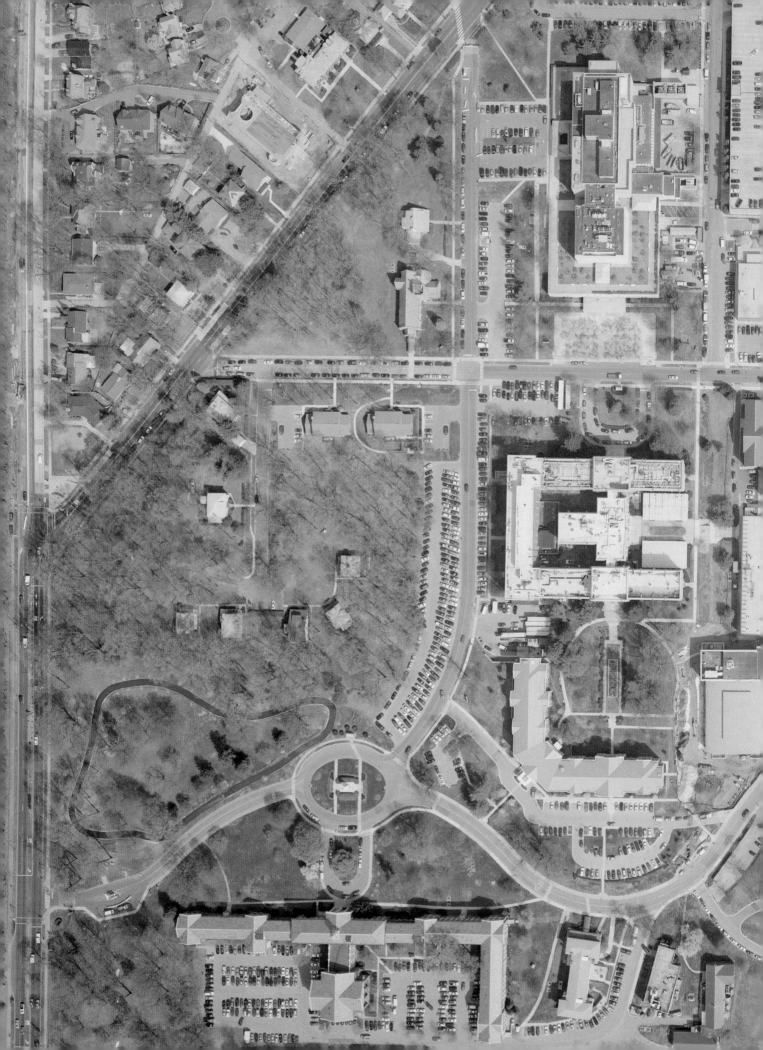

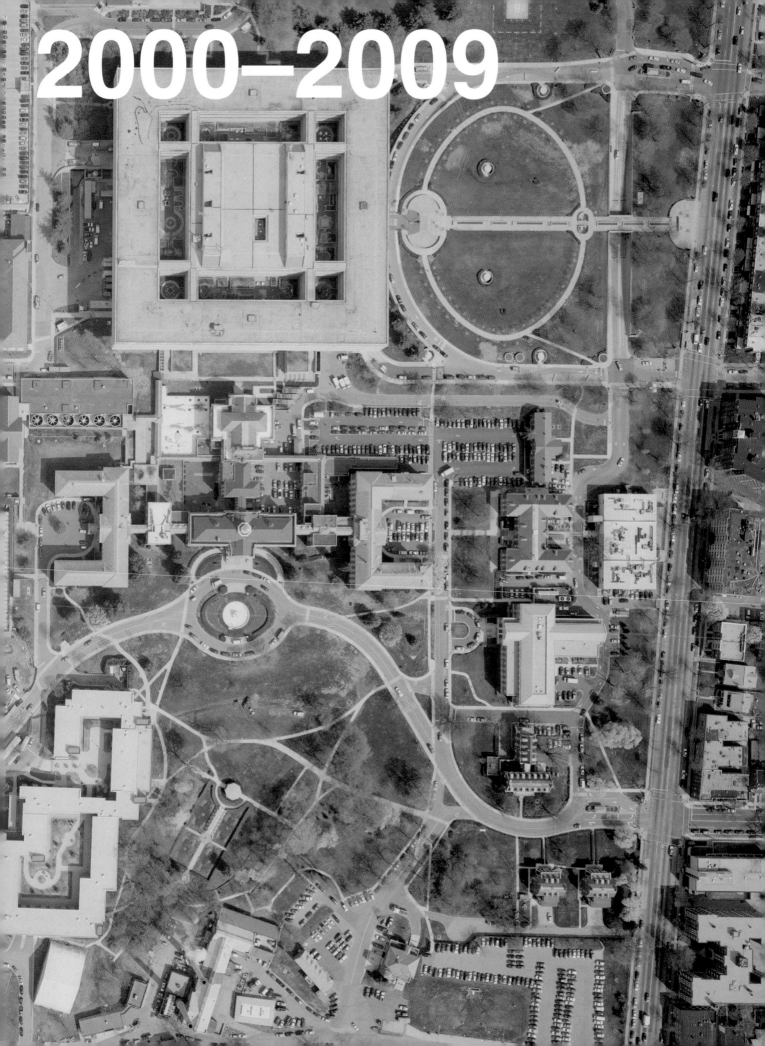

2000–2009

▶ The Hoff Fountain is especially beautiful in the spring with the tulips in bloom.
Source: Walter Reed Army Medical Center, Directorate of Public Works Archives

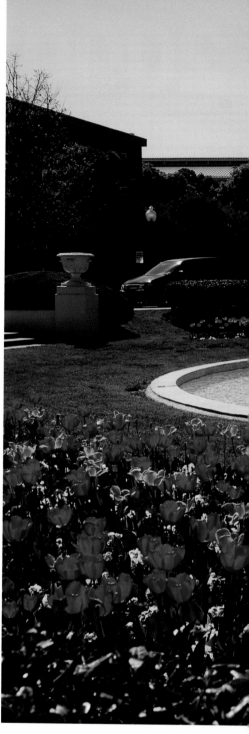

No one anticipated that September 11, 2001, a sunny day with bright blue skies, would bring such death and destruction to our country and significant change to the Army and to Walter Reed. The following Global War on Terror, with combat in Afghanistan and Iraq, resulted in many new and often severely wounded soldiers, as well as other challenges being brought to Walter Reed.

The Karen Wagner Sports Center (Building 32) was dedicated on September 11, 2003, two years after Lt. Colonel Karen Wagner was killed in the Pentagon. Karen Wagner was a 17-year veteran of the Medical Service Corps, having served in San Antonio, Ft. Lee, Germany, and Washington, DC, including a stint at Walter Reed as Head of the Personnel Services Branch. She had held personnel assignments at the Office of the Surgeon General. She was a 1984 graduate of the ROTC program at the University of Nevada–Las Vegas, where she also played guard on the university's women's basketball team.

The Wagner Sports Center includes a gymnasium, three racquetball courts, a cardio theater consisting of various pieces of cardio equipment, such as treadmills and bikes, a weight area consisting of weight-resistant equipment, an aerobics room, and saunas and locker rooms for men and women.

In addition to basketball and volleyball, a variety of other programs are offered, such as aerobics classes and walking programs, that can be done with a group or individually.

As Walter Reed Army Medical Center approached its centennial few anticipated that it would be the last decade of Walter Reed occupying its Washington, D.C., campus. The Base Realignment and Closure (BRAC) Commission recommended in May 2005 that the Army close Walter Reed Army Medical Center, and the Army agreed. However, the name Walter Reed will be carried over to the new Walter Reed National Military Medical Center on the grounds of what is now the National Naval Medical Center in Bethesda, MD. At the time of this writing, the future of the Walter Reed, Washington, D.C. campus is not known.

Despite the BRAC and it implications, war wounded continued to arrive at Walter Reed. In response to the needs of a significant number of amputees, the Army funded and built a Military Advanced Training Center (MATC) at Walter Reed that opened in September 2007. This facility, designed to augment the capabilities of existing Walter Reed facilities, has the latest in computer and video monitoring systems and prosthetics to help enhance amputee and patient care through a multidisciplinary approach, with the goal of returning multiskilled leaders and soldiers to duty. The multidisciplinary team includes physicians, nurse case managers, therapists, psychologists, social workers, benefits counselors, and representatives of the Department of Veterans Affairs.

The MATC has a Center for Performance and Clinical Research or gait lab, as well as a Computer Assisted Rehabilitation Environment (CAREN). The CAREN is designed to build a virtual environment around a patient performing tasks on a treadmill bolted

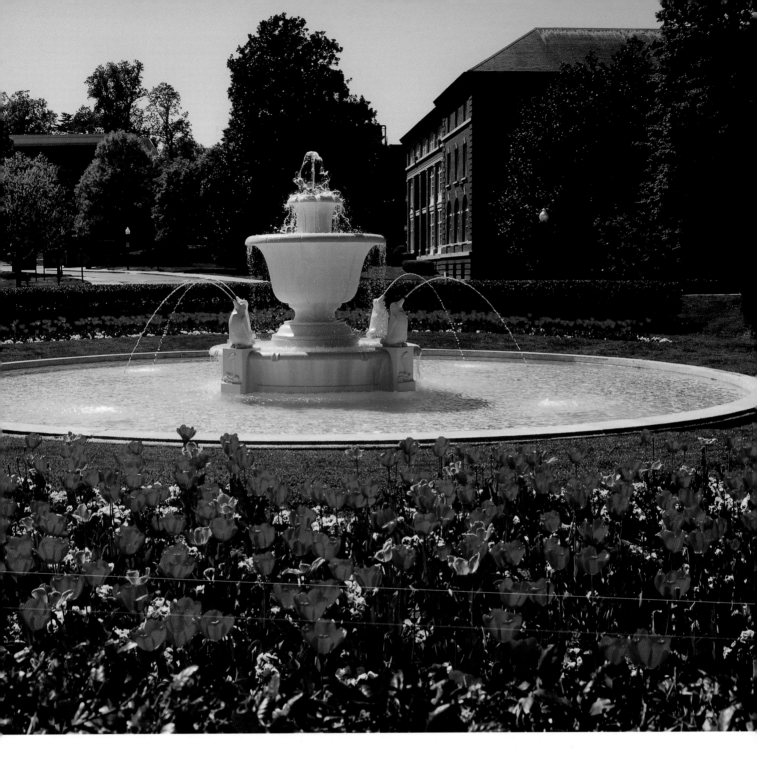

to a helicopter simulator. The CAREN uses a video capture system similar to the gait lab, but with an interactive platform that responds to the patient's every move. The CAREN can also assist warriors recovering from posttraumatic stress disorder by reintroducing patients to both simple and complex environments, and measuring their performance while ensuring absolute safety.

The MATC has a 225-foot indoor track that boasts the world's first oval support harness.

"It allows the Soldiers to walk or run without a therapist tethered to them."

Additionally, MATC includes a rope climb and rock wall, uneven terrain and incline parallel bars, vehicular simulators, a firearms training simulator, physical therapy athletic and exercise areas, and an occupational therapy clinic. The facility also has prosthetic training and skills training areas, prosthetic adjustment and fitting rooms, and separate examination rooms for all amputee-related care.

At its centennial, all who have had the privilege to serve Walter Reed Army Medical Center's most deserving patients can be proud of their accomplishments in healthcare, medical education, and medical research. Those who have provided or received care at Walter Reed understand that it is different and unique, and is known across the country and around the world.

By serving at Walter Reed during its first century, you have been and are a part of its great legacy.

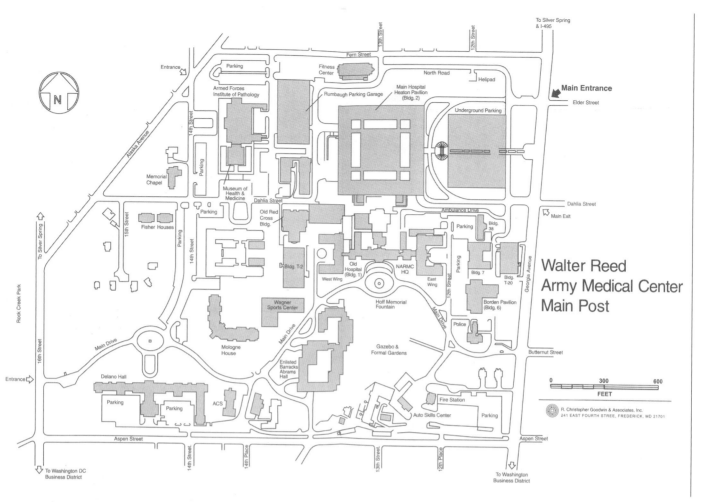

Walter Reed
Army Medical Center
Main Post

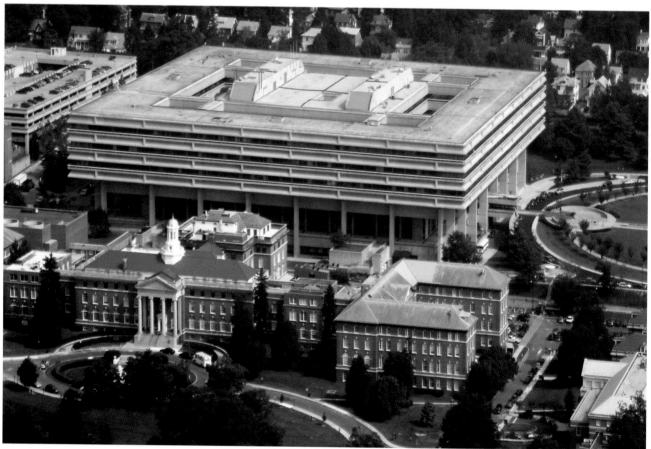

Aerial view of hospital with the finished Rumbaugh Garage on the left.
Source: Walter Reed Army Medical Center

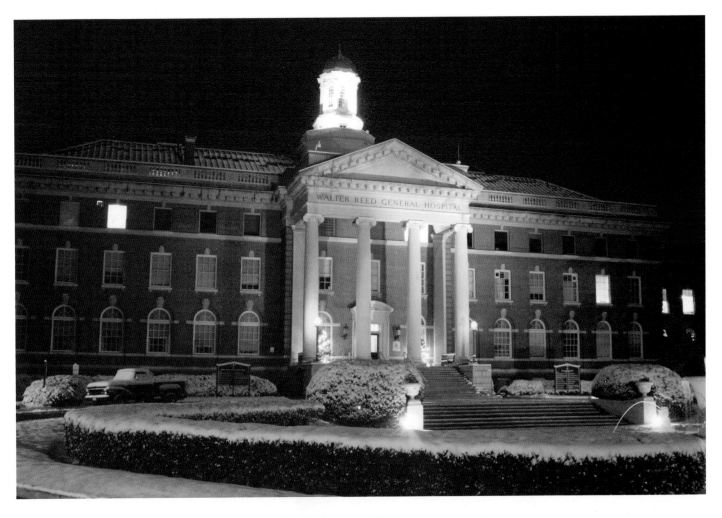

▲ Snow puts a magical glow on the campus. The first snow of 2007 was no exception.
Source: Stripe newspaper, December 14, 2007

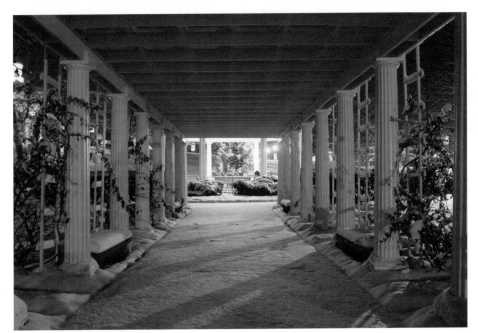

◀ The Rose Garden covered in snow provides a peaceful, contemplative escape from the real world.
Source: Stripe newspaper, December 14, 2007

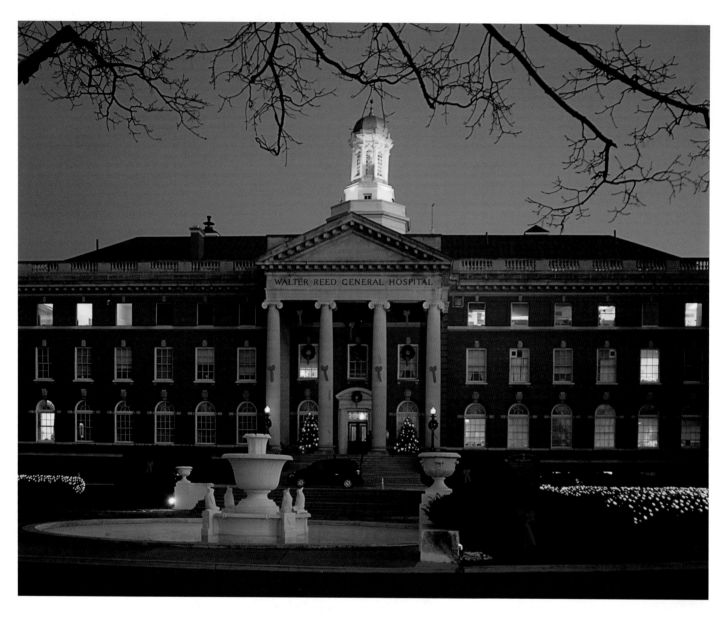

Building 1 decorated for the holiday season.
Source: Walter Reed Army Medical Center, Directorate of Public Works Archives

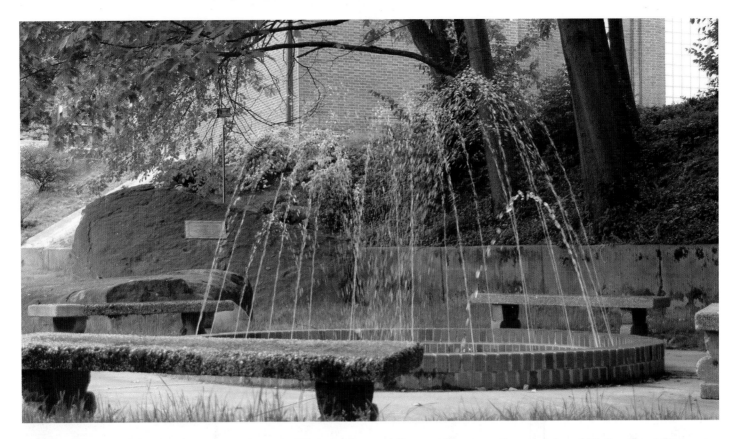

The fountain in the Rose Garden and plaque in honor of General George Glennan, Commander of Walter Reed General Hospital from 1919 until 1923 and the Army Medical Center from 1923 until 1926.
Source: Walter Reed Army Medical Center, Directorate of Public Works Archives

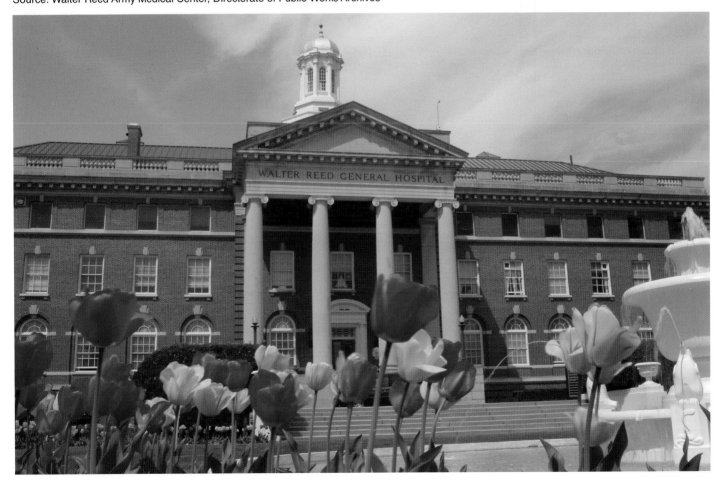

It's tulip time at Walter Reed.
Source: Stripe newspaper

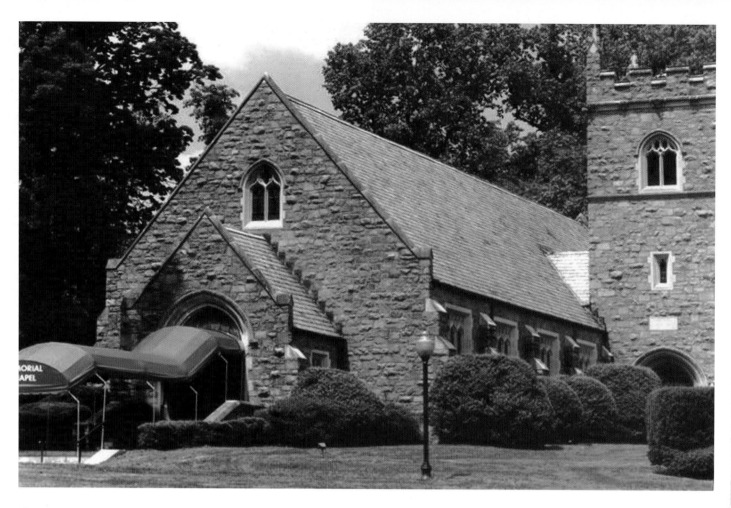

▲ Fine details of the Memorial Chapel architecture are
seen on the facing page.
Source: Walter Reed Army Medical Center, Directorate of Public Works
Archives; Kathleen Stocker - photographer

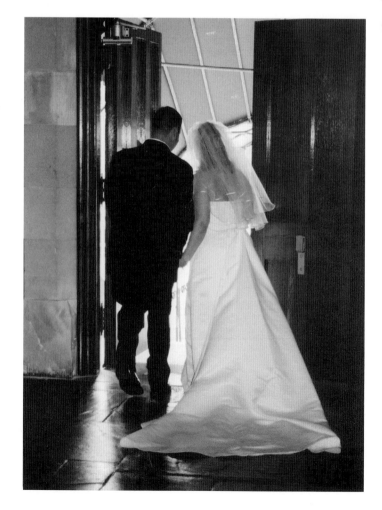

▶ A young couple, Ann Pierce and Ivan Wilson leave
the Memorial Chapel after their wedding on May 3, 2003.
Source: Pierce Collection; Elizabeth Sterling - photographer

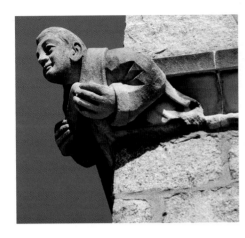

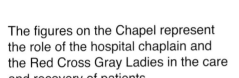

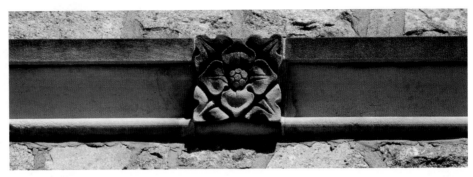

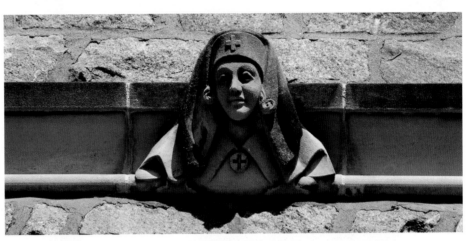

The figures on the Chapel represent the role of the hospital chaplain and the Red Cross Gray Ladies in the care and recovery of patients.
Source: Walter Reed Army Medical Center, Directorate of Public Works Archives; Kathleen Stocker - photographer

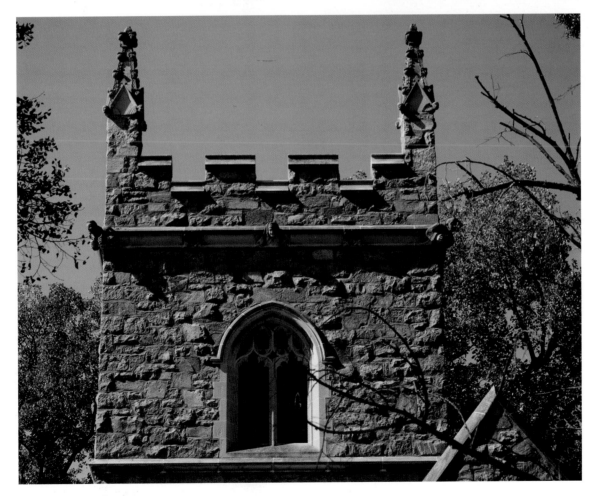

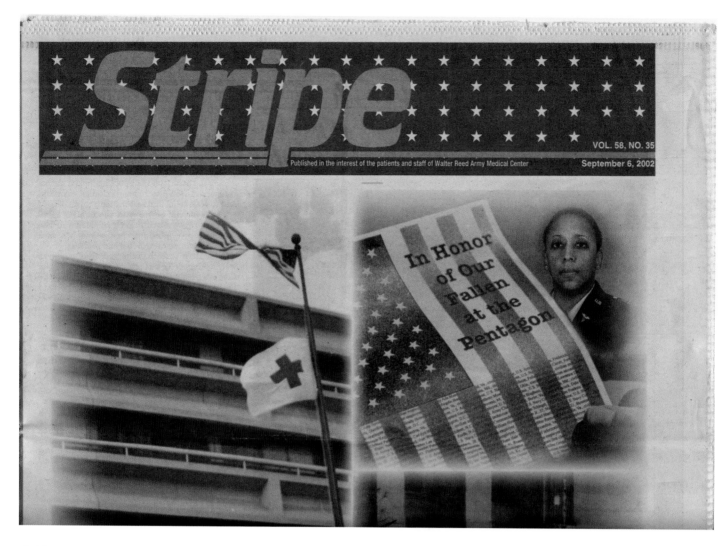

▲ The cover of the *Stripe* newspaper commemorating the first anniversary of the September 11, 2001 attacks and its victims.
Source: Stripe newspaper, September 6, 2002

▶ A sports center built for rehabilitation was named in honor of Lt. Colonel Karen Wagner (pictured above). She served as the Medical Center Brigade's Executive Officer and Secretary of the General Staff at the North Atlantic Regional Medical Command. She was the Deputy Chief of Staff for Personnel at the Office of the Army Surgeon General at the Pentagon. She served at Walter Reed for seven of her seventeen years in the Army. Lt. Colonel Wagner died in the attack on the Pentagon, September 11, 2001.
Source: Walter Reed Army Medical Center, Directorate of Public Works Archives

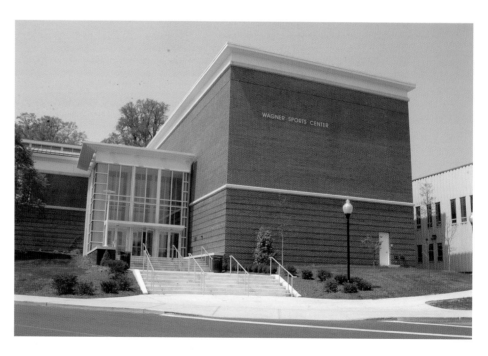

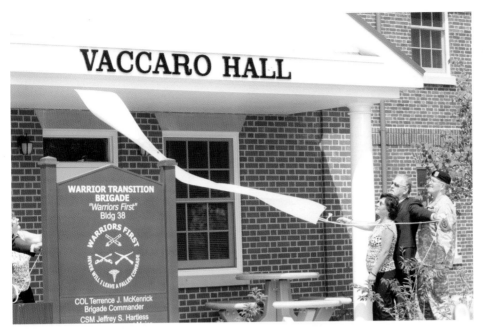

◄ Building 38 was renamed Vaccaro Hall at a dedication ceremony on August 2, 2007. Army Cpl. Angelo J. Vaccaro, an Army medic killed in Afghanistan while attempting to evacuate casualties during combat in Afghanistan, is the first service member to earn two Silver Star Medals in the Global War on Terror. The hall will serve as the headquarters for the new Warrior Transition Brigade, a center aimed at improving outpatient services. Maj. General Schoomaker and Cpl. Vaccaro's family members participated in the dedication ceremony.
Source: WRAMC History Office, PAO Historical Collection

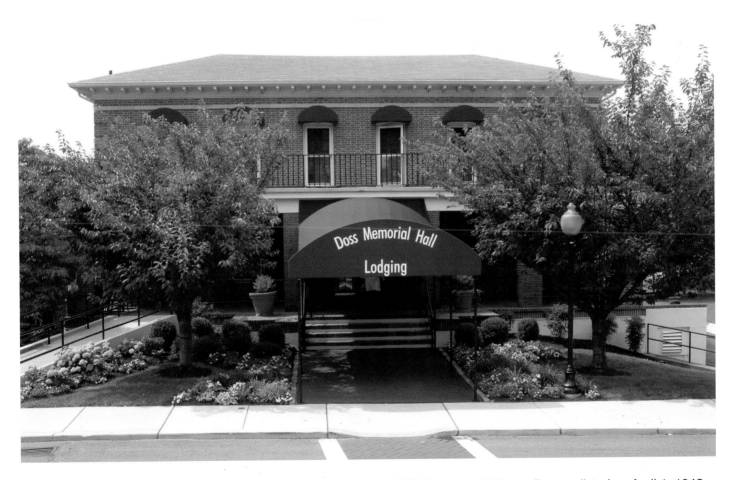

▲ The guest house, Doss Memorial Hall, was named in honor of PFC Desmond T. Doss. Doss enlisted on April 1, 1942 as a conscientious objector and served as a medic with the 778th Infantry Division. On April 29, 1945, his unit captured the Maeda Escarpment on Okinawa. Six days later, they were forced to retreat. Doss is credited with saving 76 lives by lowering his sick and wounded comrades down the cliff one by one over a period of five hours. He was the first conscientious objector to receive the Medal of Honor. He died March 2006. The house has 32 rooms for outpatients and their families.
Sources: Walter Reed Army Medical Center, Directorate of Public Works Archives; Stripe newspaper, July 3, 2008

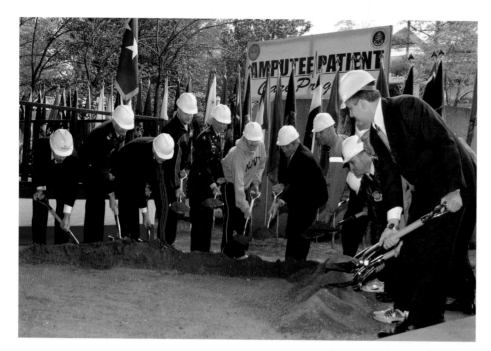

◀ Groundbreaking ceremony for the Military Advanced Training Center (also known as the Amputee Center).
Source: Stripe newspaper

MILITARY ADVANCED TRAINING CENTER

GRAND OPENING

WALTER REED ARMY MEDICAL CENTER

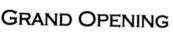

"Thriving in an Era of Opportunity"

SEPTEMBER 13, 2007
THE PARADE FIELD, WALTER REED ARMY MEDICAL CENTER

"WARRIOR CARE"

▲ Program for the dedication of the Military Advanced Training Center for wounded soldiers.
Source: National Museum of Health and Medicine, WRAMC History Collection

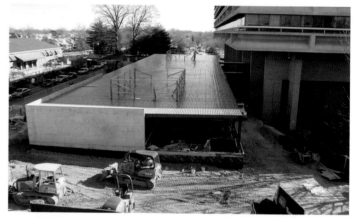

▲ One of the new buildings constructed on the campus was a new Amputee Center. The modern structure was designed to provide a focused area for soldiers to regain skills and return to active lives.
Source: Stripe newspaper, February 2, 2007

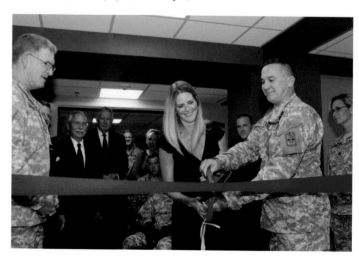

▲ Ribbon-cutting ceremony at the Amputee Center dedication with Maj. General Eric B. Schoomaker, WRAMC Commander, in attendance.
Source: Stripe newspaper

254

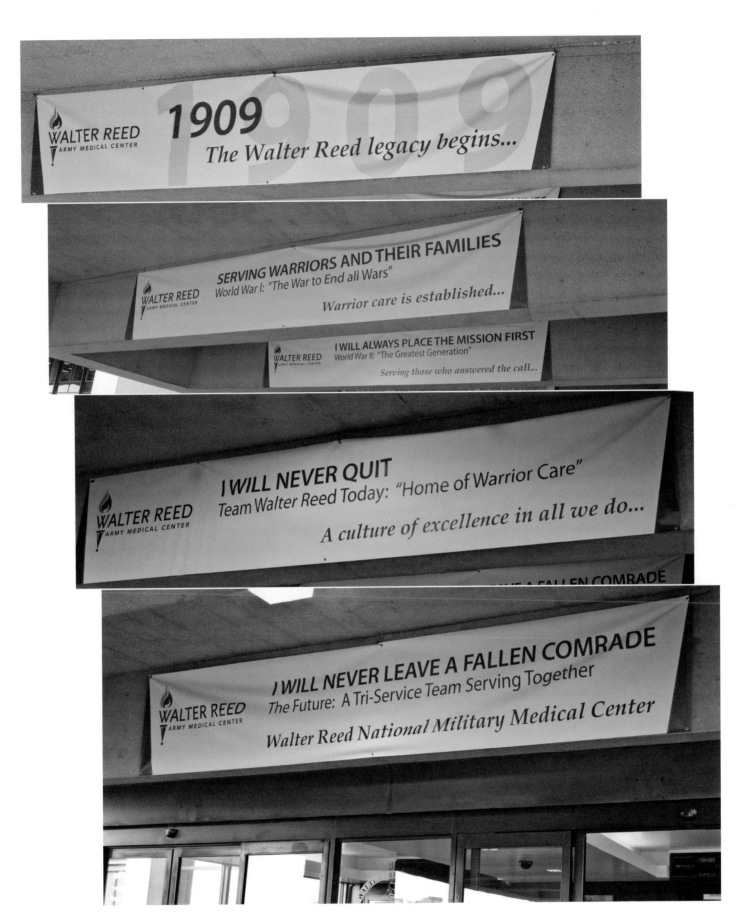

The Military Advanced Training Center was officially opened on September 13, 2007. It was designed to treat "Warriors in Transition" with limb loss or functional loss to the highest possible levels of activity.
Source: Kathleen Stocker - photographer

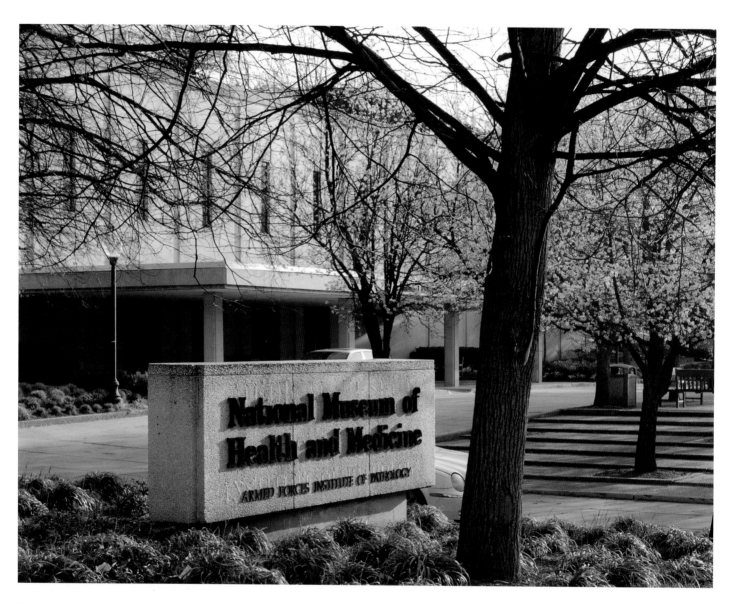

The sign at the entrance to the National Museum of Health and Medicine.
Source: Mike Rhode - photographer

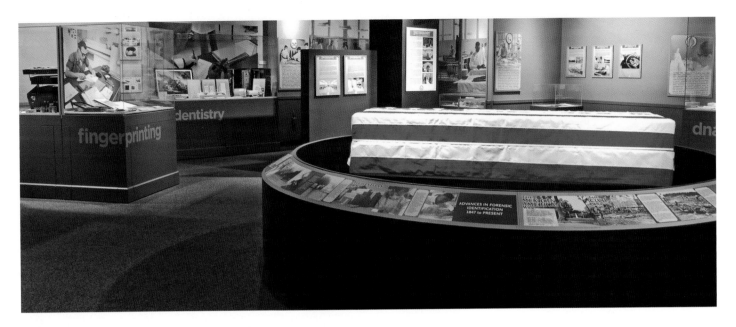

▲ Part of the display floor at the National Museum of Health and Medicine.
Source: Mike Rhode - photographer

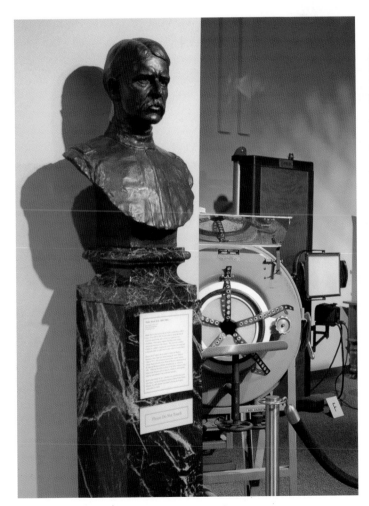

▲ A bust of Walter Reed inside the museum doors at the National Museum of Health and Medicine. An iron lung and vintage X-ray machine stand in the background.
Source: Mike Rhode - photographer

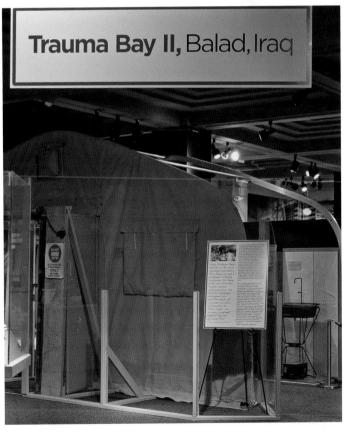

Trauma Bay II, Balad, Iraq

▲ This museum display shows a tent set up to simulate the contents of a trauma bay as it would appear in the theater of battle outside Balad, Iraq.
Source: Mike Rhode - photographer

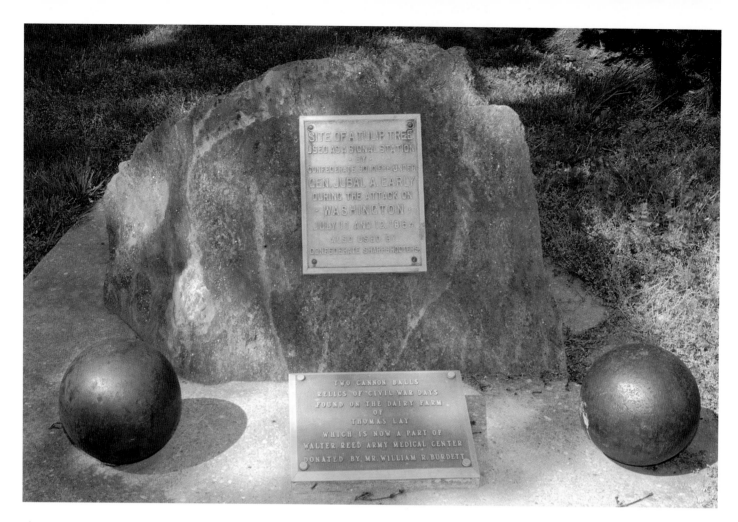

▲ In 1864, the grounds on which Walter Reed now stands was the location of Confederate General Jubal Early's troops during the Battle of Fort Stevens. This ground marked the deepest penetration of his troops into the District of Columbia. The tulip tree that stood on this spot was used by sharpshooters to fire on Fort Stevens. The cannonballs pictured were removed from the unoccupied Lay farm house on the property in 1898 by two neighbor boys. One of them, Mr. William Burdett, kept them as artifacts for most of his life but in 1963 donated them to Walter Reed and they became part of this memorial.
Source: Walter Reed Army Medical Center, Directorate of Public Works Archives; Kathleen Stocker - photographer

▶ Closeup of the plaque located opposite the officer's quarters (Building 12).
Source: Walter Reed Army Medical Center, Directorate of Public Works Archives

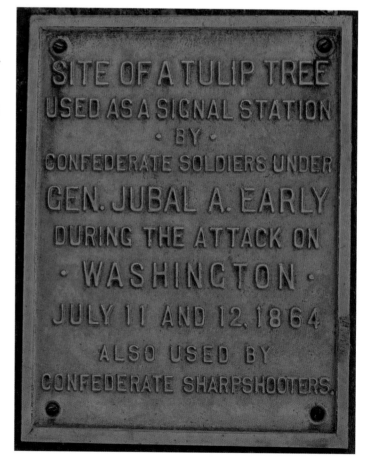

SITE OF A TULIP TREE
USED AS A SIGNAL STATION
· BY ·
CONFEDERATE SOLDIERS UNDER
GEN. JUBAL A. EARLY
DURING THE ATTACK ON
· WASHINGTON ·
JULY 11 AND 12, 1864
ALSO USED BY
CONFEDERATE SHARPSHOOTERS.

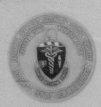
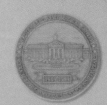

Graduate Medical Education

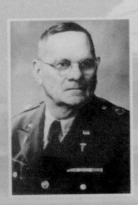

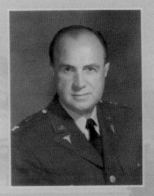

Colonel James C. Kimbrough,
the father of Army urology, served
on active duty for 36 years with
four tours at Walter Reed. The
Army Urology Course was named
for him 1956 and the new hospital
at Ft. Meade in 1961.

Colonel Ogden C. Bruton,
first chief of pediatrics and
residency program director at
Walter Reed. A renowned general
pediatrician, he reported in 1952 the
first immune deficiency disease,
now known as Bruton's Disease.

A Beginning for Army Medical Department Leaders

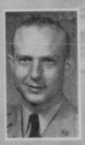

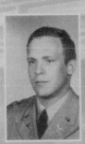

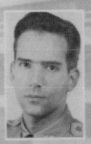

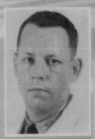

Mologne
Intern Class of
1961

Rumbaugh
Intern Class of
1964

Scotti
Intern Class of
1965

McLeod
Intern Class of
1965

Walter Reed Army Medical Center
Celebrates "Proudly Serving America's Best for Ninety Years"
1909 - 1999

This poster hangs in the hallway wall outside the Graduate Medical Education offices in Building 2, the Heaton Pavilion. The information about Colonels Kimbrough and Bruton is self-explanatory. The row of photographs are of individuals who all completed some, if not all, of their medical training at Walter Reed. Left to right are, Lewis Mologne, later a Maj. General and Walter Reed Commander; Jim Rumbaugh, also later a Maj. General and Walter Reed Commander; Mike Scotti, also later a Maj. General and Army Medical Department leader; and David McLeod, later Chief of Urology and Residency Program Director and currently Walter Reed legend.
Source: Walter Reed Army Medical Center, Graduate Medical Education

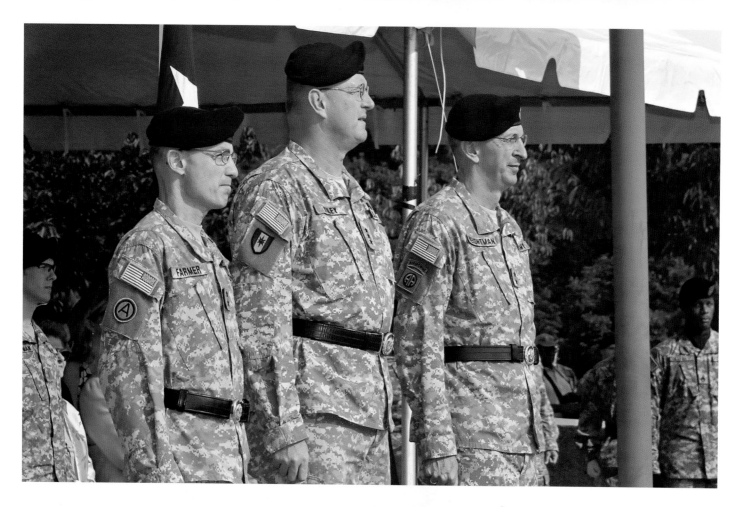

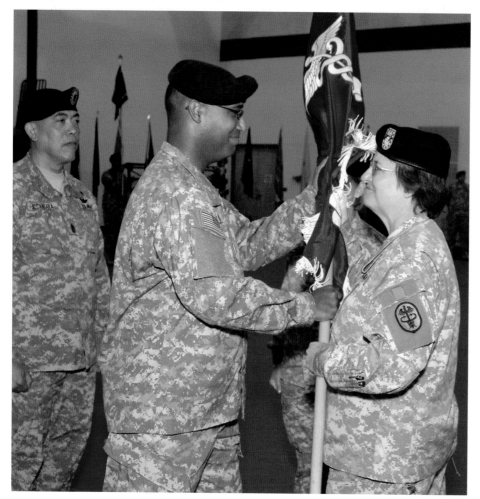

▲ Maj. General Kenneth Farmer, outgoing NARMC and WRAMC Commander; Lt. General Kevin Kiley, Army Surgeon General; and Maj. General George Weightman stand at attention during the change of command ceremony for incoming WRAMC and NARMC commander Gen. Weightman on August 24, 2006.
Source: Stripe newspaper

◄ Incoming Commander Colonel Norvell Coots (left) accepts the Walter Reed Health Care System flag from Maj. General Carla Hawley-Bowland, Commanding General of the North Atlantic Regional Medical Command and WRAMC, during a change of command ceremony July 11, 2008 in WRAMC's Wagner Sports Center. SGM Ricardo Alcantara stands behind Colonel Coots.
Source: Stripe newspaper, July 17, 2008; John R. Chew - photographer

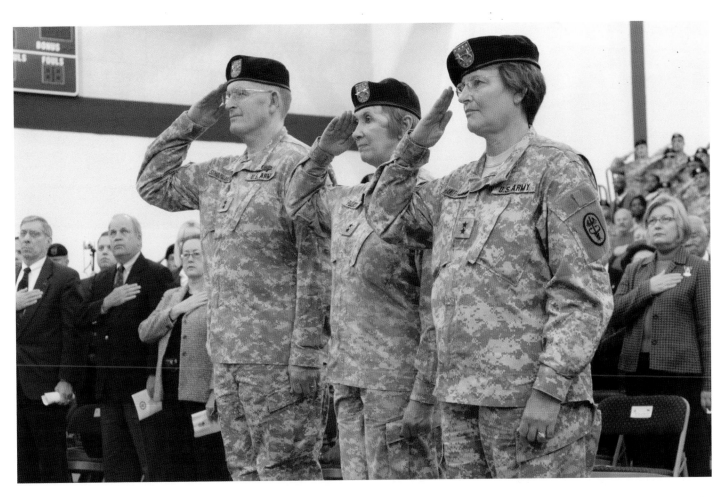

▲ Maj. General Eric Schoomaker, outgoing NARMC and WRAMC Commander and Surgeon General designee (left) with Maj. General Gale Pollock, acting Surgeon General (center) and Maj. General Carla Hawley-Bowland (right) at the change of command ceremony held December 11, 2007 in Walter Reed Army Medical Center's Karen Wagner Sports Center. Maj. General Hawley-Bowland assumed command of the North Atlantic Regional Medical Command and Walter Reed Army Medical Center. Maj. General Eric Schoomaker was promoted to Lt. General the next day.
Source: Stripe newspaper, December 11, 2007; SFC Roger J. Mommaerts, Jr., WTB - photographer

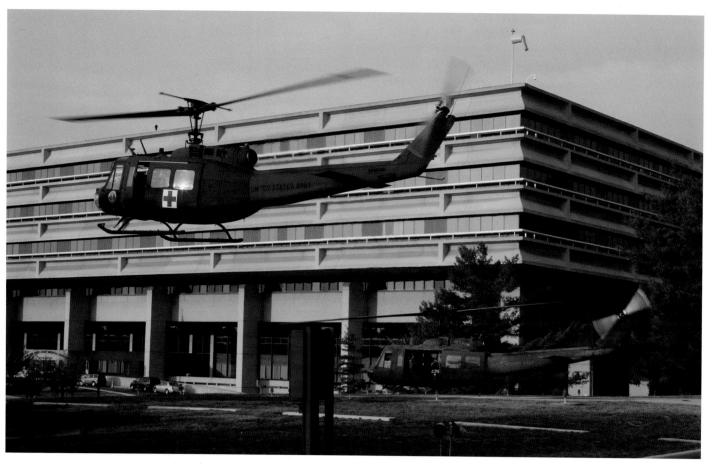

Mass casualty exercise in 2007.
Source: WRAMC History Office, PAO Historical Collection

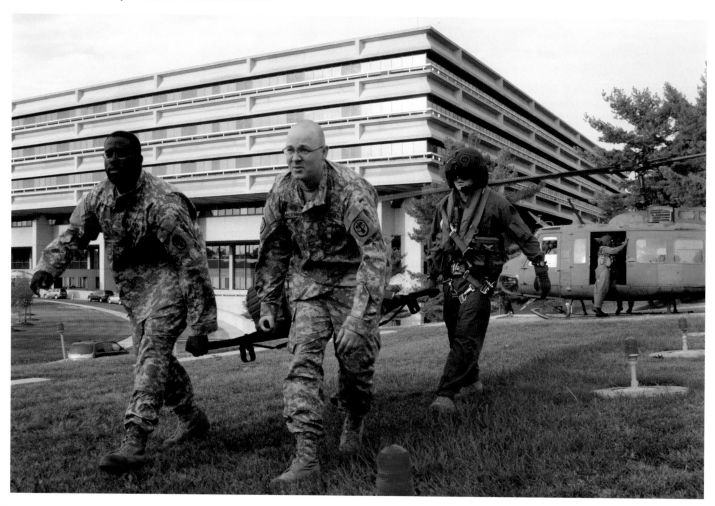

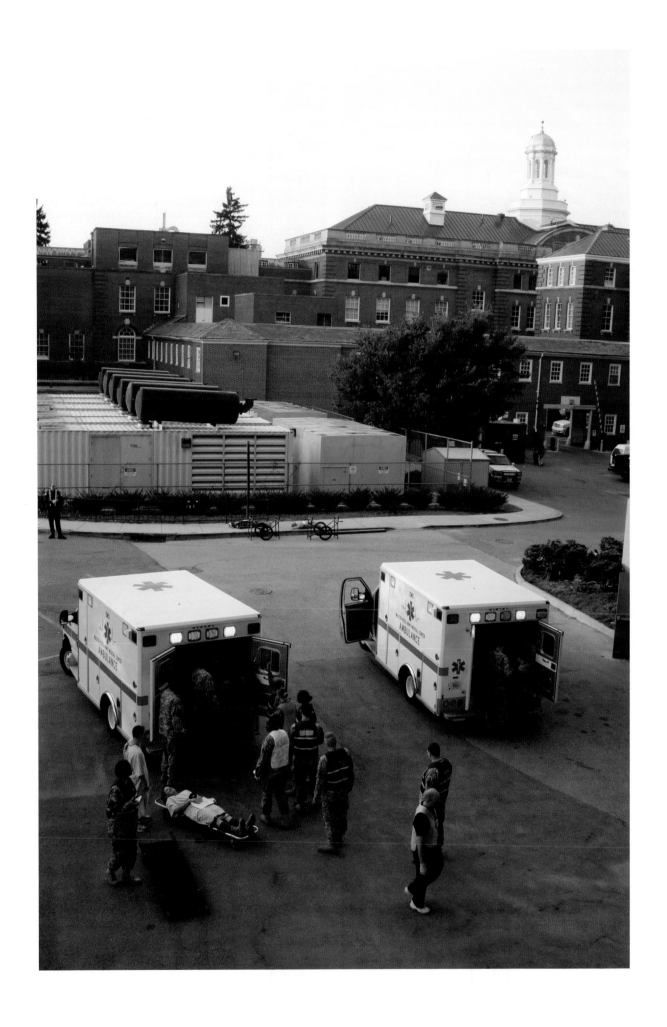

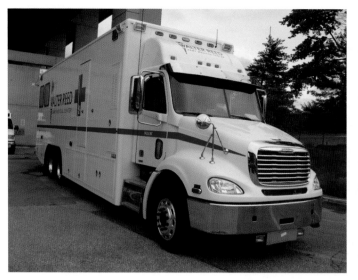
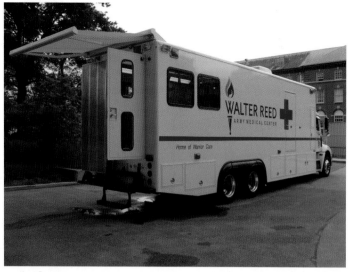

▲ The Walter Reed Army Medical Center patient evacuation vehicle (PEV), a semitrailer-sized hospital on wheels, fits up to 12 ambulatory and 16 nonambulatory patients, and allows medical personnel to administer medical treatment en route to the hospital.
Source: Stripe newspaper, April 28, 2006

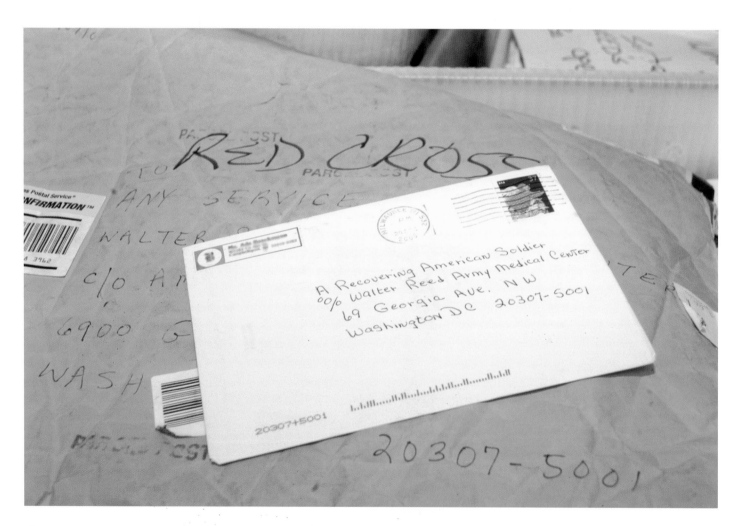

▲ Mail is a source of connection with the world outside a hospital room. It means that someone took the time to think about a patient.
Source: Stripe newspaper, January 27, 2006

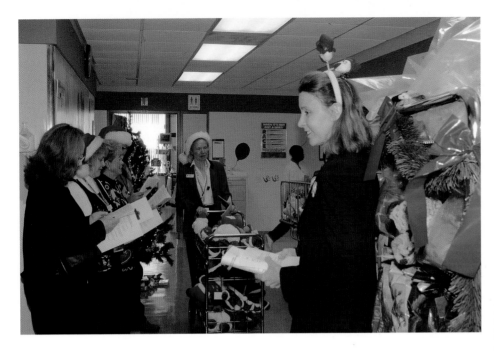

From the first Red Cross worker known as the Gray Lady in World War I to the present, the Red Cross has been a major presence on the campus of Walter Reed Army Medical Center. Whether it is sorting mail, preparing gift bags, or singing Christmas carols, the Red Cross volunteers are always there to encourage and cheer the patients and assist the staff.
Source: Stripe newspaper, 2005 and 2006 issues

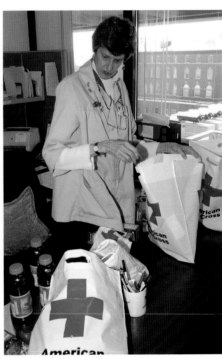

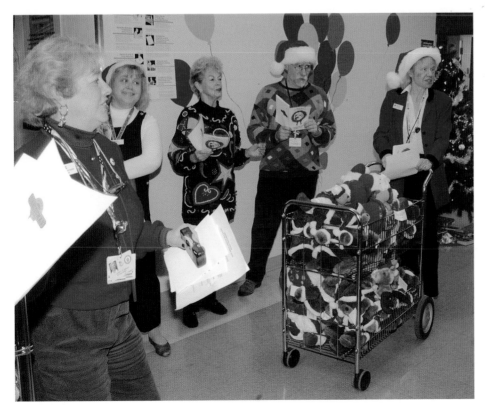

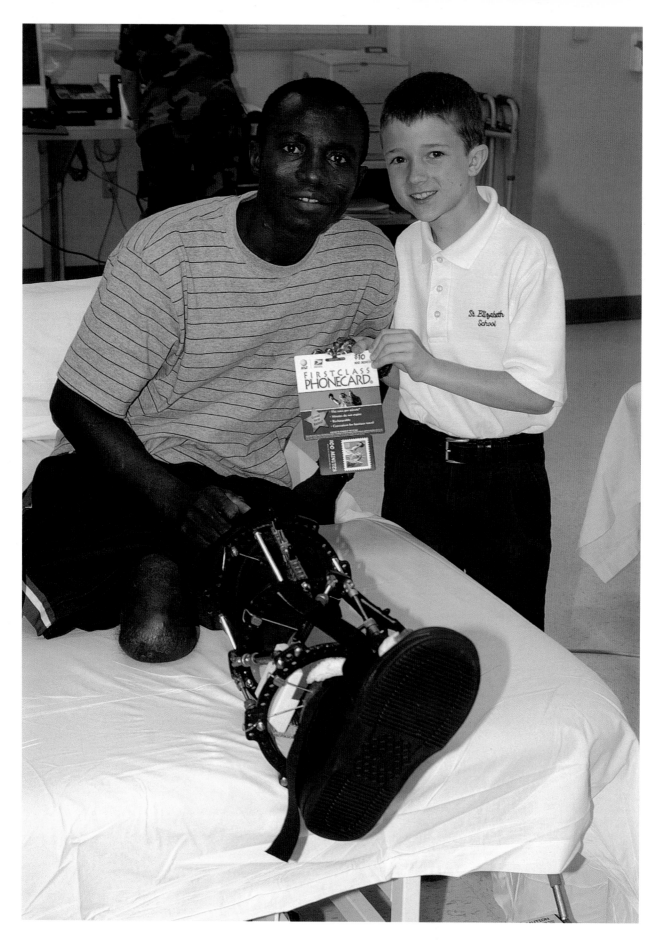

Sometimes it's the little things that speed recovery. Here, a young boy shares his birthday presents by bringing phone cards to patients in the hospital. The boy had requested his guests to bring him gifts of telephone cards.
Source: Stripe newspaper, August 29, 2005

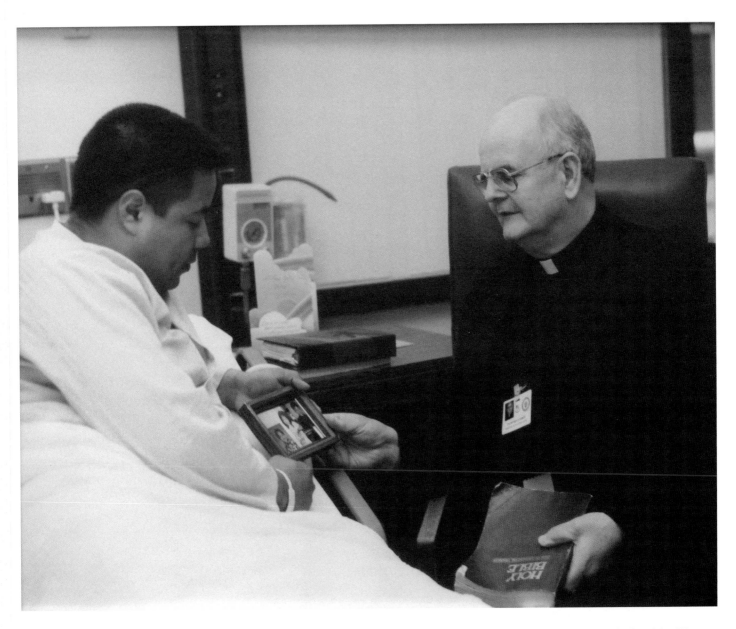

Father Patrick Kenny visits with an inpatient. It is estimated that he has visited over 150,000 patients during his 27-year tenure at WRAMC. All who know him speak of the man who makes them smile.
Source: Walter Reed Army Medical Center, Graduate Medical Education

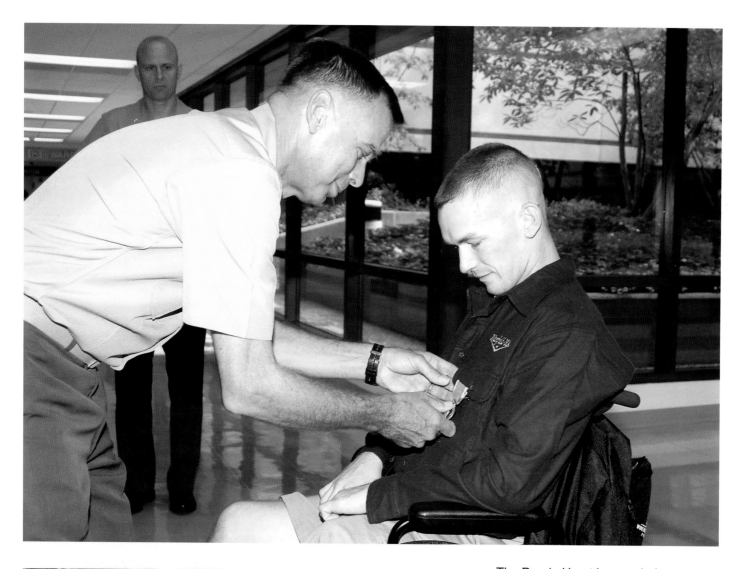

The Purple Heart is awarded to members of the military who sustained wounds in combat.
Source: Stripe newspaper, November 17, 2006

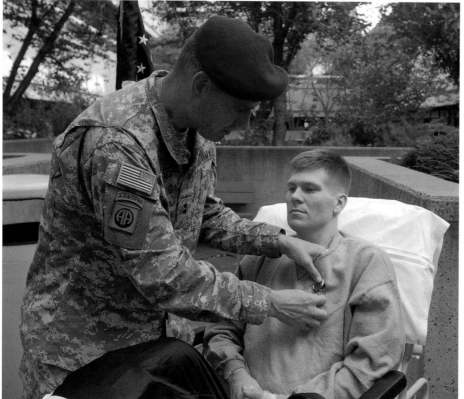

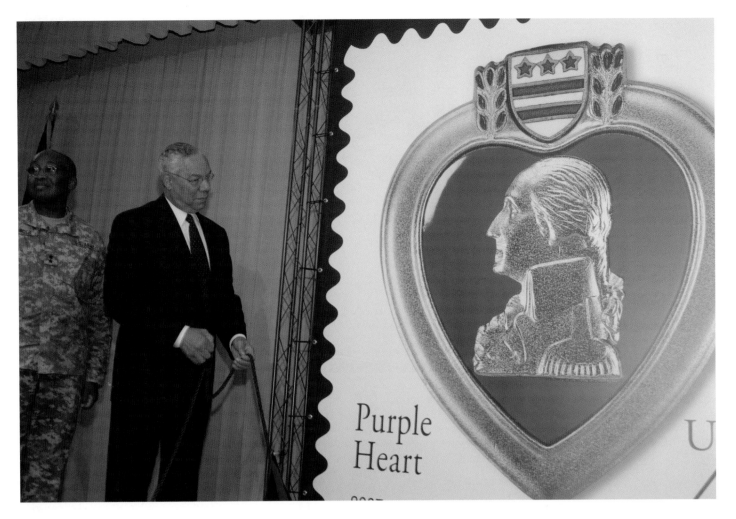

▲ The U.S. Postal Service dedicated the new Purple Heart stamp during a ceremony at Walter Reed Army Medical Center where two wounded soldiers were awarded Purple Hearts by General Colin L. Powell (Ret.). Maj. General Elder Granger (left) participated in honoring service members at the Purple Heart ceremony on the 75th anniversary of the Purple Heart medal. August 7, 2007.
Source: Stripe newspaper

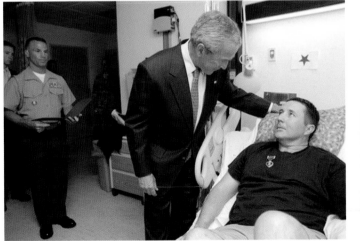 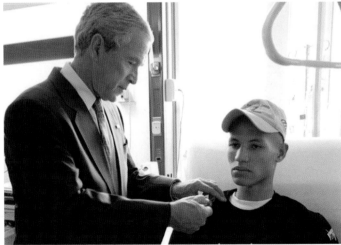

▲ President George W. Bush continues the practice begun by President Harding to visit the wounded warriors at the hospital. Here, he is presenting wounded service members with their Purple Hearts.
Source: Stripe newspaper

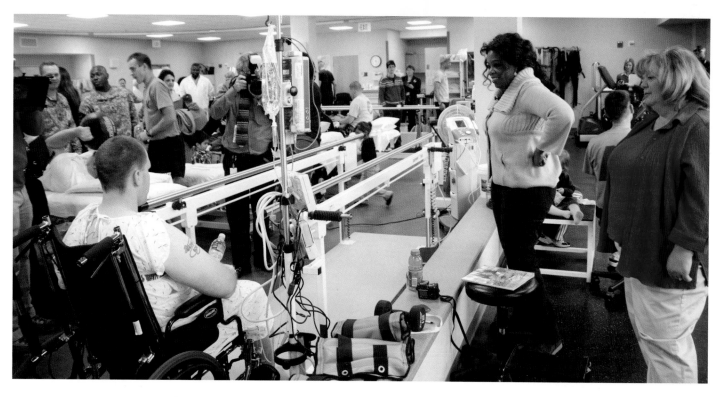

▲ Talk show host Oprah Winfrey visits wounded soldiers.
Source: Stripe newspaper

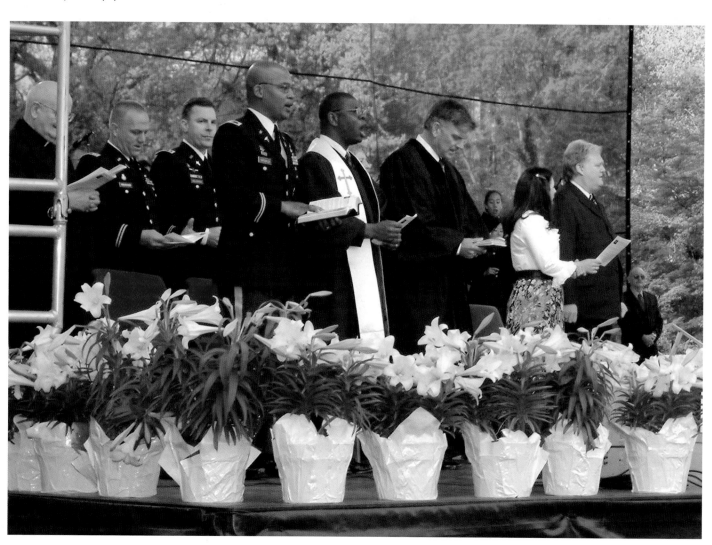

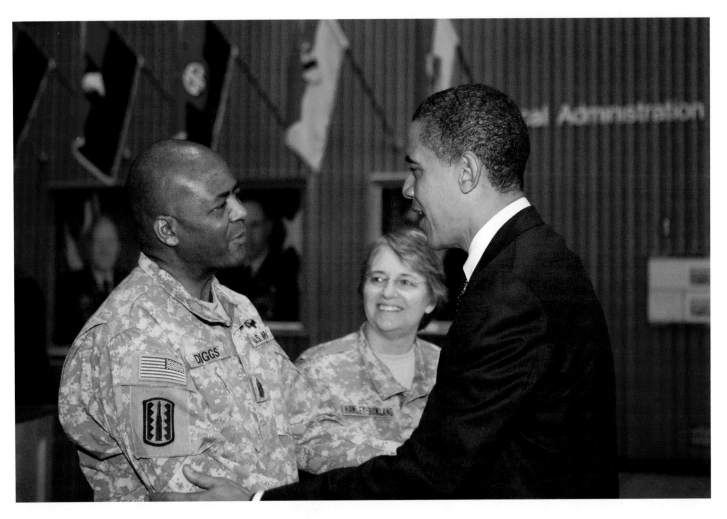

▲ President-elect Barack Obama meets with CSM James E. Diggs and Maj. General Hawley-Bowland during his visit to Walter Reed Army Hospital in the days leading up to his inauguration.
Source: Stripe newspaper

▶ The variety of visitors to Walter Reed Hospital continues. Here, cartoonist G. B. Trudeau poses for photo with a fan during a visit to the hospital in February 2006.
Source: Stripe newspaper, February 3, 2006

◀ The annual Easter Sunrise Service continues to be a major event in the life of the Walter Reed Army Medical Center. In April 2006, Franklin Graham conducted the service much as his father had done years earlier. The service was held in the Garden near the Pavilion and broadcast on a jumbo screen. Ricky Skaggs, Grammy winning Country music artist is on the right.
Source: Stripe newspaper, April 21, 2006

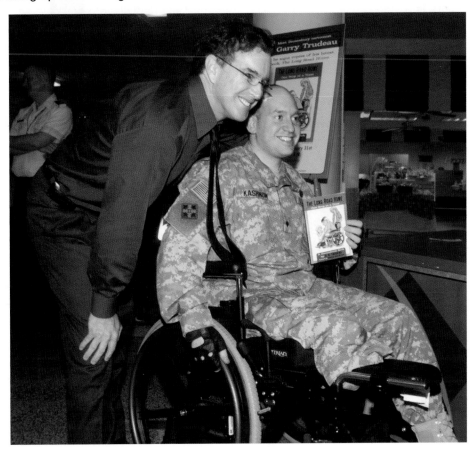

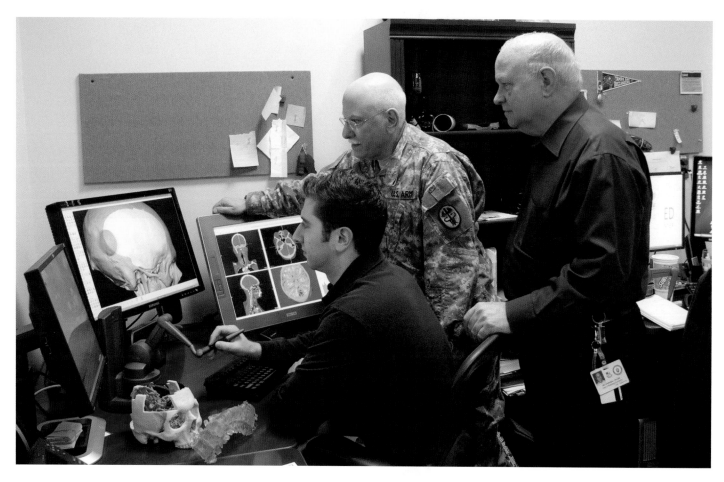

▲ The 3D Medical Applications Center provides physical anatomical models and cranioplasty implants using medical imaging data, and is used by physicians, surgeons, and dentists in many diverse specialties. The models have proven to be invaluable for presurgical planning on complex cases, allowing for rehearsal of surgery, prebending of plates, and intraoperative reference, which results in reduced surgical time. Here, Chief of Radiology, Col. Mike Brazaitis and Col. (Ret.) Steve Rouse, confer with Peter Liacouras, PhD in the design of a skull plate.
Source: 3D Medical Applications Center

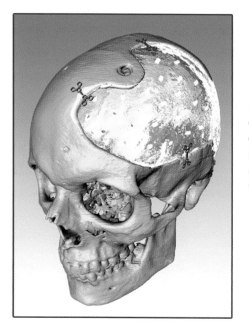

(Left) A computer model of a skull based on CT scan data. (Right) An acrylic skull created on a rapid prototyping machine based on computer data similar to that shown above and on the left.
Source: 3D Medical Applications Center

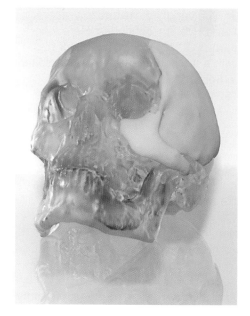

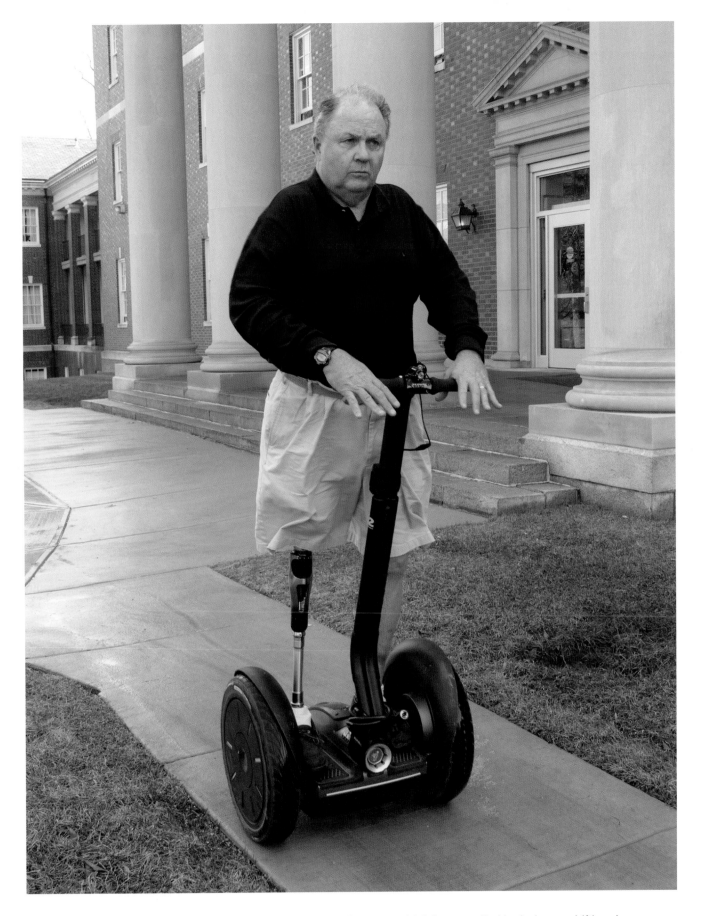

Judge John J. "Jack" Farley, III, tries out a Segway. The Segway, which is controlled by balance shifting, has proven to be a useful device in helping wounded soldiers improve coordination while having fun. The nonprofit group Disability Rights Advocates For Technology (DRAFT) has donated more than 150 of these devices to military amputees. Farley, wounded in Vietnam, was a patient on the orthopaedic ward known as the "snake pit" after sustaining wounds in Vietnam in 1969.
Source: Douglas Wise - photographer

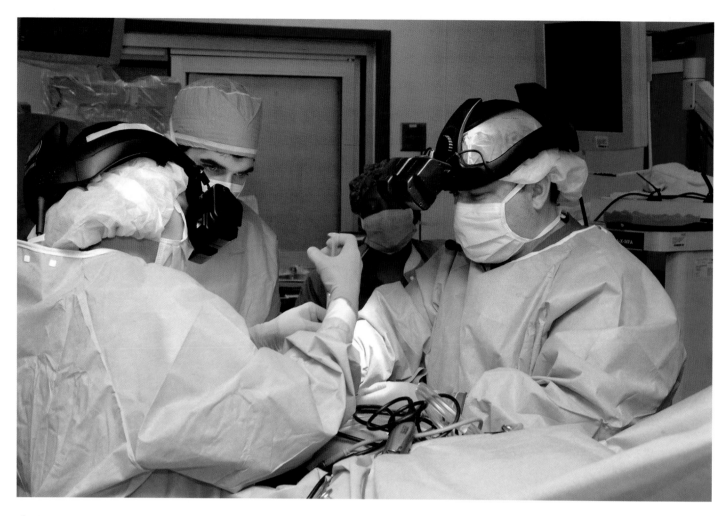

▲ Surgical techniques in the operating room have changed over the years. Here, a team works with 3D headsets to perform the latest surgical techniques.
Source: Stripe newspaper, March 30, 2007

▶ Prosthetics should look as natural as possible. This frequently means that artists need to paint the devices to match the skin tones and other coloring features of the patient. The image shows cosmetic hands before and after color match artistry.
Source: WRAMC History Office, PAO Historical Collection

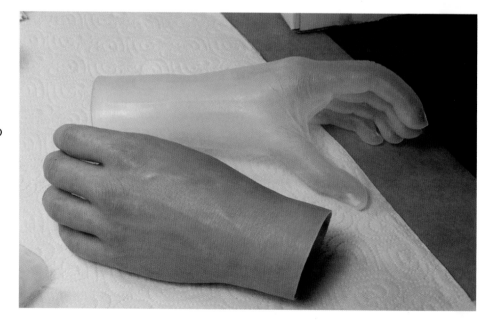

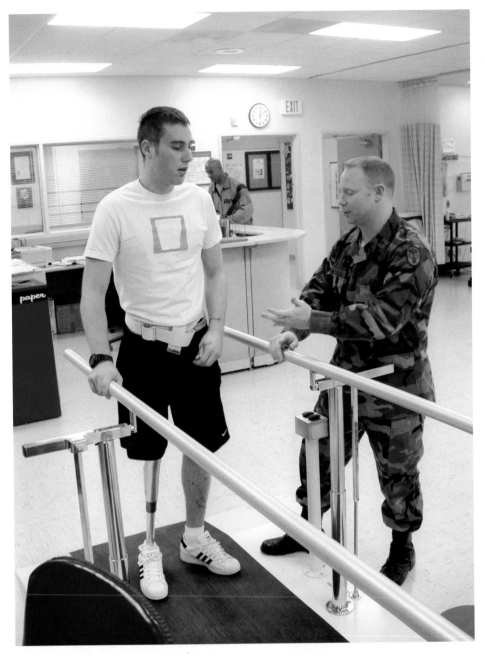

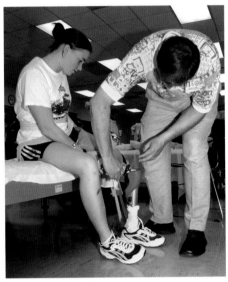

PFC Tristan Wyatt practices gait in the physical therapy clinic.
Source: Bruce Maston - photographer; National Museum of Health and Medicine, AFIP, NCP 4159

▲ Physical Therapist Bob Barr adjusts the C-leg of Lt. Melissa Stockwell.
Source: Stripe newspaper, February 28, 2006

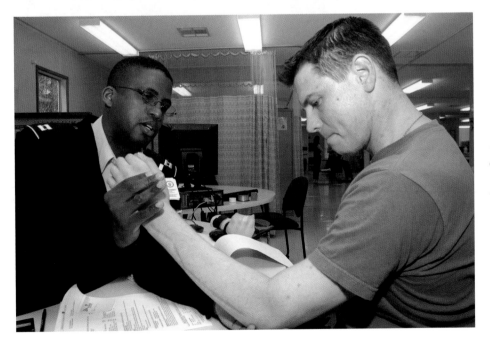

◄ It takes a lot of concentration to make the arm do what should be so easy. Occupational Therapist Capt. Smith-Forbes provides encouragement.
Source: Stripe newspaper, April 7, 2006

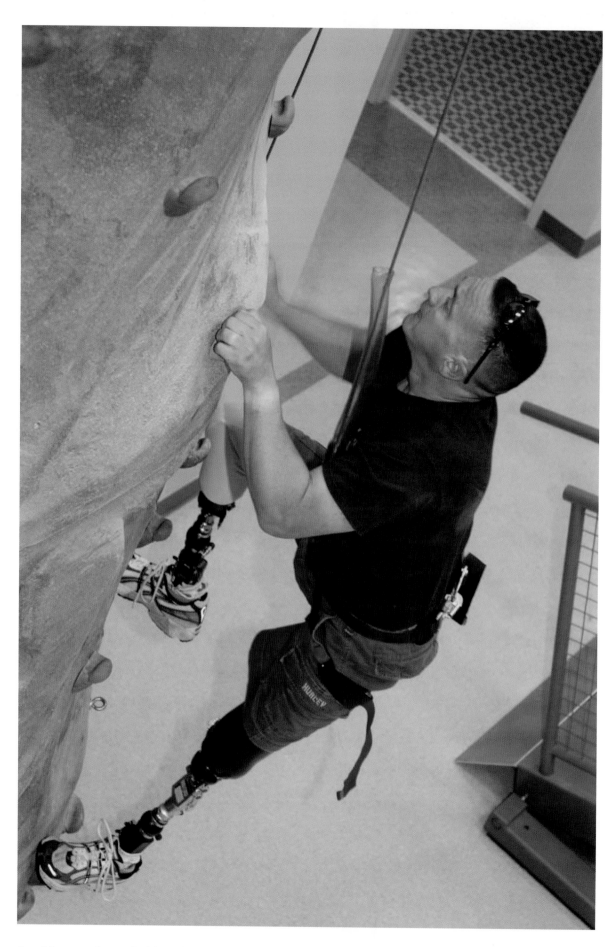

A soldier practices climbing skill on the rock wall located in the Military Advanced Training Center.
Source: WRAMC History Office, PAO Historical Collection

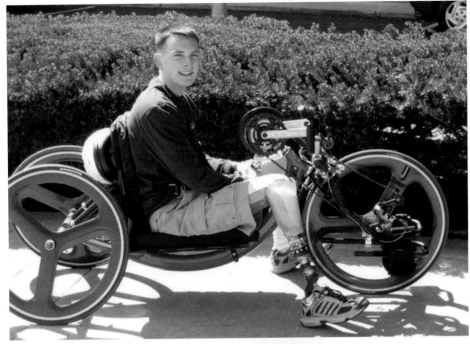

Use of a hand-crank bike contributes to the development of confidence and ability, allowing continued participation in leisure activity.
Source: WRAMC History Office, PAO Historical Collection

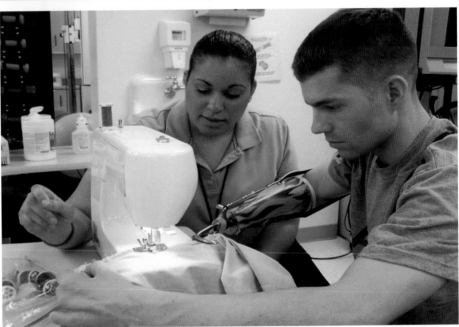

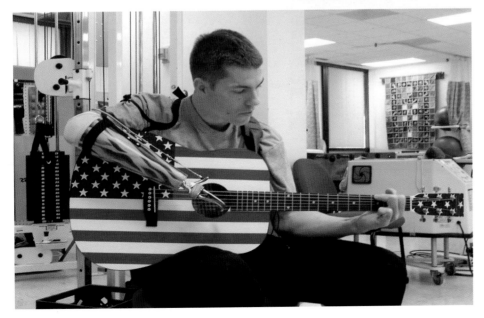

As in the past, integration of a range of functional activities during rehabilitation is an ongoing goal in the occupational therapy clinic. While durable prosthetic design from earlier years is used today, recent research in prosthetics has lead to the development of lighter weight components, customization with computer aided design, advancement in myoelectric controls and cosmetic enhancements.
Source: WRAMC History Office, PAO Historical Collection

277

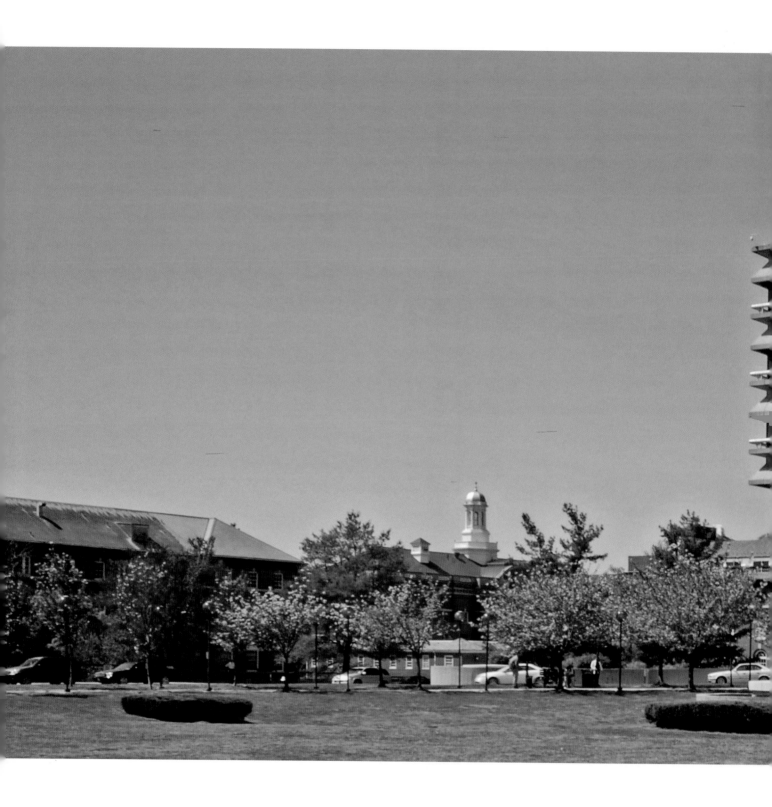

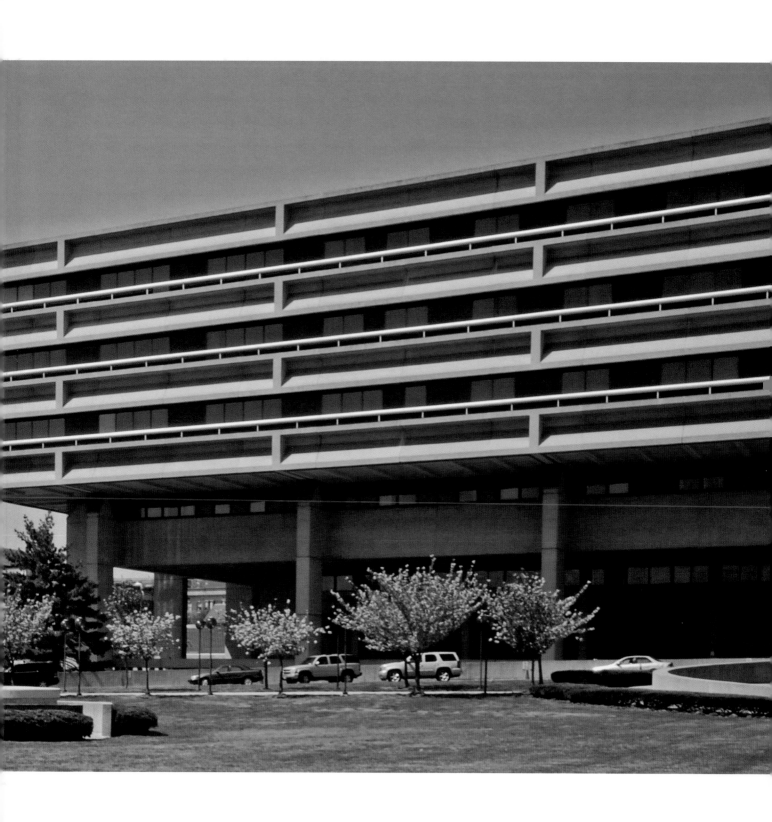

Heaton Pavilion, Building 2, in the spring with the cherry trees in bloom.
Sources: Walter Reed Army Medical Center, Directorate of Public Works Archives; Kathleen Stocker - photographer

ISBN:978-0-9818228-3-9